In Remembrance of Linda

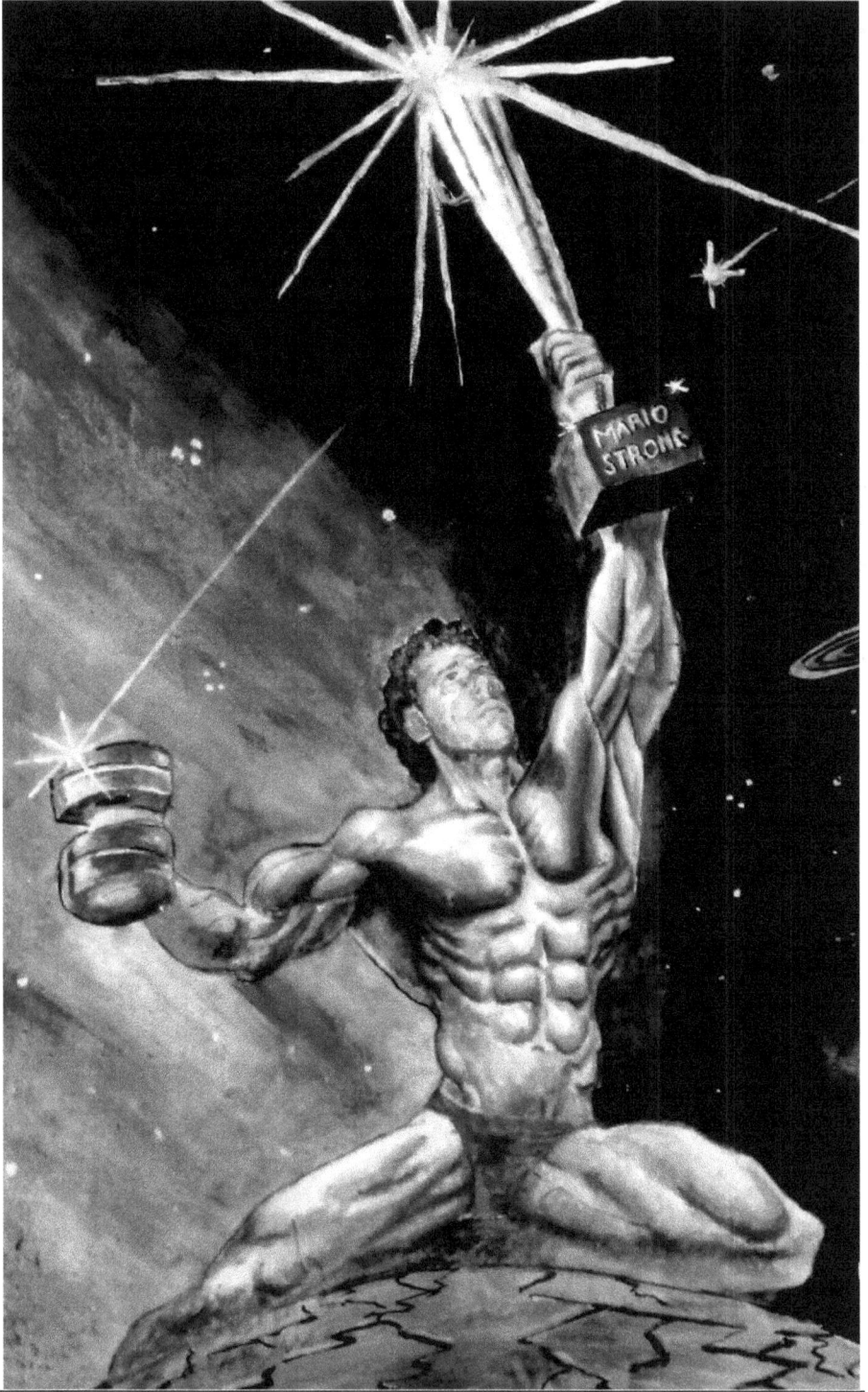

MARIO STRONG

REFLECTIONS OF A
NATURAL BODYBUILDER

Copyrighted Material

Notice

This book is intended as an instructional, entertainment, and reference volume only, not as a medical manual. The information here is designed to help you make informed decisions about your health and fitness. It is not a substitute for any treatment that may have been prescribed by your doctor. If you suspect you have a medical problem, we urge you to seek competent medical help. The information in this book is intended to enhance proper exercise training. All forms of exercise and dieting pose some inherent risk. The author and publisher advise readers to take full responsibility of their safety and know their limits. Before performing any of the exercises in this book make sure the equipment you use is well maintained, and do not take risk beyond your level of experience, aptitude, training, and fitness.

The exercises, diets, and fitness orientated advice, as well as bodybuilding programs given in this book are not intended as a substitute for any exercise routine or diet regimen that may be prescribed by your doctor. Please consult with your physician before starting any of the exercise or nutritional programs within this book. Have your physician give you a complete medical checkup and seek his or her advice on following any such prescribed fitness orientated programs, especially if you are overweight, have not exercised in a while, have had any health problems, or if there is any history of health problems. We also recommend that you then visit your physician on a regular basis and report any problems that may occur.

Mention or display of specific names, images, companies, organizations, or authorities does not imply endorsement by the author or publisher, nor does mention or display of specific names, images, companies, organizations, or authorities imply that they endorse this book, the author, or publisher.

While every effort is made to insure that the information and advice provided in this book is correct and precise, we make no guarantees as to the accuracy and are not responsible for any mistakes or misprints.

ISBN 978-0-615-30639-1

Library of Congress Control Number: 2008903136

Official Web site: MarioStrong.com

To
My father for teaching me discipline
My mother for giving me love
Aida for sharing my life

And to all those that dare
to live long and be strong
naturally

MEN OF IRON

What is this quest of men and steel

Flirting with danger on a daily basis

Pushing themselves to the max and beyond

These men of iron and the suffering they endure

What force ignites their hunger to succeed

As they journey onward through time

Along the unforgiving highway of pain

Through years of sweat, strain, and tears

For what is their reward

What is their goal

But to live for another day

Of iron pumping madness

CONTENTS

THAT WHICH DOES NOT KILL YOU MAKES YOU STRONGER

ACKNOWLEDGMENTS

The pure bodybuilding lifestyle is one of solitude. Although we train among others that share the same passion as us, it is nevertheless our own burning desire that gives us the strength, courage, and fortitude to workout throughout the months, years, and decades. Whether we are competing on a stage or just taking a stroll along the beach, our living sculpts of muscular art are with us every step of the way. But, as much of a self-propelled sport as bodybuilding is, there are those that have encouraged, motivated, and inspired us along the way.

For me, my first inspiration came as a child when I would sit back on a chair and watch my father train with the barbell set he purchased while overseas during his stint in the military. In my eyes, my father was Hercules, and I would dream of the day when I would be as big and strong as he was. For my tenth birthday, my father, who had noticed my desire, designed a simple weight-training program for me to follow. The seed had been planted deep in my heart. For the next several years, I trained in the basement of my home and yearned for the time when my goals would become reality. In the years that followed, my brothers, Johnny and Domenic, came of age and joined me in the basement. As time went by, we continued to equip our home gym with additional pieces of exercise machinery and plates of steel to help our bodies meet the daily demands that we placed on them. Our little corner of the universe was filled with inspiring photos of bodybuilding champions such as Arnold Schwarzenegger, Franco Columbu, Sergio Oliva, Larry Scott, Dave Draper, Frank Zane, and dozens more. These images, along with the inspiring stories written in the physique publications, helped motivate us to push and pull the steel with every ounce of energy we had. Eventually, I opened my own bodybuilding club and began to train those who shared my same passion. In the gym, I learned from the thousands of students that trained under my guidance, and ultimately I penned many of my findings and concepts in various newspapers and bodybuilding publications. Thanks to Dan Lurie's *Muscle Training Illustrated*, I got my first opportunity to voice my opinions on physical culture to a vast bodybuilding audience. In time, my name became synonymous with bodybuilding and eventually I was able to give back to the sport that had given so much to me.

It is mostly through my experiences in bodybuilding that this book has become a reality. Because of men like Leon Brown, Joe Carrero, Jerry Valente, Patrick DeLuca, Frank Rapacciulo, Carl Stair, Tommy Kirdahy, Tony Bartollotta, Myke Decembre, Bruce Newburgh, Mark Delio, Gill Rios, Joe Rivera, and the many other muscle builders who have crossed my path and have inspired me over the decades, I was able to accomplish most of the goals I set for myself. Training alongside men such as these ignited the fortitude and determination within me to become relentless in my search for ultimate health, greater size, and strength in the sport that I loved.

My life in bodybuilding has spanned more than four decades and in my eyes, this is just the beginning of a wondrous trip. From the day I first picked up a barbell to the many times I stood onstage in front of sold out audiences, my time in bodybuilding has been marvelous, and I smile whenever I reflect upon the fulfillment it has brought me.

I would like to give a special thank you to the artistic imagination of Bernie Schuman, whose talent not only graces the pages of this book, but also my Web site: MarioStong.com.
Bernie's drawings can be viewed on pages 6, 184, 224, 239, 246, 257, 267, 287, 296, 305, 317, 320, 332, 400, 426, and in the chapter titled: Anatomy of a Bodybuilder. To see more of Bernie's talent go to: MyCaricatures.com
Book cover design by Kristy Buchanan
Painting on book cover by Hugh McMunn
Drawing on page 178 by Gregory Baker
Photo credits: Dan Lurie (pg. 23), Keith Miguel (pg. 60),
Jack Orr (pg. 122-23), Debra Rei (pg. 128), Chet Yorton (pg. 397)
All photographs courtesy of the author, except for those previously mentioned.

Thanks Aida for helping to smooth out the rough edges of this book

PREFACE

LET ME INTRODUCE MYSELF

I am a natural for life bodybuilder! Some prefer the term physical culturist. I have never used steroids, growth hormones, diuretics, or any drug – illegal or prescribed – for the purposes of building muscle, getting ripped, or gaining strength; and I never will. In fact, I have never used drugs to get high, drank alcohol to get a buzz, or smoked cigarettes to look cool. My main reasons for bodybuilding are health and vitality. The cosmetic side of the sport is secondary to me. Sure, I like having baseball size biceps and superhuman strength. However, for me there is the bigger picture, one that is much greater and long lasting. For decades, I have poured gallons of sweat at the gym and have followed a natural bodybuilding lifestyle with several main goals in mind. Those goals are the quest of vibrant health, fitness, muscle, strength, and longevity. These are the goals I reached for since I first picked up a barbell, and they remain like a fire within my heart that still rages today as I continue on my life's journey.

It has been more than four decades since my father first showed me how to lift weights. Like all new trainees, my working knowledge on the subject of weight training was very limited in those early days of my muscle-building career. Through the years, I studied and applied different theories related to physiology and nutrition and applied them to my bodybuilding regimen. Over time, it became clear that all my efforts brought valuable gains and rewards my way. Eventually, my knowledge on the subject of physical culture peaked and I began to teach others the benefits of living a natural and healthy lifestyle. I was, and remain someone who practices what he preaches. I am a representation of my practice, and I motivate others to aim toward a healthier way of life.

For years, I flirted with the idea of writing a book on the subject of natural bodybuilding but never had the focus and desire to dedicate my time to such a lofty project. That all changed in 2007 while attending John Carrero's NGA California Physique Championships. Suddenly, a fire was ignited within me, encouraging me to put on paper what I had experienced in the sport. I had already created a popular bodybuilding Web site that was loaded with pages of entertaining and informative material, but now, I felt it was time to create something more substantial. I wanted to create something a person could hold in his or her hands and look to for guidance and reference, and then share what they learned with others. I wanted to write a book about my history in the sport of bodybuilding and describe in detail some of the muscle building principles I have discovered and have found useful. I also wanted to send a message to those that believe drugs are necessary to be successful in bodybuilding. This book is such an animal!

Through my involvement in the sport of bodybuilding, I have made many good friends as well as a few archenemies along the way. I have been a gym owner, trainer, competitor, judge, author, promoter, and just about everything else related to this wonderful sport. I have had the pleasure to workout with some of the biggest names in bodybuilding and have judged those that have judged me. I have trained thousands of students and have learned that each and every one is unique with different needs and goals to meet. I have traveled the country to participate in physique competitions and have enjoyed meeting the many faces of bodybuilding. I have learned much over the decades and have lived the very words that I preach. For the most part my memories in bodybuilding are ones that I cherish: they bring a smile to my face whenever I reflect upon them.

As I look to what has changed over the last forty years in bodybuilding, I sometimes relish the days of true Guts and Glory, when camaraderie existed among the bodybuilders and when there was hope that our sport would one day become a recognized Olympic sport. That hope has long vanished because of the greed and egos of those unable to see the truth of their ill-gotten gains. Outside the natural bodybuilding movement, the sport has become nothing more than a sick lie. Today, the forefathers of physical culture must be turning in their graves, because the enormous anabolic cloud that has darkened the sport of bodybuilding rains with the blood of those too weak to escape its deadly grip. Some people recognize the term *natural bodybuilder* as describing someone who does not take steroids, growth hormones, or diuretics for the purpose of building muscle and gaining strength. In my eyes, it goes even further than that. I believe that a natural bodybuilder is one that not only shuns muscle-enhancing drugs, but also follows a lifestyle that brings him somewhat closer to nature. We are all from this earth and it is paramount that natural bodybuilders make a conscious effort to attain radiant health by means of living a healthy lifestyle through the proper application of nutrition, exercise, rest, and positive thinking. It is mostly through these basic key factors that optimum health and fitness can ever be realized.

This book is a guiding light for those seeking a healthy alternative to the anabolic scene. It has definitely been a labor of love in expressing my feelings and beliefs on paper. If one person in a thousand can understand my words then the effort has been well worth it. In this book, you will find some funny stories as well as some tragic ones about some of the experiences and people who have crossed my path in this complex sport. Not every person mentioned in this book is a natural bodybuilder. Some are friends that I have come to know through my involvement in bodybuilding, while others are mentioned as a reference. Some of the names in this book are fictitious, while others have been omitted to avoid litigations. Since I am realistic, I know that there are those who may not follow the same philosophy towards bodybuilding that I do, but nevertheless, have something positive to offer. Most importantly, we all share a great passion for the sport.

This book, *Reflections of a Natural Bodybuilder*, is a natural muscle building and fitness-training guide mixed with nostalgia, sport, personality, story, and humor. I have created this unique book for bodybuilders, physical culturists, athletes, and the average laymen seeking muscular development, strength, health, and longevity. In this book, two main themes prevail. One is living a healthy and long life through natural bodybuilding, and the other focuses on the dangers of drugs within the sport. It is disappointing that the latter has to be discussed in a book that is meant to be a guiding light towards health and longevity, but that is just the reality of the times. It is my hope that the knowledge and experience presented in this book enrich the reader's life.

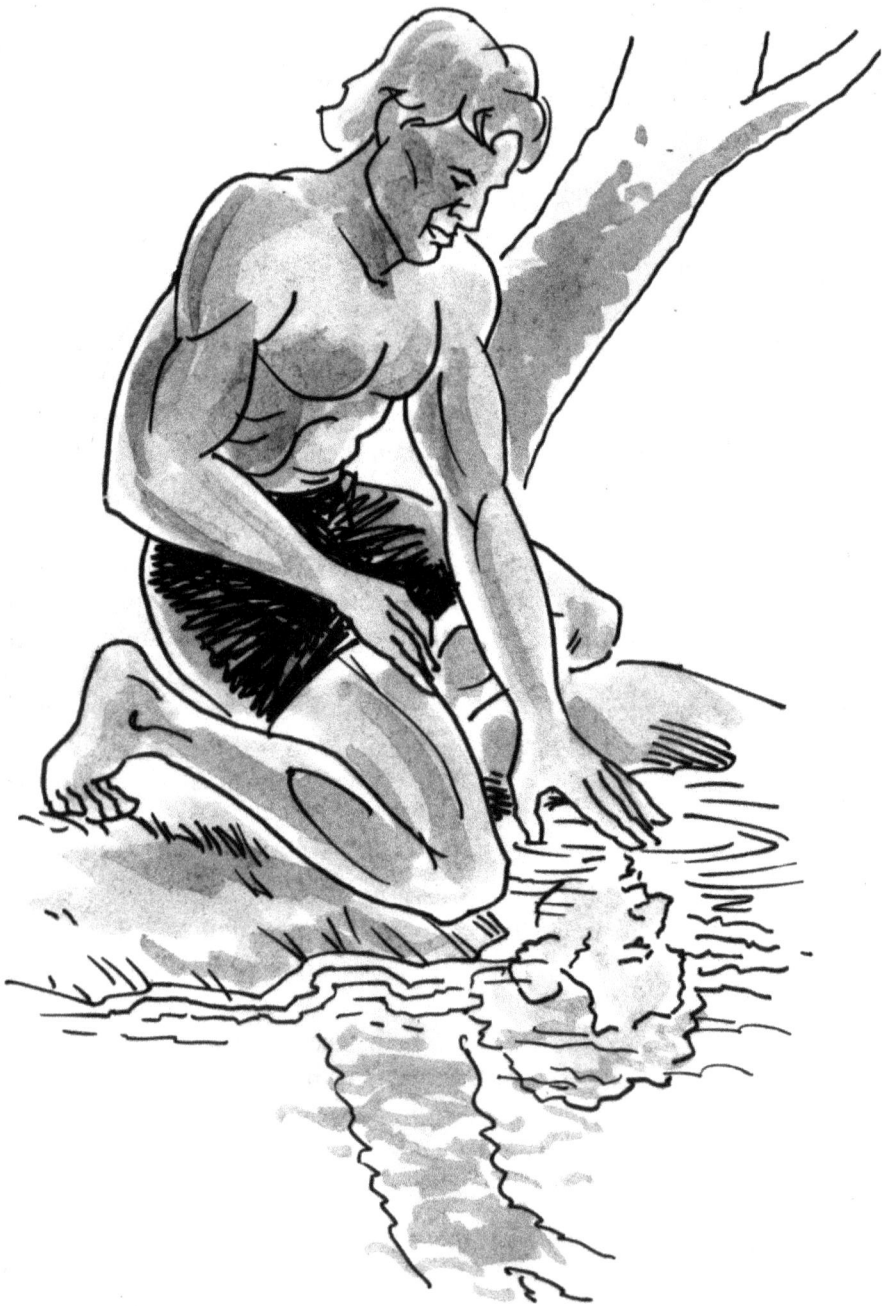

PART 1

REFLECTIONS OF A NATURAL BODYBUILDER

THE EARLY YEARS

GETTING STARTED

Before I was strong, I was weak! I was born during the hot summer of 1955. It was the season that saw Mickey Mantle hit his 100th career homerun and the beginning of an era for my parents, Mario and Carmela, young newlyweds from Brooklyn. They raised a family of six children, starting with me, Mario Jr., and went on to live the American dream. I was an average child, thin in structure and not very strong. I caught the common cold, had the measles and mumps, and even suffered from pneumonia twice. I was also born with a spinal condition in my lower back that would plague me for life.

The first time I ever laid eyes on a barbell was before I could even walk. My father trained at home with the free-weights he purchased while serving overseas during the U. S. occupation of Germany in the early 1950s. When he was discharged from the military, he brought the weights with him to America so he could continue with his training. The weights were dark brown in color and nameless. They were intimidating to look at, but aroused my young curiosity. As a child, I would sometimes pick up the small weight-plates and roll them around my house; occasionally a plate or two would make their way down the basement stairs. I even tried picking up the heavier weight-plates and once attempted to place a twenty-five pound disk onto a barbell. This did not go as planned when the cold steel weight-plate slipped from the barbell and fell onto my little fingers, giving me my first taste of pain.

As time went on, I would watch my father train with his free-weights. To me, he was a giant among men. I would watch in amazement, as he'd load all the big weight-plates onto the bar and then proceed to press it over his head several times. He was a superman! In reality, the weight he lifted was only about 150 pounds but to me it was a million pounds. I continued to watch my dad exercise and I yearned for the day when I could lift the same heavy steel and become as big and strong as he was.

However, before I could begin to pump the iron, I first had to address the lower back problem that would constantly make my legs give out and cause me to collapse. My physical impairment was so bad that my family, relatives, and friends would call me Boom-Boom on a regular basis. After a while, that nickname stuck to me like glue and it would take many years before I could free myself from it. I was always falling and during my early school years, I was fitted with metal leg braces (the same type and color that Forrest Gump wore) to help me stand and walk correctly. I also received treatment at Bayley Seton Hospital on Staten Island, twice weekly. Like clockwork, a therapist would pick me up at 2 PM every Tuesday and Friday from school and drive me to the hospital for treatments. There, he would put me through a series of painful torso and leg stretching movements to help alleviate my somewhat crippling condition. The stretching felt like torture but it did help stabilize my ability to stand and walk with limited falling. After each therapy session, I would go into a playroom to be with the other kids who also suffered physical ailments. While we played, the therapist constantly flirted with the nurses but was never able to score.

My serious disability diminished a bit through the years. I knew I needed to cure myself if I was ever going to be free of this curse and live a normal life. I was eager and ready to begin a life dedicated to health and fitness. But I didn't know where to begin.

THE GODFATHER OF FITNESS

As a youngster during the early 1960s, I would watch a fellow that wore a fitted jumpsuit, and who occasionally was accompanied by his wife and dog. During the daily morning program, he would jump up and down while inhaling and exhaling to musical sounds. This person intrigued me and every morning I would join my mother in performing the exercises that this fitness buff was demonstrating. Each morning before school, I would get a couple of chairs and place them in front of the black and white television set in the living room. When the show began, we were ready to perform the various exercises exactly as directed by this robust individual. For me, it was my first attempt at any form of proper exercise. I was just a kid and the only exercise I ever got was playing ball or running from my father when I did something wrong. However, this man made me curious and I began asking myself what this exercise stuff was all about. He always seemed cheerful, vibrant, and full of life. This is something that I also wanted to possess and as the years passed, the seeds of fitness he planted inside of me grew into a strong oak tree that still flourishes today. More than a half century after this natural for life bodybuilder first became a household name, Jack LaLanne, is still going strong as he and his wife, Elaine, continue to inspire millions of people worldwide as to the benefits of proper exercise, nutrition, and good, clean living. Thanks, Jack for being a shining inspiration when I needed it.

TIME FOR PAIN

I first began to weight train on my tenth birthday. My father's weight-plates that I had rolled around as a child soon would bring me pain I had never experienced before. My father designed a simple beginner's workout for me. It consisted of the Military Press, Barbell Curl, and Barbell Reverse Curl. The first week consisted of each exercise done for one set of ten repetitions, using only the barbell's resistance, which was twenty pounds. The second week I did two sets per exercise and the third week, I did three sets. I followed this program for several years and as time went on I increased the poundage but did little else in the way of additional exercises.

When I became a teenager, I was finally able to free myself from the unsightly metal leg braces that were once my cross to bear. I now wanted more in the way of physical development and sought new exercises and methods to build up my body. One day in early 1970, I came across a copy of *Muscle Builder & Power* that had bodybuilding champion Dave Draper on its cover. In amazement, I stared at his Herculean physique. "How was this possible?" I asked myself. How could anyone be so muscular and look so powerful? As I flipped the magazine's pages, I became even more amazed. Pictures of Larry Scott, Chuck Sipes, Sergio Oliva, and other muscle builders astonished me. I had found what I was looking for, and from that point on, never looked back. I began purchasing the muscle magazines whenever I could find one and absorbed their words in order to transform my learning into new muscle. I took the recommended weight gaining products, protein powders, and vitamin supplements that these champs endorsed. My brothers, Johnny and Domenic, and I started buying additional pieces of exercise equipment for our home gym. Before bodybuilding gyms became popular in America, most guys just trained at home with limited equipment. When my brothers and I started training in the mid 1960s, there weren't any bodybuilding gyms on Staten Island, so, the home gym it would be until the 1970s. During this period, we amassed several hundred pounds of steel as well as some primitive (by today's standards) exercise machines to train our bodies. Our gym was a small, 8'x12' brightly lit room, located in the basement of our home. On its walls were pictures of the champs from floor to ceiling. As we got bigger and stronger, we purchased more equipment and hung newer pictures of the latest bodybuilding stars. Occasionally, friends would stop by to pump some iron and share ideas on how best to reach our goals. We were all relentless in our quest to succeed and made every effort possible towards greater gains in both muscle mass and strength. In our eyes, the world stood still, as we marched through our lives with focus, purpose, and the determination to achieve.

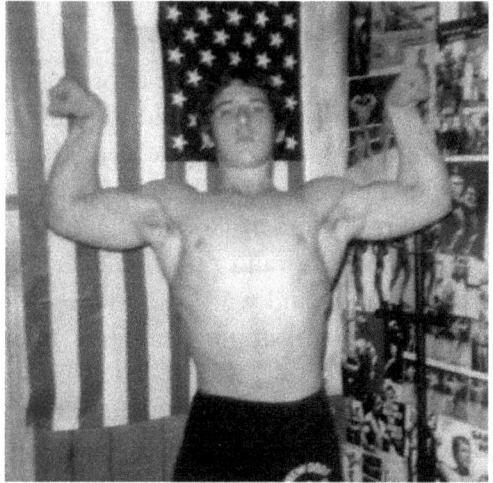

SPREADING THE WORD
During the early 1970s, I began to consume only natural foods. No more artificial foodstuffs for me. If it contained more than one ingredient, I wouldn't eat it. Out were the candies, sodas, cakes, breads, pastas, milk, and sugar products. In were fruits, vegetables, nuts, grains, legumes, chicken, and spring water. I began my nutritional transformation in 1969, the same year the New York Mets won their first World Series, and now I was going full steam ahead towards my ultimate goal of lasting health and vitality. I learned in detail of the pitfalls within the American diet. I wanted to teach what I

practiced and needed an outlet to do so. While attending classes at New Dorp High School on Staten Island, I became somewhat of a controversial figure. During my senior term, my physique reflected the years of my hard training and everyone took notice. My school had a newspaper titled, *The Pioneer*, and one of its editors was in my English class. One day, he approached me about my training and asked what kind of advice I could give him to develop his upper body. After writing a diet and exercise program for him, he then asked about my opinions on nutrition. Immediately I started ranting about the dangers that were on supermarkets shelves. At the time, I was fanatical about proper nutrition and preached whenever I could about the benefits of natural foods and warned about the poisons being sold to the public. I gave him few simple examples about food additives and explained their possible side effects. The following week, I read my comments – word for word – in the school's newspaper, and found myself on the defensive end among the students and staff. During class, teachers who seemed doubtfully interested in what I was up to constantly questioned me to the reasoning behind my way of life. The cafeteria was no better, as students that were having greasy burgers and fries challenged me on the "sacrifices" I was making. Eventually, I won over some of them with my concepts of health and vitality, and curiously watched as others began to take notice. This was back in 1972, and these types of experiences helped me create the foundation for what was to come years later. They helped me learn to better communicate my concepts to any ears that would listen.

ANABOLIC WHAT?

The first time I ever heard about steroids was from a friend who was on the New Dorp High School varsity football team. My friend was a big, burly sort of guy who was scary to look at but friendly in his mannerisms. One day, while on the bus ride to school, we discussed training and supplements. Mysteriously, my friend looked around to see if anybody was watching and pulled out a bottle of blue tablets from his jacket. He said they were called Dianabol and had helped him gain size and strength. He also went on to say that many members of the football team were using them for the same purpose. He recommended that I go see his friend and get some Dianabol to help me with my bodybuilding. After classes were dismissed for the day, I walked to the local health food store and spoke to a man named

Charlie Siegel who was the co-owner of Family Health Foods. I figured if anyone knew about the benefits of Dianabol it would be Charlie, since he was a former bodybuilding champion during the 1950s, and was as big as a house. Charlie grabbed me by the collar and warned me that Dianabol was an anabolic drug. He stated that many bodybuilders who used the drug had damaged their major organs and went bald before they were thirty. I didn't want any of that! I was training not only to build muscle, but also for health and longevity. I took Charlie's words to heart and the next day I told my friend about the dangers of the drug and that he should stop taking them before he suffered some serious side effects. He just shrugged me off, saying, "I need them for football and don't care about any possible future side effects." This was in 1971! Not much has changed since.

GETTING STRONG NOW

During the summer of 1972, I trained at my Uncle Sal's, *Flamingo Pool & Health Club*, on Staten Island. The club was located far from my home, which meant several long train rides (to and from) each week. During the 1950s, my Uncle Sal was into fitness and was a star baseball player for the Wagner College Seahawks on Staten Island. His health club's gym had a couple of benches and a cable machine. It also had a set of chrome dumbbells and several hundred pounds of free-weights that felt as good as they looked. A year earlier, bodybuilding champion Leon Brown won the title of Mr. Staten Island, which was sponsored by my uncle and held at his club. Now I was there to workout and make some serious gains. Other than training in my basement gym or on the Universal Machine at school, it was the only other location that I had ever trained at during my high school years. Probably the one thing that motivated me most that summer was the sexy fitness instructor that hung around the gym watching the guys train. Being a red-blooded American teenager, I pushed and pulled the iron with my ego and watched in amazement as my strength made some decent progress. My bench press went from 160 to 205 pounds in the three months I spent there and my bodyweight began to climb as I gained twenty pounds of solid natural muscle.

When I returned to New Dorp High School that same year, my friends could not believe how much I had grown and how strong I had become. This only served to motivate me even more and by the end of my senior year, I was weighing a muscular 200 pounds and lifting steel I never thought imaginable. In the high school gym, I was banging out full stacks of weights on the Universal Machine and at home I took on the motto that, "If it wasn't bolted down I'd lift it." My enthusiasm was soaring high and I was on my way.

During the early 1970s, high school coaches discouraged their athletes from training with weights. They actually believed that lifting weights would make the athletes slow and muscle-bound. On several occasions, I tried out for, and made, my school's baseball and football teams, only to find myself at odds with the coaches regarding my weight training. I was a bodybuilder and there was no way I was going to alter my training just to be on a team. The coaches wanted me on the field while I wanted to be in the weight room. On the field, I was fast, had a great throwing arm, and could easily hit home runs or throw touchdown passes. In gym class, I was able to climb the ropes in perfect L-form, perform chin-ups with one arm, and sprint with explosive force. These were some of the benefits of lifting iron. The coaches wanted me to stop lifting and spend more time on the field. I felt this would impede my progress, both as a bodybuilder as well as an athlete, so, I opted not to be on the teams. Decades later, the benefits of weight training have become apparent as high schools throughout America now incorporate it into their sports programs. I guess I was just a little ahead of my time.

STAYING HUNGRY

During my mid-teen years in bodybuilding, I was big on supplements. I read every muscle building publication available and hungrily studied the training and nutrition secrets of the champs. I wanted to be as big as Arnold, as strong as Franco, and as popular as Draper. I was driven to succeed and bought into the supplement industry's marketing that to get big and strong, XYZ supplements were the way to go. My bedroom's dresser-top made Lou Ferrigno's dresser in the movie *Pumping Iron*, look vacant. Every square inch was filled with large bottles and canisters of the latest vitamins, enzymes, oils, proteins, and weight gain powders. There were Joe Weider's Multi-Vitamins, Bob Hoffman's Energol, and Dan Lurie's Crash Weight Gain Formula, just to name a few. You name it I took it. I must have been consuming fifty tablets, along with three to four mass-building drinks daily to help wash them down. I was determined to get big and strong; if this was the path the champs took then that was good enough for me.

During my high school years, my bodyweight went from a lean 160 pounds to a powerful 200 pounds. I performed total body workouts in my home gym three times a week. At times, my training sessions would last up to four hours. If there were an exercise I could perform, I would add it to my workout. I was game for anything and everything, and tried my best to improve a little bit each day.

It would take me several years to wise up and realize that although supplements do work to some degree, the best way to lasting muscle and health was through proper nutrition. During my senior year in New Dorp High School, I eliminated all supplements from my diet and totally relied on natural foods for continued gains. Almost instantly, I began to see improvements in my physique and strength. Getting all my calories and nutrients from real foods shocked my body into never before realized levels of mass and power. Before I knew it, I was training harder, getting bigger, and lifting poundage I never dreamed possible. Since that time, I have not taken any form of supplement and to this day, continue to enjoy great gains at the gym.

THE FIRST SHOW

By the time I became a senior in high school, I had several years of consistent weight training under my lifting belt. For years, I slaved with the iron in the basement of my home alongside Johnny and Domenic, in hopes of realizing greater size and strength. We bought all the bodybuilding magazines available and dreamed of the day when we would have physiques equal to those of the images that appeared in those publications. Up until that time, my brothers and I had never attended a bodybuilding competition. The sanctioned physique shows were sparse in New York and never took place on Staten Island. That all changed during the last week of February 1973, when I learned that a physique competition was going to be held at one of the high schools on the Island that coming Saturday. The show was titled the AAU Mr. Sr. Metropolitan Bodybuilding Championships. It was held in conjunction with an official AAU Olympic Weightlifting competition that was billed as the main event.

On the day of the competition, my father drove my brothers, a couple of friends, and me to the show. Since this was our first time attending such a competition, we were extremely eager and arrived at the school before most of the competitors, judges, and audience. One by one, the competitors for both competitions slowly strolled into the school, as we all visually scrutinized their physiques. For the most part, none of the athletes looked overly massive but some were quite muscular and seemed a bit tense. After registering, the competitors proceeded to a section of the school where tons of iron was assembled so the Olympic lifters and bodybuilders could warm up before stepping onstage. Back in the 1970s, AAU physique competitions took a back seat to Olympic Weightlifting and this day was no different, as the bodybuilding portion of the day's events would have to wait until every lifter completed all his attempts.

Finally, by 6 PM, the Olympic lifters completed their portion of the day's competitions and exited the building. The much-anticipated moment had come, when we all would witness for the first time in our lives actual raw muscle being flexed right in front of our excited eyes. As the MC announced their names, the anxious bodybuilders with their Herculean forms stepped onto the stage and faced the screaming fans. There were six physique competitors in all that evening, and each bodybuilder came to the show toned, polished, and well oiled. In amazement and awe, I watched as the athletes flawlessly transitioned from one pose to another, while following the judges' directions to position their physiques into the mandatory poses. As these muscular he-men flexed their superhuman forms, I studied their proportioned anatomies and envisioned myself one day competing in the same manner, while standing in front of a cheering crowd. As the bodybuilders flexed hard and squeezed every drop of sweat out of their pumped physiques, their bulging, fibrous muscles striated into overwhelming disbelief. One bodybuilder in particular stood out from the rest. His name was John Boos. As soon as John stepped onto the stage, you knew he was the man to beat. He had perfect symmetry, proportion, muscularity, presentation, and was well tanned. John was a seasoned competitor, who was well known among the East Coast bodybuilders. He already had a string of victories under his training belt and on this night he would add one more to his trophy shelf.

This was the real deal; these guys were huge with muscles popping out in areas that I didn't even know muscle could exist. Being the motivated seventeen-year-old bodybuilder I was, their physiques inspired me to chart my own road towards success, and before the night was over, I would learn every exercise and nutritional tip possible from these muscular athletes. In the days, weeks, and months that followed, I continued to train with great intensity. I knew deep inside my heart that one day, I too, would stand on a physique stage and achieve the goals I hungrily sought. I had the patience and belief, now it was only a matter of time.

STING LIKE A BEE AND DANCE LIKE A BUTTERFLY

On occasion, during my high school years, I would be taunted by others who knew of my bodybuilding but who were bigger than I was and wanted to test my will. I never paid much attention to their stupid antics until one day while hanging out with some friends at a local shopping center after school. One individual in particular, who I thought was a good friend of mine, crossed the line when he unexpectedly pushed me to the ground and challenged me to a fight in front of everyone. Now, I don't know what he was thinking, but he made a big mistake. Although he was taller and outweighed me by at least thirty pounds, he was no match for me, since I was in excellent physical condition from all my years of weight training and martial arts. As I rose to my feet other students ran over to watch what was about to unfold. I was furious at the cheap knockdown and let loose with a barrage of punches and kicks that sent my former friend bouncing off parked cars and into the street. All of my training came into play as I found myself easily winning the fight, which was vicious and painful for my opponent. After I finished pouncing on the poor fool, I asked some of the other instigators if they wanted to trade fist with me.

As I headed in the direction of another kid, someone started to frantically scream. "Stop! Stop fighting now!" the voice demanded. As I turned around, I looked in disbelief as my mother and Cousin Linda came running towards me in an effort to cease my actions. By coincidence, they had been shopping in the area. My mother clamped her arms around my torso and wrestled me to the ground. She held me there for a minute or so until I calmed down and then let me up while maintaining her tight grip on me. She scolded my so-called friends for what had transpired and warned them that she would be speaking to their parents (which she did) later that day. Although I had won the fight, I was humiliated that my mother was throwing me around like a rag doll in front of my schoolmates. The one positive thing that came from the incident was that it served as a warning to others that I was not like them. Unlike most other high school kids, I had spent thousands of hours training to become muscular, strong, and fit. If need be, I was capable of instantly defending myself like a war machine. I felt like Bruce Lee and Muhammad Ali wrapped into one. I was mobile, hostile, and agile. I stung like a bee, danced liked a butterfly, and began to realize my potential.

FOLLOWING A DIFFERENT PATH

By the time I was seventeen it was obvious to my family and friends that I was leading a different life. At family parties, I would always bring my own nourishment and would constantly preach to my many relatives about the benefits of proper nutrition and exercise. As much as I tried, my well-intended advice went in one ear and out the other. My extended family knew what I was about and although they commended me for my efforts and wished they could do the same, they never found the fortitude within themselves to go the distance.

The same applied to the students I knew in school. They were following the same path as most of the other kids by not being physically active in sports or self-conditioning. They obliviously ate their junk food and drank soft drinks. They also smoked their cigarettes to look cool and gulped bottles of beer to be part of the crowd. It was the same story with recreational drugs. As a teenager, I had many friends and had some great times with them. They were friends with whom I traveled to school, played baseball, and went fishing. We were a close-knit group and did everything together like normal teenagers, until the tide began to turn and they started to experiment with recreational drugs. Luckily, I was intensely into bodybuilding during that period of my life and did not follow the same road as my friends. I'd preach to them on how they were ruining their health by getting high on drugs, but they would just laugh at me saying I didn't know what I was talking about. The drugs ruined our friendships, as some became addicted and lost control of their own lives. It would take them several years to break the chains of addiction, but the damage was already done. Not only were our friendships strained, but also their health has never been the same since. Now, I am not much of a religious fellow but I do know right from wrong and do not need the fear of God in me to make me do the right thing. Why many of this generation's teenagers experiment with recreational drugs and sports enhancement pharmaceuticals, is beyond my realm of reasoning. I wonder what the thought process is for some of these individuals, if any. We live in a world where everything you need to know about the dangers of drugs is right at our fingertips, and yet, the denial that not only our youth, but also society lives with is disturbing. I am afraid nothing is going to change anytime soon. All I can do is keep up the fight and hope that my words will be heard once in a while.

Fortunately, during my senior year of high school I was able to help one individual break the drug habit with the help of bodybuilding. I designed an exercise program for a friend and monitored his progress throughout the year. Every so often, he would get sidetracked with drugs and I would find it necessary to reel him back onto the correct course. By the time our graduation came around, he was in great physical condition and finally drug-free. Years later, he would thank me for changing his life as he went on to be a husband, father, and successful businessman. To me the effort was well worth it and I realized that this bodybuilding thing I was into could be put to good use to help others. I knew I could make a difference in the lives of those that would listen to my words. The trick was to find those whose ears were open to new ideas.

THE FAMOUS MR. UNIVERSE
In 1971, I took a ride with my father and brothers to Union City, New Jersey to visit the Weider Headquarters. I had heard that Dave Draper was an employee there, and we were all eager to meet the Blond Bomber as well as Joe Weider. At the time, Joe Weider was the most recognized and respected name in bodybuilding. When we arrived at our destination, we were disappointed to learn that Joe Weider had recently moved his entire operation to Woodland Hills, California. However, our disappointed soon changed to joy when the remaining Weider staff advised us that the 1971 IFBB Mr. World Competition would be televised that afternoon on the Wide World of Sports. Being the avid bodybuilding fans that we were, we became ecstatic and rushed back to Staten Island to watch the previously taped program. The IFBB Mr. World competition was the first professional bodybuilding competition ever aired on national television. When the competitors stepped onto the stage, my brothers and I were stunned by the massively proportioned physiques. There they were, Herculean forms of muscle and flesh that we learned to admire through the physique publications. Arnold Schwarzenegger, Sergio Oliva, Dave Draper, and Dennis Tinerino all flexed their muscles as they vied for top honors. It was the first time we had ever witnessed the big-named

bodybuilding stars compete against one another. We were in complete awe at the display of sheer muscle that flashed across our television. Arnold won that day and it would not be until 1973, during my senior year, that I would once again see him flexing his winning form on the tube.

I idolized Arnold Schwarzenegger and nearly fell off my chair one day while watching a commercial for Holiday Health Spas. The commercial featured actor Bob Cummings as host for the health club chain. After Bob mentioned a few words about the club, he would say "And here I am with the famous Mr. Universe, Arnold Schwarzenegger." The camera would then pan over to the left and the Herculean champion appeared before my eyes, flexing his mighty physique for the world to see. Being the hard-core bodybuilding enthusiast that I was, I watched in pure amazement as Arnold displayed his Mr. Universe physique. I had idolized his physique for years and now I was witnessing what I so deeply sought. The commercial aired at 12:35 PM every day. During my senior year, I was on the school's early morning program and was released each day at noon. Immediately after the last class, I would run to the bus stop to get home in time to see Arnold flex his biceps. Every day when I arrived home, I would turn on the TV to watch the commercial and found myself becoming more motivated than ever to hit the steel. After watching Arnold flex, I would spend several hours in my home gym, exuding the same confidence that my idol winningly displayed. I was determined to succeed and trained as if there was no tomorrow, in the belief that one day, I too, would be crowned champion on the physique stage. It was only a matter of time.

ALL WORK AND NO PLAY

My life has not always been just about building big biceps and lifting heavy steel. From grammar school to college, my days off from classes were spent working at a women's wear factory owned by my father. My father was a pattern designer by trade and for years owned his own clothing factory. The name of the company was Angela Sportswear and it was located in the south side of Manhattan. From the young age of seven, I would accompany my father to his factory to work beside him to learn the complexities of the business. At first, I just cut threads off garments and swept the floors. As the years went by, I got more involved in the business and eventually started designing my own garments as well as maintaining the company's books. Although it was not hard work, it was, nevertheless, time consuming, cutting into my training time. Working with my father meant waking up at 6 AM and not returning home until 10 PM or later. The man was a workhorse, and whenever I had a day off from school, or was not studying for an exam, I was by his side at the factory absorbing his focus and determination to succeed in life. It is from watching my father's drive in the business world, through both the good times and bad, that I have remained disciplined in bodybuilding through all the obstacles and setbacks the sport can bring. I am extremely grateful to my Dad.

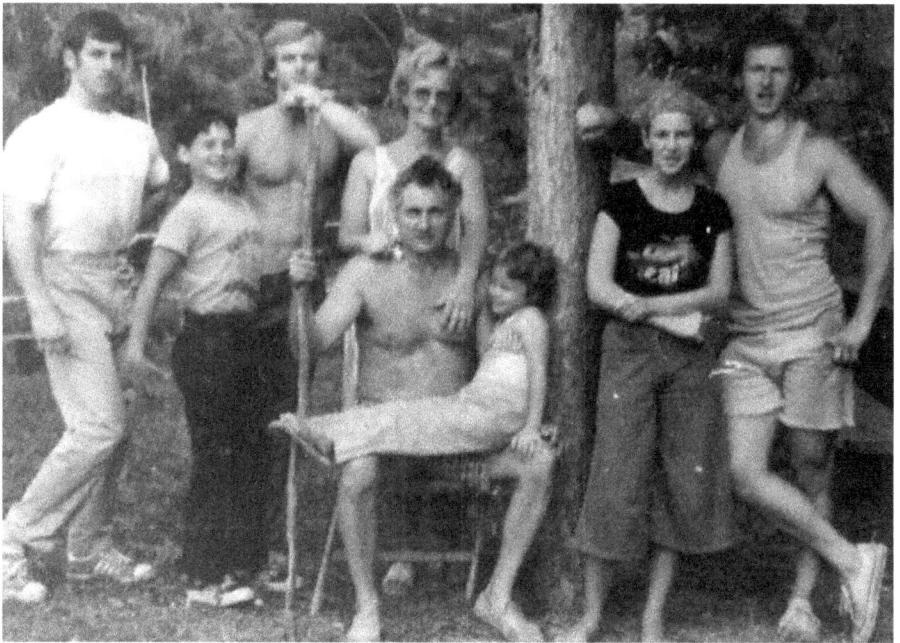
The Strong family gathers at their Catskill Mountains home – 1978

GREEN ACRES IS THE PLACE TO BE

Early in my life, I was very fortunate to have a father, who not only worked hard, but also loved the outdoors. When I was a youngster he would frequently take me on big-game hunting trips (I never killed a wild animal) in blizzards and sub-freezing temperatures. Through my father, I learned to love the ruggedness of the wilderness and was overjoyed in the early 1970s when he purchased 150 prime acres in the Catskill Mountains to build a second home. The property consisted of a five-acre lake and an equal amount of open space to build a log cabin as well as a stable for several horses and cows. We also had a section for chickens, turkeys, goats, rabbits, and just about every other form of livestock my father could find. The rest of the land was trees, shrubs, hills, and boulders. In my eyes, it was The Garden of Eden, but in reality, it was hard work.

There were tons of trees to saw, boulders to carry, and acres of grass to cut. Caring for the property was endless work, but I enjoyed the challenge because it brought me closer to nature. It was great to be in such a natural environment. Each morning, I would breathe in the fresh air as I listened to the chirps of the birds above. We even had a running path around the lake that measured a quarter mile in length on which I ran barefoot whenever possible. The path was rocky and rough and helped me build such thick calluses on my soles that after several months of running in this fashion I was able to run barefoot on snow and ice without the threat of frostbite. Also on the property was a small cemetery dating back to World War I. It contained about 30 graves and was a constant reminder of the certain end we would all face, but that I was trying to avoid.

HEALTH IS YOUR GREATEST WEALTH

As a teenager, I subscribed to several bodybuilding magazines, one of which was Dan Lurie's *Muscle Training Illustrated* (*MTI*). Dan's magazine was full of stories about the bodybuilding champs of the day and served as a catalog for his exercise equipment. One day, my father drove my brothers and me to Brooklyn to visit the Dan Lurie Barbell Company on Utica Avenue. This would be the first of many such visits and the most memorable. Outside Dan's establishment was a huge vertical sign that displayed an image of him flexing his biceps in his famous strongman pose. As we walked into the building, we became mesmerized by giant posters of past and present champions covering every square inch of wall, from floor to ceiling. Posters of Arnold Schwarzenegger, Sergio Oliva, Steve Reeves, Larry Scott, and every champion imaginable hung there before our hungry eyes. Behind the shop's counter was Tony Badel, a local bodybuilder employed by Dan, who was occasionally featured in *Muscle Training Illustrated*. As we looked around, we saw mountains of weight-plates, some taller than us. There were exercise machines everywhere and racks of current and old copies of *Muscle Training Illustrated* and books related to the art of muscle building. After a short while of touring the shop, Dan smilingly walked towards us and asked if we needed any help. It was great to finally meet him after having read his publication for so many years. He was very helpful that day in giving my brothers and me some beneficial training advice as he demonstrated several pieces of equipment for us. Dan Lurie (see photo) was a legendary bodybuilding promoter, who in earlier years, competed successfully in the AAU Mr. America and later became a Sealtest Circus Strongman on TV; his motto was, "Health is your Greatest Wealth." That was something I also prescribed to and it was good to see Dan looking and feeling the part he portrayed. That day, we bought an adjustable bench along with every past issue of *MTI* we did not already own. On the trip home, my brothers and I read the magazines in detail as we studied the photos of the great legends, and read the informative training programs for mass and strength. By the time we arrived home, we were psyched and headed for our gym. We had fire in our blood and were ready to hit the steel with a vengeance, as we were more determined than ever to become bigger and stronger than we ever dared to imagine.

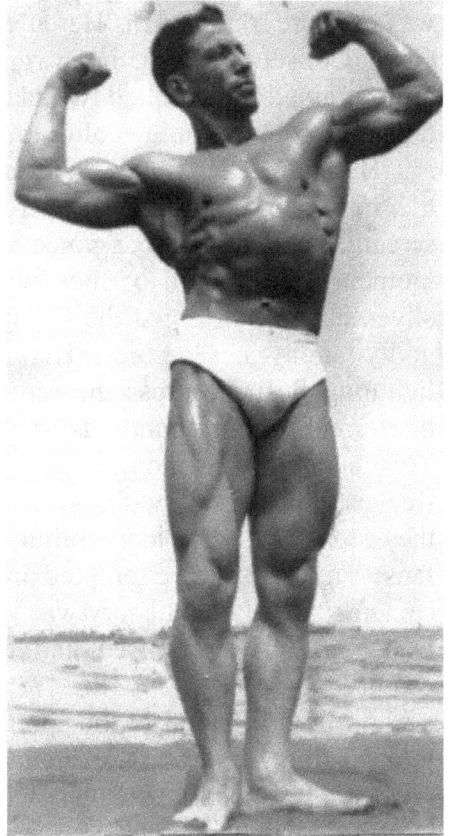

A HERCULEAN MOMENT
On September 8, 1973, I had the pleasure to attend Dan Lurie's big WBBG event in New York City. The show featured guest posers Sergio Oliva, Frank Zane, Dave Draper, and Kenny Hall. Chris Dickerson (Pro Mr. America) and Boyer Coe (Pro Mr. World) were among the dozens of competitors that evening. It was a great thrill to see all the champs flex their stuff at the event. However, they were all overshadowed by a legendary figure that was to appear onstage that evening.

Towards the end of the evening, the much-anticipated event that drew thousands of muscle builders from all over the country had finally arrived. Dan Lurie's heavily promoted appearance of the legendary Steve Reeves at the 1973 WBBG World Bodybuilding Championships was about to become a reality. Those loyal to this legend held tight onto their seats as a stage-wide movie screen lowered to the floor. All eyes stared ahead, not daring to miss a second of this historic moment. Suddenly, the screen filled with images of the movie *Hercules Unchained*, revealing this perfectly developed being whose symmetrical structure could have only been created by the gods. He was no mere mortal. This Herculean figure stood at the entrance of the Great Coliseum. There he was this mighty being, whose muscular arms strained as he pulled two massive chains that wrapped around the tall stone columns at the coliseum's entrance.

Hercules!, the filmed echoed loudly across the theater, bringing the now standing-room-only crowd into a near frenzy. Hercules!, screamed this thunderous voice again as it sent legions of fans into a moment of disbelief, as they witnessed this immortal figure on the silver screen pull down the Great Coliseum walls with his seemingly godly strength. Hercules, Hercules!, roared the film, as jolts of lightning flashed across the screen, electrifying every muscle in the house and sending hundreds in attendance rushing towards the stage. Then suddenly the moment of a lifetime had come. Dan Lurie, Steve Reeves, and Steve's wife, Aline, walked towards center stage. There they stood, side-by-side, smiling and waving at this sea of admiring fans. The vast crowd erupted into a chorus of cheers and flashing cameras; they knew history was happening right in front of their eyes. Dan Lurie had promised and delivered the greatest show of the century!

As the trio stood in the spotlight of admiration, a massive fellow jumped from the seating area and onto the stage and rushed towards a startled Mr. and Mrs. Reeves, who were both understandably shaken by this unwelcomed intruder. Acting with instinct and without fear for his own safety, Dan Lurie immediately ran in the direction of this crazed man and blocked the path to the couple. Dan then knocked the lunatic to the floor and gave him a mighty thrust off the stage and into the hands of the waiting security personnel. The crowd cheered and applauded wildly with relief as Dan, Steve, and Aline walked towards the microphone to address the still standing room audience. It was a moment in time to last for generations, which motivated me beyond belief to train harder and with more focus than ever before. I was hungry to succeed and began to vision my own Herculean future in the realms of Muscledom.

MOM SAVES THE DAY

In the early 1970s, there were no commercial bodybuilding gyms on Staten Island, so it was up to the individual bodybuilder to buy and equip his own home gym. Because of this, my brothers and I primarily trained at home. Our homemade gym was equipped with over a thousand pounds of steel and had a variety of machines and benches to fulfill our needs. Its well thought-out design assured us that no body part was denied its share of work as we were afforded the ability to perform a wide array of exercises.

One day, while training alone in my basement gym, I was performing the Bench Press movement with a respectable weight. As I banged out several sets, I gradually increased the resistance to 250 pounds, which was not bad for a seventeen-year-old bodybuilder in those days. At the time, I did not have a power-rack to catch the weight in case I got stuck, so performing the exercise alone was a little dangerous, to say the least. After completing my last rep, I missed placing the barbell back on the bench's weight-rack and it crashed onto my chest, causing a severe injury to my right shoulder. I was pinned with little strength to move the bar and realized I was in some serious trouble as the bar slowly crept towards my neck. Desperately I yelled for help. Luckily, my mother was home on the first floor. She hurried down the steps and ran into the gym. In horror, she looked at my peril and without pause stepped behind the bench and grasped tightly onto the barbell. With one mighty heave, she pulled the barbell from my chest and placed it back on the rack. Just like me, my mom had great physical strength and saved the day and my life!

That was certainly not the first time my mother acted heroically. In 1963, when I was eight years old, my father took us on a trip to see Niagara Falls. It was a hot steamy day and the car ride to Buffalo from Staten Island took about eight sweaty hours. Our car had no air-conditioning and by the time we arrived at a lodge to rest I was in need of some relief. Luckily, the lodge we stopped at had an outdoor pool, and it looked very inviting. As my parents were unpacking the car, I decided to take a cool dip in the pool while still wearing my shoes and clothes. I lost my footing and my body began to slide towards the deep end of the pool. I was sinking below the waterline. As I struggled to keep my head above the water, I remembered watching cartoons on TV where the characters would raise their fingers above the waterline as a signal to others that they were in serious trouble. I did the same and caught the attention of a passerby who yelled out to my mother that someone was drowning. Without knowing who was in trouble, my mother jumped into the pool and put her arm around my torso, then pulled me above the waterline as I frantically gasped for air. My mother saved my life! But, as horrifying as the experience was for me, it paled in comparison to the explosive reaction my father had when he discovered what I had done.

FILBERTS, BANANAS, AND CARROTS

Everyone has made mistakes throughout the course of history. But I guess failing is a part of learning. In my senior year of high school, I was very much into nutrition and looked for the perfect diet. During this time, my diet was void of all candies, soft drinks, cakes, and just about every other artificial manmade food item available. I was living on only basic natural foods and doing quite nicely until one day I got the bright idea to start eliminating some natural food items from my nutritional program, with the concept of sustaining my health and strength with a very limited number of foods. The first food items banished from my diet were the flesh foods: beef, chicken, fish, and pork. I had already eliminated milk and eggs, so this meant that I would no longer be consuming protein from any animal sources.

Over the weeks and months to follow, I began to exclude foods from the vegetable, fruit, and grain groups until my only sources of nutrition were from filberts, bananas, carrots, and spring water, which I bottled at my home upstate. I was buying bunches of thick organic carrots from Family Health Foods on Staten Island and 50-pound sacks of filberts from a vendor in Manhattan who saw me so often that he knew me by my first name. The bananas were purchased at the local food market. Together, I was consuming tremendous amounts of these three items to help me compensate for the protein and calories I was denying myself from other food sources, in particular, the flesh foods. For a while, I thought I had discovered the perfect diet as my training was still going strong and my physique remained muscular.

After three years on this strict regimen, my personality became more passive and my endurance became diminished. My skin color had turned orange from all the carotene consumed. The so-called perfect diet had failed me in terms of weakened health and strength. The turning point came when my father, who had seen enough of my deterioration, decided to dump about 100 pounds of filberts that were stored in my dresser, into the sewer on the street corner. He expressed his disapproval of my limited diet and made his point very clear with this action. I knew he was right, so it was back to the drawing board to rebuild my body. I soon reintroduced chicken back into my diet along with a wide spectrum of vegetables, fruits, grains, and legumes. Not before long, I was back on the saddle, riding bronco. Although the experience had temporarily weakened me, it made me stronger for the future, as my knowledge in nutrition continued to grow.

REACHING A MILESTONE

After training for many years in my home gym, I found that my progress was beginning to slow down as the equipment I had to train with became somewhat limited. I needed more in the way of heavier steel and machinery and began to seek other venues to pump iron. Back in 1975, Staten Island had little to offer for weight training. There was the local YMCA that had a Universal machine and some dumbbells, but not much else for a bodybuilder. Probably the only halfway decent gym was located inside the Berry Homes in Dongan Hills. It was owned by the city and managed by a fellow named Gerald Troshane. The small gym had a few steady members that shared a key to the place, but it too, was limited. I needed more! I needed a gym that was well equipped and had an atmosphere that produced results.

Fortunately, the answer to my prayers was located across the Verrazano Bridge in Brooklyn. On Christmas Day of that same year, I took a trip to Brooklyn with my then-girlfriend, Denise, to visit the new Bath Beach Bodybuilding Gym. The gym had just moved from its original location on Bath Avenue to Avenue U and had a special promotion of $100 for a whole year of pain. When I arrived there, my muscles drooled with excitement as I gazed across the spacious gym floor and marveled at the tons of free-weights and rows of benches and exercise machines. Everything imaginable was there before my eyes. The gym was owned by a bodybuilder who knew what it took to become a champion, and was equipped with the tools to make it happen. As a Christmas gift, Denise bought me a membership to the club, and happily, a milestone in my life's journey was at hand.

John Barberro was the owner of Bath Beach Bodybuilding. John was a true bodybuilder at heart and trained hard to build a physique worthy enough to step onto any local physique stage. His gym was designed to produce results and that was exactly what I got from my time there. My first few workouts at Bath Beach were a little intimidating, since I had never really trained at a commercial gym before and now found myself working out alongside seasoned bodybuilders and powerlifters that lived for the gym. As the months toiled by, I learned a great deal from watching the Brooklyn muscle builders as they became bigger and stronger with every rep and set they performed. I was motivated, applied my newfound knowledge into my own training program, and soon found myself making enormous gains in a relatively short period. The limits of my home gym were now gone and I began to crash through barriers that once held me back. As my physique became more muscular and my strength levels increased, I found others seeking my muscle building advice and happily wrote exercise and nutritional programs to help them reach their own goals. I felt comfortable in the role of helping others with their training at Bath Beach Bodybuilding. On May 1976, to earn a few extra bucks I started to train people at a small garage gym I opened on Staten Island. Word soon spread about my local neighborhood gym and before you knew it, my garage was filled to the rafters with biceps and pectorals. The demand for my knowledge and time was at a fever pitch and I began to dream of opening Staten Island's first professional bodybuilding gym. But where and when would history begin?

THE BEGINNING OF AN ERA

THE STATEN ISLAND BODYBUILDING CLUB

For years, I trained consistently and with great ferocity to develop a muscular body that was as strong as it looked. During my intense transformation, I also acquired a mountain of knowledge on the sport of bodybuilding. I had read every physique publication available and began training muscle builders at my garage gym using the knowledge and experience I had gained. I had become a living chemistry set, fine-tuning my physique through proper nutrition, resistance training, and positive thinking. I lived a clean life. I never drank alcohol and never smoked or took drugs to get high. I had no vices! Since an early age, I always walked a straight line when it came to my health, thanks to the path I followed in bodybuilding. It was a way of life I believed in and I wanted to share it with everyone else. I was ready to take on the challenge and make the Staten Island Bodybuilding Club a reality.

On September 7, 1976, after several months of searching for a location to build a gym, and after acquiring exercise equipment from various sources, I opened Staten Island's first bodybuilding club in the heart of the Island on New Dorp Lane. The gym was appropriately named the Staten Island Bodybuilding Club, and was equipped with Weider, Lurie, and York Barbell free-weights, benches, and machines. It also featured a complete set of solid Jackson dumbbells that dated back a couple of decades. The Staten Island Bodybuilding Club had two brightly lit floors to workout on and was designed for maximum results. Its high mirrored-walls were encased with dozens of bodybuilding posters that helped to create a unique atmosphere and welcomed everyone who came there. This motivating atmosphere would inspire thousands of bodybuilders to excel and achieve their goals in the decade to come.

In 1976, bodybuilding was still somewhat of a sub-culture. It was the running era and weight training for sports was forbidden at many high schools and universities. Arnold Schwarzenegger had already won six Mr. Olympia titles, but was virtually unknown outside the bodybuilding world. The physique publications of the day were rarely found on newsstand racks and the public at large laughingly frowned upon women training with weights.

On Staten Island, there were several well-known bodybuilders. Names such as George Orlando, Larry Powers, Jerry Valente, and Leon Brown were recognized throughout the muscle-building world. The Island had a few local garage-type gyms and a small YMCA. There was a serious void on Staten Island for bodybuilders wanting more and I eagerly stepped in to fulfill their needs.

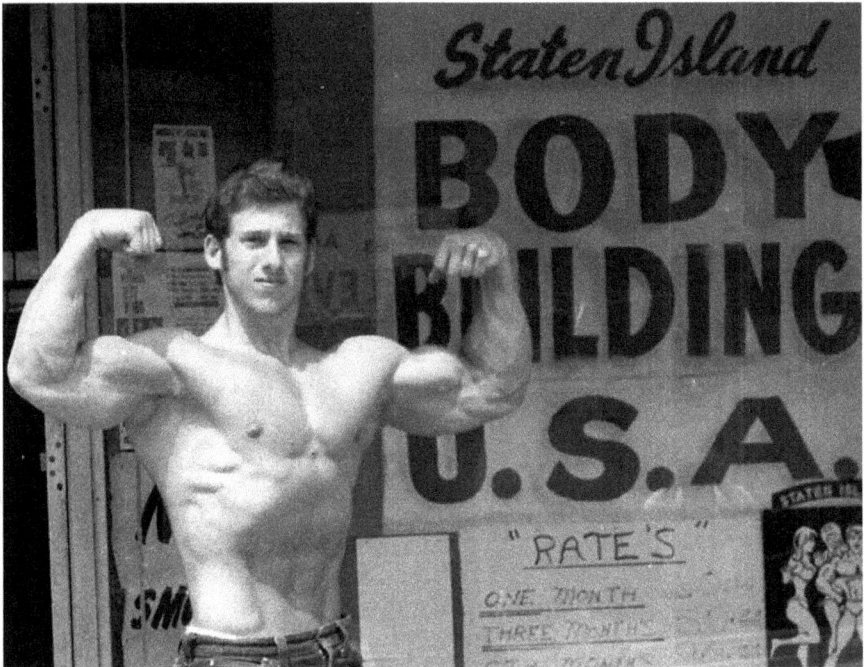

Mario Strong poses in front of his Staten Island Bodybuilding Club - 1977

Membership levels were low during the first few months of the Staten Island Bodybuilding Club's existence. Other than the few hard-core Island muscle builders, the demand to body build by the locals was not there. Staten Islanders were yet to discover the benefits of training with weights and it would take several shockwaves to awaken this sleeping town. On a national level, the first wakeup call came from the movie *Rocky*. Released on Thanksgiving weekend in 1976, *Rocky* captured the fighting spirit of the American man. The movie inspired thousands of men nationwide to become more fit, and on Staten Island, my gym received its share of new members because of it. However, as popular as *Rocky* was with the general public, it would pale in comparison to the direct shockwave the sport of bodybuilding was about to experience.

PUMPING IRON

In 1974, the book *Pumping Iron* hit stores nationwide and became an instant bestseller among the world's muscle builders. The groundbreaking bodybuilding documentary gave a first hand account of the lifestyles of Arnold Schwarzenegger, Lou Ferrigno, Mike Katz, and others to show the sacrifice, pain, and calculation of competitive bodybuilding. It was the first book of its kind and I eagerly read my copy cover to cover as I absorbed every word and image within its pages.

As the years rolled by, bodybuilding remained a subculture within the American fabric of society. Arnold Schwarzenegger was still largely unknown to the public and training with weights was still believed to make you muscle-bound. Bodybuilding competitions during this era were rare by today's numbers and the popularity of the sport was limited to those who trained for their own self-satisfaction. That was all about to change.

In 1977, the long awaited movie version of *Pumping Iron* hit the theaters. It was in limited release, playing only at the Plaza Theater in Manhattan. The premier was on a Thursday night, and while at my Staten Island Bodybuilding Club that historic evening, my members and I unanimously decided to go attend the premiere. Therefore, I locked my gym's door early and led a caravan of several cars loaded with motivated bodybuilders to Manhattan. Outside the Plaza Theater was a large billboard with an image of none other than Staten Island's very own Leon Brown, shown flexing his muscular back. There were also large posters of Arnold Schwarzenegger and the other bodybuilding champions in the film, which were spaced along the sidewalk to inspire the crowd. Fans everywhere flashed their cameras to capture the images of the heavily muscled celebrities as they entered the theater on this eventful night. The sidewalk was filled with pectorals and biceps as the line of bodybuilders waiting to see the movie stretched around the corner. It was a who's who of bodybuilders as local and national champions waited patiently in line to see the film.

Once inside the spacious theater, my friend Jerry Valente introduced me to Lou Ferrigno. Lou was one of the stars of the film and was big as a house, weighing what seemed close to 300 pounds at a height of 6'5". He and Jerry were former training partners at the R&J's Bodybuilding Gym in Brooklyn and it was good to see the both of them ecstatic about their reunion. A short while later, the lights went dim as everyone took to their seats. As the film began to roll, images of the legendary Eugene Sandow filled the screen, showing this pioneer of bodybuilding at his classical heights during the sports early days of the 1900s. Arnold was the main star of the film and he was portrayed as an extremely goal oriented, confident athlete who was determined to win at all cost. The evening as a whole was a remarkable occasion, for it would prove to be a major turning point in the sport's history.

From that day forward, the sport of bodybuilding would grow in popularity. Through time some of the film's characters would become mainstream; Arnold Schwarzenegger would begin to set his eyes on conquering Hollywood, Lou Ferrigno would become known as The Incredible Hulk, and Franco Columbu would actually become a movie producer as well as a fine actor. The film also boosted increased memberships in health clubs and larger sales of the physique publications. The demand for tons of steel and exercise machines also soared to record highs as home trained bodybuilders spent truckloads of cash to equip their own gyms with the necessary tools to help build their bodies in much the same way as the legends they so admired. There was no turning back for the sport of bodybuilding.

The impact of the next shockwave would create a series of events that would define the course of my life. Staten Islanders were about to be awakened to the world of bodybuilding.

PATH TO VICTORY

I was a bodybuilder. I trained religiously, followed a natural diet, practiced my posing, and looked like a real he-man. I also admired the bodybuilding champs and it was my dream to compete on the physique stage one day. In May 1976, I attended Dan Lurie's WBBG Mr. Staten Island Competition and witnessed a future member of my club easily win the show. His name was Russell Cunningham. Russell was a rough sort of character, with thickly proportioned muscle who was as strong as he looked. I remember watching him pose and vowing to myself that, I too, would one day win the coveted championship. Over the next several months, I became relentless in my training and on Valentine's Day of 1977, I made the decision to really *Go For It*. In preparation for the upcoming show in May, I increased the intensity of my training and began to workout more frequently. Since I owned my own bodybuilding gym and spent most of my day there, I had plenty of time to bomb and blitz. I designed a regimen where I would workout three times a day, seven days a week, working each body part every other day. It was over-training, but I was so determined that I worked past the pain and fatigue. And train I did, pushing the cold steel several times a day, sometimes with partners, sometimes alone, but nevertheless, pumping the iron without pause. As the months went by, I gradually reduced my calorie, fat, and carbohydrate intake to bring out my muscular striations. Whenever possible, my good friend Jerry Valente, who was also a member of my club, would bring a posing dais to my gym to help me with the art of muscle display. Jerry was no stranger to the competitive stage. During his prime, he trained with Lou Ferrigno and competed against some of the biggest names in the sport. I was glad to have his help.

On Saturday, May 28, 1977, after fourteen weeks of competitive training, it all came together for the show. Dan Lurie was a major physique promoter in the 1970s. He also published several magazines including *Muscle Training Illustrated*. The Mr. Staten Island competition, as well as the other four borough shows, was being held with the Mr. New York City and Eastern America championships, in one big World Body Building Guild (WBBG) production at Washington Irving High School in Manhattan. One of the qualifications for registering to compete in a borough competition was that the athlete actually had to reside in that borough. During the morning registration process, I, along with other Staten Island bodybuilders planning to compete, saw several faces that were unfamiliar to us. These guys were not from our hometown but were registering for the Staten Island competition. They were able to do so by falsely providing the addresses of family members that lived on the Island as their own which the person in charge of the registration process had no way of verifying. Instead of challenging the process, we just looked at each other and shrugged our shoulders, not realizing we'd be competing with even more people than we originally thought.

The Staten Island prejudging was the first event held that day. One by one, the athletes walked on stage and flexed their stuff for the judges. The comparison rounds were tough since we posed on demand and squeezed our fibrous muscles into sinew. Fifteen competitors vied for top honors in the Staten Island competition and the results wouldn't be known until the evening show. Back in 1977, there were no class divisions in local physique competitions. Everyone was grouped together in one division and competed against each other. For me that meant having to flex against all fifteen bodybuilders to see who would be that year's top gun.

Standing on a physique stage in front of an audience of a thousand or more cheering people and wearing nothing more than your posing suit can be somewhat intimidating, even for the most seasoned bodybuilder. This was my first competition and as I stood there onstage in the prejudging lineup, I felt butterflies racing through my stomach as I saw both the judges as well as the audience analyzing my physique. Bodybuilding is such as subjective sport, that the ability to deliver a winning look requires not only a well-developed physique, but also a positive attitude that transcends to the judges' scorecard. After the initial butterflies subsided, my ego awakened and I got the crowd into an uproar by jumping in front of the other competitors to hit a few 'most muscular' poses. This electrified the other competitors and before we knew it, we were having a pose-down before the scoring even began. As the competition heated up that morning, I became more confident onstage as the audience reacted favorably to my physique and as the judges continued to call out my number for comparisons. After twenty minutes of battling with the other competitors, the judging had been completed for the title of Mr. Staten Island. The scores were tallied and the results would not be revealed until the evening event.

After the prejudging, I joined a group of fellow competitors and took a walk to a nearby park to relax and let the time stroll by. It was a hot sunny day and temperatures were well into the 90s. While hanging out in the park, we received a lot of strange looks and stares from the local patrons. Who could blame them? There we were, this group of well-tanned muscular he-men, whose skin was paper-thin and whose veins were gorged with blood. We definitely stood out amongst the everyday folk and enjoyed the attention as we anticipated what was to come at the evening show.

When we returned to the school later that afternoon, a crowd had gathered to see the competitions. Friends, family members, and fans had come to cheer on their favorite bodybuilders. It was a large crowd, which meant the evening event would witness another WBBG standing-room-only production. As the crowd stood around mingling, a large chartered bus pulled up in front of the school with an enthusiast group carrying pom-poms and cheering loudly. They were from Staten Island and had come to the show to cheer for me as well as support the other Staten Islander bodybuilders. At 6 PM, the doors to the high school finally opened and the crowd of more than two thousand took to their seats as the competitors went backstage in preparation of the upcoming competitions. Dan Lurie had a live band at the show to entertain the audience as well as perform for every bodybuilder that flexed their stuff that evening. After the *Star Spangled Banner* was sung and opening remarks were given, the bodybuilders from Staten Island eagerly walked onto the stage. One by one, they posed, receiving applause and cheers from the enthusiastic crowd.

I was the 8th competitor to walk onstage that night. When the MC announced my name, the band began to play my selected song, which was *The Impossible Dream.* As I stepped onto the posing dais, a massive ear-shattering roar filled the auditorium. Without pause, I began to pose, slowly transitioning my body from one angle into another. There I was onstage, flexing my muscular physique to the crowd's delight. I had trained and dieted to the max for several months in anticipation of this moment and I absorbed every cheer and applause that came my way. As cameras flashed away like charges of lightning hitting my body, the thunderous roar of the crowd became louder and more deafening with every oil-filled pose I gave.

The Staten Island fans had been previously orchestrated by me to give it their all, and give it they did; swaying pom-poms in the air and cheering my name loudly as they produced such a ear-shattering scene that the NYPD officers posted outside the school ran into the building to see what was happening. Backstage, fellow competitors from all the upcoming competitions flooded the sides of the stage to see what was causing the commotion. It was a crazed scene that had produced the effect I wanted, and would later be written about in the physique publications. Decades later, I still smile when I think about it.

After all the Staten Island competitors finished their individual posing routines, the top five athletes were asked to step forward from the group to receive their awards. I was in that group and gave a double-biceps pose when my number was called. The other four competitors jumped in to match me and soon we were posing down with every ounce of strength and sweat left in our bodies. The screaming audience, whose frenzy electrified everyone onstage to give it their all, continued with their chorus of cheers as the band played to its chant. As the MC pleaded for silence, the top five competitors began to receive their placing. After the fifth and fourth place finalists received their trophies, it became apparent to everyone in the audience that I was going to win the show. The other two competitors, while well proportioned, did not have the same mass, symmetry, and quality muscle as my physique displayed. As the deafening roar of the crowd hit a high-decibel level, I stepped onto the winner's portion of the trophy platform and posed my heart away. In my mind, I had already won the show and I began to congratulate myself on the victory. Then third place was announced and I said to myself, "Something's wrong." The guy deserved second, not third, and the audience showed its displeasure at the placing with angry boos. As I stood there in disbelief, I told him that he was robbed and then without notice I heard my name announced as the second place finisher. I felt like a ton of bricks had just hit me. It was bad enough that the remaining competitor did not even reside on Staten Island, as the rules stated was essential to be allowed to compete in the borough's competition, but to add insult to injury, this guy was not even close to the condition that the third place finisher or I were in. I, along with the other previous place finishers wondered what was happening. However, I had my chance earlier in the day to file a grievance about where some of the guys' really resided, but didn't do anything. I waved to the crowd, accepted the trophy from the renowned bodybuilding author Leo Murdock, and left the stage. This did not sit well with the Staten Island fans that were in the audience. They stood up, stamped their feet, and began shouting fowl towards the judges as the rest of the crowd joined in to demonstrate their dissatisfaction towards those responsible for this debacle. As it turned out, I should have given more attention to what was going on around me and not have been naive as to the games in bodybuilding. After all, the 1977 Mr. Staten Island competition had at least six competitors in it that were not from the Island, and I, along with the other local muscle builders, should have demanded that this wrong be righted before the show began. Nevertheless, the damage was done, so I accepted the outcome and went backstage with the rest of the competitors to plan for the next year's competition.

While sitting in a dressing room backstage, I listened as the word spread among the other competitors as to the incident that had occurred. Suddenly, several bodybuilders that were scheduled to compete in the other four borough competitions began to express their concerns to whether they had gotten a fair deal on that day. As this was occurring, my father, who was in the audience, also learned that the first place victor didn't reside on Staten Island and began to petition the judges to award the first place trophy to the real winner. As the show continued, the capacity crowd watched my father argue his point with the judges. Gradually, the audience once again joined in the argument and rose to its feet, while insisting upon the judges to correct what was wronged. It had been nearly twelve years since my father introduced me to the world of bodybuilding and he was not about to watch me be denied the title I trained so hard for. As the clock ticked, the incident slowly transcended into scandalous overtones as the audience demanded that the real winner be awarded the title.

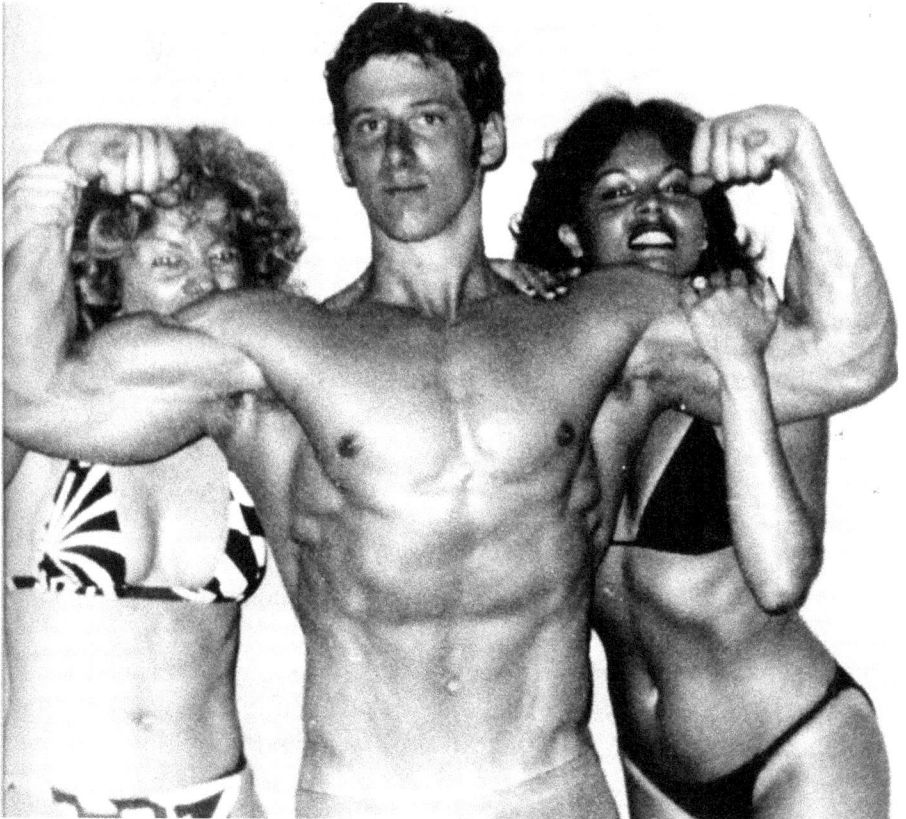

Mario Strong backstage at the 1977 WBBG Mr. Staten Island competition

Finally, Dan Lurie, who had been busy elsewhere and oblivious to what had happened, entered into the chaos. After learning about the incident, Dan located the previously announced Staten Island victor and took the first place trophy from him. As my father continued to express his displeasure towards the judges and as the audience shouted for justice, Dan Lurie walked into the auditorium and handed my dad the first place trophy. Then Dan led my father backstage to wait behind a curtain.

While still backstage, I had no knowledge of what had occurred between the judges, my father, or Dan Lurie. Other than hearing the near riot pandemonium of the crowd that continued to shout for justice, I was blind to what was about to happen. Without warning, Dan Lurie came into the dressing room, grabbed my right arm, and told me to go with him. As he brought me onto center stage, he directed me to step onto the winner's platform and hit a few poses. A few minutes earlier, I had been on this same spot, but now, the outcome was going to be much different. As I stepped onto the platform, I listened and watched as the crowd went into a thunderous cheer of approval. Dan then called my father from behind the curtain to present me with the overall Mr. Staten Island trophy. As my father joined me on the winner's platform, I felt a sense of accomplishment as he raised my right arm and the trophy in a victory salute. Then, for the first time at a bodybuilding show anywhere in the USA, the newly-released theme song *Gonna Fly Now* was played by the live band to help celebrate the occasion. It was an historic moment in my life and I was ecstatic to hear the trumpets play, while I flexed for the cheering crowd and watched as dozens of flashing cameras electrified the stage to capture my somewhat tarnished but much deserved victory.

I was shocked, relieved, and thankful at the outcome of events as they unfolded and was especially grateful that I was going to be able to take the Mr. Staten Island trophy home to my gym where it rightfully belonged. The media coverage of my winning the Staten Island title would compare it to a scene right out of the movie *Pumping Iron*, where Lou Ferrigno's father was shown to be constantly by his son's side, guiding him on to victory. Like big Louie's father, if it was not for my father's guidance early in my bodybuilding career, and for his efforts that evening, I would have never reached the winner's platform on that historic day. Now, after all the sweat and pain, my father was there onstage with me to share in something he began a long, long time ago, and I couldn't have been happier for him.

In a way, all the craziness of the evening made for great entertainment and would become folklore among the many legendary stories of the Staten Island bodybuilding community. The one good thing that came out of all the madness that night was that bodybuilders competing in future Mr. Staten Island shows would be guaranteed that every competitor registered would be personally screened by me to make sure they lived on the Island. In the weeks and months to come, I found myself to be a local celebrity of sorts. The local media featured my victory in its newspapers, and soon strangers came to my gym to meet with me and perhaps get an autograph for their kids. Winning the title meant a lot in 1977. Back then, being Mr. Staten Island was an honor that was respected by not only the local muscle builders but the public as well. On Staten Island, it was like being the heavyweight-boxing champion of the world. Wherever I went, whether it was shopping at the mall or getting a haircut at the local barber, the subject of my victory and what it took to get there became the topic of the day. I even experienced my own club's members seeking my advice more readily, as bringing home the title to the gym made them not only feel proud of their club, but also made them believe in my bodybuilding concepts even more. It was my first competition, my first win, and my first award to be placed in my gym's trophy case. I had won the title fairly and now it was time to build on this victory.

STRONG MARKETING
I have never been one to shy away from publicity and in 1977 that became very apparent. Winning the Mr. Staten Island title was like getting the Good Housekeeping Seal of Approval. It was a respected title among my bodybuilding peers and sounded impressive when introduced to local Islanders. Suddenly I was in demand. I had something to sell and began to market myself as Mr. Staten Island. My gym had two large windows facing the main street that would be used in the promotion of my victory. I had a life size black and white picture made of myself winning the title and placed it in one window. In the other window, I had a giant poster painted in red, white, and blue with OWNED AND OPERATED BY MR. STATEN ISLAND - MARIO STRONG – BUILDER OF CHAMPIONS. The gym was on a heavily traveled road in the middle of Staten Island. Eventually, if you lived on the Island you had to see it and wonder who Mario Strong was. The strategy worked well and brought the curious and brave into

my gym to learn about the benefits of joining. Membership was starting to soar and the best was yet to come.

I wanted to take advantage of my popularity. The summer was approaching fast and with it the release of the blockbuster film *Star Wars* in July. I began to plot my next move. *Star Wars* was contracted to play exclusively at the Fox Plaza Cinema on Staten Island, which was only a few blocks from my club. To create additional revenue, the theater showed advertisements of local businesses before the feature films. I had a friend that worked there at the time and she suggested that I create an ad about the gym to play on the big screen as a way to attract new members. Immediately the wheels began to turn in my cerebrum. I hired a professional photographer for a photo shoot at my club that coming Saturday. I also arranged for about a dozen members to show up with their girlfriends to act as models. The guys wore just shorts and the gals wore bikinis. The idea was to sell muscle and sex appeal. The gym's door remained locked to the public as the photo session lasted a couple of hours. The session went smoothly until the photographer decided to have all the guys lift as much steel as they could in different positions for one great photo. Pound by pound the members picked up tons of steel and held it steady while waiting for the camera to flash. As sweat poured from their straining flesh, they fought the pain and prayed for the picture to be taken. The photographer took his time, aiming to get everyone in the picture. Finally, the flash went off, and immediately tons of steel came crashing to the floor as the straining members released their weights in one big, thunderous, loud boom. The vibration of the falling iron sent fluorescent light bulbs on the gym floor below us crashing down.

By the end of the photo shoot, we had our pictures and off they went to a movie producer to create a one-minute feature on the Staten Island Bodybuilding Club. The ad consisted of twelve photos with captions and played in a slideshow format as the theme song from *Rocky* blasted in the background. *Star Wars* was a big hit that summer as tens of thousands of Islanders saw the movie and my gym's commercial along with it. For weeks, the gym was packed with new members wanting to be big like the guys in the ad. It was a great marketing ploy that caught the attention of the *Staten Island Advance*, which was the Island's main newspaper and whose readers termed the ad, "A motivating and exhilarating sixty seconds." Decades later, I would post the ad on cyber space for the world to enjoy.

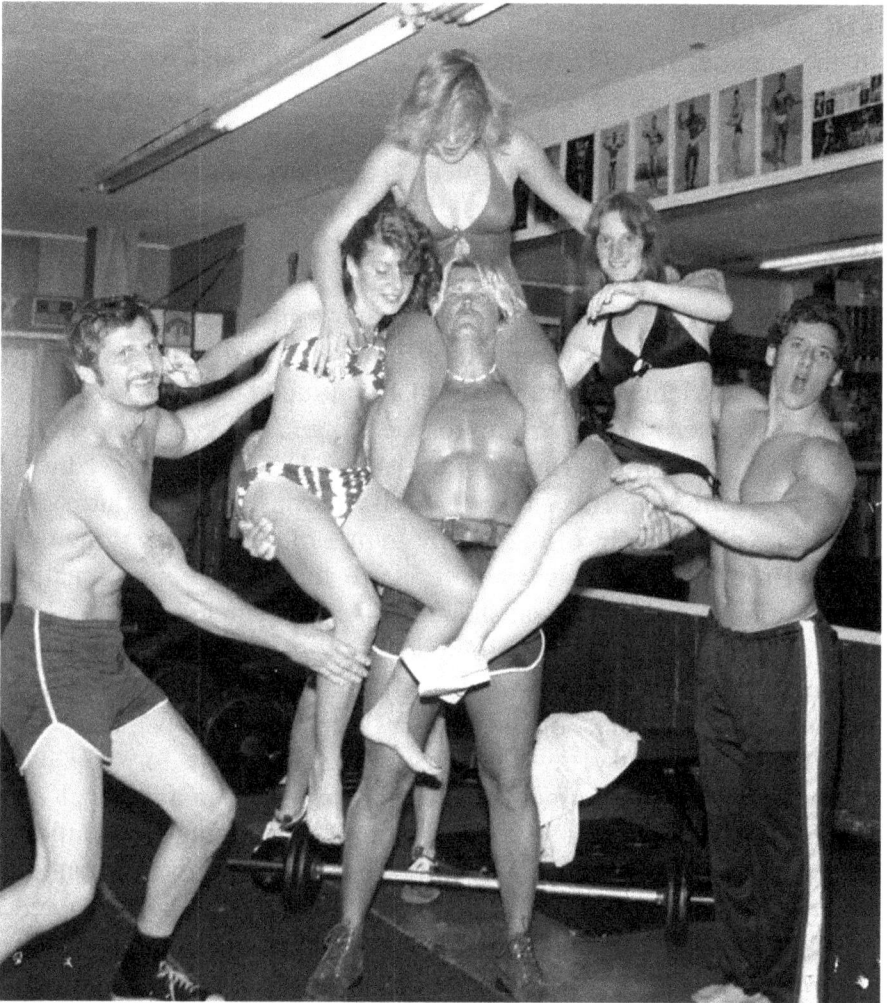
Mario yells to the photographer to wait while getting everyone in position

While creating the movie ad that summer, I also employed another method to promote my club. I had 200 sheets of plywood painted white, with red and blue-stenciled lettering painted over the white background. The wording on the billboards advertised the name and location of my gym. I hired a crew to hang them twenty feet high on telephone poles in key locations throughout the Island. The marketing worked well and brought in business. After hanging for several weeks, the signs also brought the NYPD into my club to serve me with a summons for unlawful posting. Luckily, my gym was full of NYPD officers and I was able to avoid the summons as long as I had every sign taken down in 24 hours. It was a long night!

THE AUTHOR

In the summer of 1977, a member of my gym who worked for the *Staten Island Advance* asked me if I would be interested in writing a fitness-related article for the newspaper. I said, "Sure," and wrote an informative piece on nutrition titled, "The American Diet." The article was well received by the readers of the newspaper and I was asked by its editors for more fitness articles, which I happily penned. As time went on, the Staten Island Bodybuilding Club became the place to be if you had any aspirations of building muscle and becoming a physique champion. My reputation as a knowledgeable trainer was soaring as the demand for my expertise continued to grow.

A year after I began writing for the *Staten Island Advance* a fellow named Denie Walters came to my gym. Denie was the editor of *Muscle Training Illustrated* (*MTI*). His purpose at my club was to perform a photo shoot of one of my gym's more prominent members, Leon Brown. Leon was training hard for an upcoming national competition and was in great shape for Denie's camera lens. As Denie shot pictures of the Brown Bomber, he noticed some articles that I wrote for the *Staten Island Advance* hanging on a wall in the gym and he took a few moments to read them. Liking what he saw, he asked me if I would like to try my hand at writing an article for *MTI*. Once again, I obliged. In no time, I was being published on a national scale. My first article for the magazine was titled "Beginning Bodybuilding" and was a fitting start for many more to come. For years, I continued to write many articles for *MTI* and soon found myself being quoted in other physique publications as bucket loads of fan mail found their way to my gym's door. One year, after penning the original series, *Journey to the Olympian Zone*, I was fortunate enough to find my name included on a list of the top three bodybuilding authors as voted on by the readers of *MTI*. The seeds of my muscle building philosophy had been planted throughout America and now it was time to branch off in other directions.

LIGHTS, CAMERAS, ACTION

In September of 1977, I found myself in another role in the bodybuilding spectrum. To date, I had been a gym owner, trainer, competitor, and author in the sport that I loved. Now, I was being asked by Dan Lurie to be a judge at his big annual event, the WBBG American, World, and Olympus Bodybuilding Championships held at

Madison Square Garden. It was an offer I could not refuse and eagerly took my place among the other well-known physique artists of the day to judge some of the greats in bodybuilding. In a sense, it was somewhat surreal. For years, I had read and followed the careers of the muscle champs and now here I was judging them for history's records.

Judging a physique competition is serious business. It is a responsibility that should be left only to the very skilled. Bodybuilders train hard, probably harder than any other athletes on the planet do. They spend years at the gym, pouring sweat onto the weights to create physiques worthy enough to step onto a posing platform, and be judged by their peers. For competitions, they diet away every ounce of unwanted body fat and continuously practice posing in hopes of presenting a polished look. Judges have the thankless task of fairly evaluating each competitor's overall appearance and presentation. Sometimes, especially with national and world-class bodybuilders, the judging can be extra tough as these athletes have little, if any, weaknesses, and their presentations are usually first rate. Judges themselves are usually bodybuilders who have trained endlessly in the gym and perhaps competed several times on the physique stage. For them bodybuilding is a meaningful way of life and it is their desire to give back to the sport that was good to them. I myself have judged more shows than I can remember and have always respected the time and effort of every competitor.

After the morning pre-judging was over, I went outside Madison Square Garden to talk with some friends. While in conversation, one of my friends told me to turn around and look at what was taking place behind me. As I turned, I saw a local TV news team beaming in on me with a video camera. I had been wearing a tight brown t-shirt that day which showed my physique in an impressive way and this caught the eye of the cinematographer and reporter. The TV crew then walked over to me and before I knew it, I was being interviewed for the eleven o'clock news. Even though the news team caught me off guard, I was thankfully able to answer all their questions about myself and about the competitions in a calm, professional manner. As the crowd watched, I began to ham it up for the camera and began flexing my arms for its lenses. It seemed that this was the body part they were most focused on anyway, so I gave them a few of my best poses and forgot about the interview until later that evening.

At the evening show, I had a pleasant surprise. While in the judges section I had the good fortune to be sitting in front of the honorary guest of the evening, Mr. Steve Reeves. During the evening intermission, I introduced myself and broke into a conversation with the legendary Hercules. One of the topics I recalled Steve Reeves passionately opposing was the use of anabolic steroids in the sport of bodybuilding. Mr. Reeves was very much against the use of drugs for sports enhancement and told me that he believed bodybuilding would evolve into two different philosophies: natural and unnatural. He told me that bodybuilders who continued to abuse chemical agents to enhance their physiques were risking their health and were asking for early deaths. And he was exactly right. Years later the predictions of this Herculean legend sadly came true as many amateur and pro-bodybuilders alike became ill and died long before their time. While talking to Steve Reeves I felt the passion he had for the sport. He was a bodybuilding pioneer that inspired millions to take up weight training. I felt very fortunate for the few moments I had to converse with him and can only hope that more bodybuilders follow in the footsteps of this natural bodybuilding legend.

After the show was over, I joined Dan Lurie, along with what seemed to be every muscle builder in New York City, at a celebration party held in a restaurant across the street from Madison Square Garden. As everyone gathered around the restaurant's main TV, Dan asked the manager to tune it to the news channel that covered the day's WBBG events. As this was happening, I advised Dan that I was also included in the interview. Sure enough, as soon as the broadcast coverage began, there on the small screen for the entire metropolitan area to see, was a news-promo of the competition, with me flexing my arms in a double-biceps pose and the reporter stating, "Here I am with Mario Strong at the 1977 World Body Building Guild Championships at Madison Square Garden." I was somewhat stunned and delighted to see myself for the first time on a TV program. Halfway into the news broadcast Dan Lurie, Steve Reeves, and I were shown being interviewed while several competitors posed throughout the story. The whole news piece lasted about two minutes and captivated everyone's attention. Dan was very pleased at the positive publicity his show had received and thanked me for sharing the spotlight. I was also pleased with the coverage and thoroughly enjoyed myself that evening as the group of muscle builders in attendance cheered along.

I DON'T WANT TO BE AS BIG AS ARNOLD

Every single day of my club's existence prospective members would walk through its door seeking to learn about the fitness programs offered. As I talked to these individuals, I would occasionally hear "I don't want to be as big as Arnold" or "If I get muscle-bound I won't be able to play baseball." It was always something along those lines that made me talk to myself. If these guys only knew how hard and how long it took to become a muscular marvel, I doubt if most of them would have even joined my gym to begin with. Upon hearing these statements I use to reply with something like "Don't worry, I'll design a personalized exercise program so that doesn't happen to you." Meanwhile, my gym was geared towards getting big and strong, which meant that every new member followed the same basic result-producing program. When these members started seeing their arms getting bigger and their strength increasing, they suddenly became intensely motivated with the desire of becoming more muscular and stronger. They were hungry and wanted more!

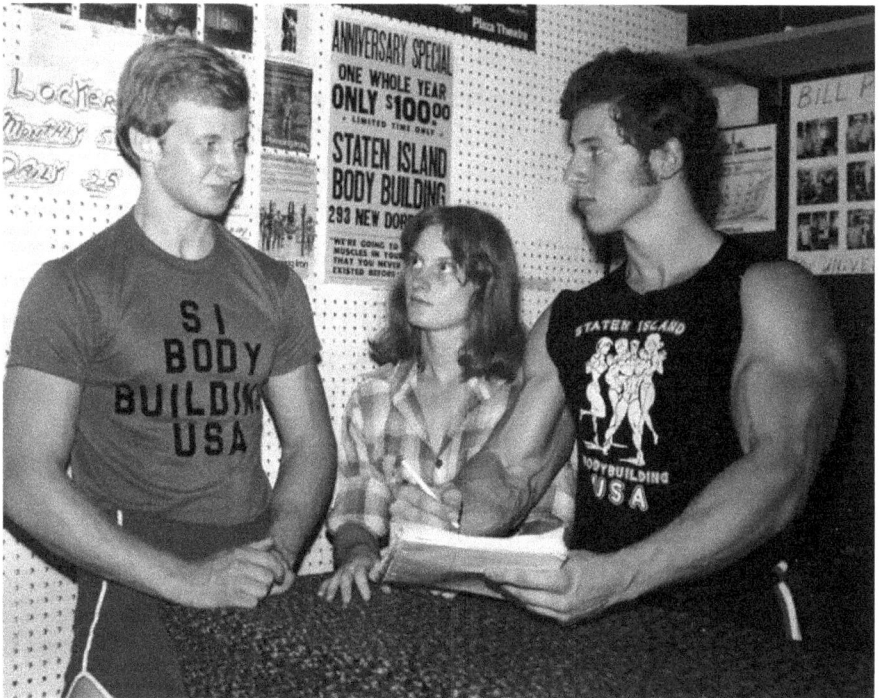

Mario Strong was always ready to help members with their training programs

Before long, they were seeking new exercises and my advice for greater gains. I happily guided them further in their progress while always jokingly reminding them of their earlier quotes when they first entered my gym. After a while, some of these members packed on so much muscle that their wives complained to me about their husbands not being able to fit into their shirts and that some of their men were spending more time admiring themselves in the mirror than looking at them. As time went by, some of my students, who originally did not want to be big like Arnold, actually built bodies good enough for the physique stage and eventually brought a few championship titles to the gym. I guess there is a little bit of he-man in all of us.

THROUGH RAIN, SNOW, AND DARKNESS

My members were naturally hard-core. Not only did they train hard and heavy, they were consistent. The world could end and they would still find a way to get to the gym. On several occasions, they proved their worthiness as they overcame Mother Nature and man's failures as they fought the odds to accomplish their workouts. In the winter of 1978, Staten Island experienced back-to-back blizzards within a few days of each other that left mountains of snow everywhere and brought commercial transportation to a standstill. Walking through the snow it would take me two hours to reach my gym, which was only three miles from my home. Unbelievably, when I arrived at the club after each blizzard, I would find some of my members standing and shivering outside its door, waiting patiently to get their muscles pumping. To make matters even more difficult, the gym's heating system was always shutoff at night, so that left them with ice cold steel to lift for the first hour or so. However, that did not matter. They were driven by purpose and wouldn't let little things like record blizzards and subfreezing temperatures get in their way.

In the summer of the same year, the city experienced a record heat wave. My gym was packed with members and it seemed like business as usual. Unexpectedly, the lights went out. There was no power, no air-conditioning, no fans, nothing. The lower level of the gym was in complete darkness. Several times, I called for my members to come up and out of the pitch-blackness for their own safety but they refused. When I went down the stairs, I couldn't see anyone. It was black as midnight, and the only way you could tell anyone was down there was by the heavy breathing and moans of pain as the members continued to workout in complete darkness. They were determined to get their workouts in and trained on as the night crawled by. There are many stories of obstacles that were overcome at my gym but all had similar endings. It never mattered if Mother Nature brought blackouts, blizzards, hurricanes, floods: my members remained dedicated to their cause of muscle and strength and I was always there at the gym to make sure they did their best.

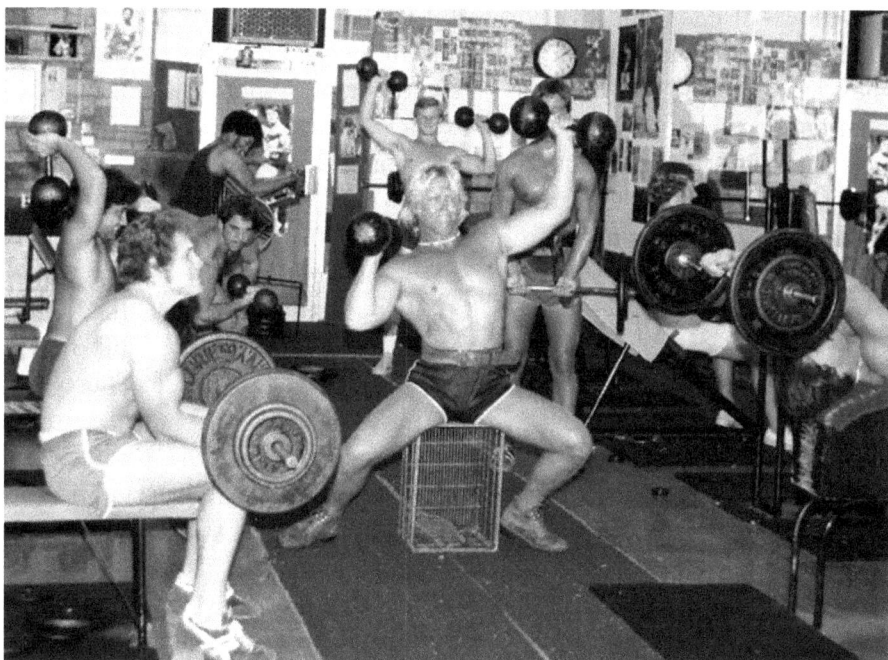

Staten Island bodybuilders training like there is no tomorrow – 1977

THE PERSONALITIES

The training floor of the Staten Island Bodybuilding Club was just over 2,100 square feet and contained a variety of benches, machines, and steel. There was a motivating atmosphere within its walls that came from the members who were there to succeed. Throughout the course of any given day, loud groans, thuds, and clanging of weight-plates could be heard in tune with every set and rep that was performed by the Island's elite muscle builders. There was little conversing and no idle chatter among these men of iron. They gathered at my gym for a reason and inspired each other beyond mortal limits. To them, training was serious business as they were focused on their goals and trained with every once of might they had strained to acquire. When the Staten Island bodybuilders trained, they moved heavy poundage in every direction possible with the purposes of enlarging their physiques, increasing their strength, and building their confidence to gargantuan proportions. They all had strengths and weaknesses to overcome, aches and pains to endure, and hopes and dreams to be reached. The camaraderie of the club always seemed to simmer just below a boil, as the body-men were hungry for steel and got their fill each and every day by lifting tons of raw iron, side-by-side, while on their quest to Muscledom. Nevertheless, as hungry as they all were, they never viewed each other as competitors, challengers, or rivals. They were allies united by a bond. That bond was the passion they shared for the sport of bodybuilding. To them it was no special thing, but to the average folk they were a rare breed yet to be discovered, yet to be archived, and yet to be imitated.

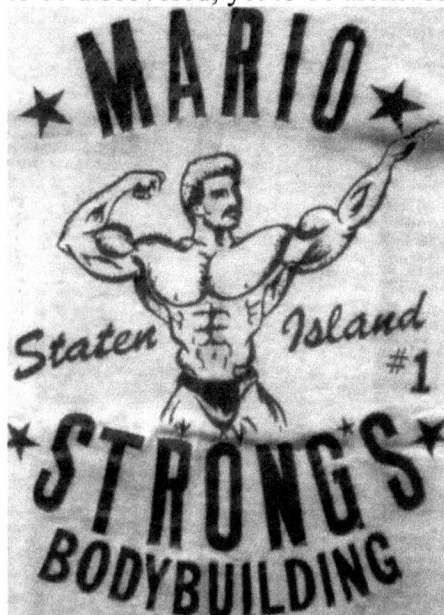

Like many other gyms throughout America, the Staten Island Bodybuilding Club had its share of personalities. There were those who would try to lift the impossible and others who would do a couple of light sets and then pose in front of a mirror for an hour or so. We also had plenty of the standard gym-rats. You know the kind, those muscle-heads that are always at the gym no matter what time of the day it is. There were also the standard heavy bench press addicts and big arm curlers who could not recognize a squat rack if their lives depended on it. We had the supplement poppers who swore by the latest fad and those who timed their rest periods between every set to the second. There were those who wore their tank tops two sizes to small and those who hid their muscles under triple-X sweatshirts. You name it and my gym had it, which helped to create an interesting mix within the club.

As many members as my gym had over the years that's how many different personalities there were with unique stories to match. Being a gym owner, manager, and trainer requires a certain level of finesse and psychology to keep things running smoothly. For the most part, the members were a great group of guys and gals. Occasionally, a fellow would join and become a nuisance to the more serious-minded members. Because of this he would eventually find himself on the receiving end of a kick in the butt. There were plenty of times when some of my members would get on my nerves and push me to the limit. You have to remember, back in the 1970s hard-core gyms primarily consisted of guys in their twenties who were self-consumed egomaniacs. On more than one occasion, I had to get physical with some of them to make sure they did not forget whose gym it was. Rarely, I had little choice but to disallow a member from returning to my gym. This served as a reminder to the rest of the group and kept things running smoothly. There were also those that would stupidly stand in front of some guy doing heavy laterals or whatever and find themselves with a sore foot after one of the dumbbells hit its desired target. To most of my members, the gym was a place of serious business. They came to my club to get the most out of the time they invested there and it was my job to see that their gains were realized.

Being a managing gym owner also meant being a psychologist to some degree. Remember, you have hundreds of members entering your establishment throughout the course of any given day. Each member is unique with his or her wants and desires. Some come to the gym with problems on their minds. Others just come to hang out and pass the time. Always being present at the gym put me in the center of each individual's needs. Besides helping my members with their training and diets, I found myself quite often giving advice to help them with their personal problems. When they saw me, they saw someone they could open up and vent to, someone who would listen, and perhaps someone who would have a solution. At times, I felt like a priest during confession. You would not believe some of the stuff that was confessed to me. Stories involving adultery and even criminal activity were revealed to me. Sometimes as a joke, I would tell the member giving their confession to kneel at the squat rack and sing *Gonna Fly Now* as penance for their sins. After many years in the business, I became quite good at giving sensible advice and probably helped save a few lives along the way. I guess it was just part of the job. When you joined my club you not only got a first rate gym to train at, you also got some sound advice on how to handle your personal life as well as build your body.

It was always a pleasure to be a part of my Staten Island Bodybuilding Club. Every morning, I would find several members eagerly waiting my arrival to open its door for the day ahead. When it came to muscle building the gym had trainees from many walks of life. At anytime of the day you could find police officers, doctors, lawyers, students, firefighters, etc. All were welcome. We even had some local Tony Soprano-types that were dedicated to their training and would "make you an offer you couldn't refuse" if you were in their way. For the most part, I got along well with the members and did my best to help them achieve their desired goals.

One day, a well-known Soprano-type of fellow, who was a member at my gym, was nice enough to make *me* an offer I could not refuse. Although I cannot recall any names, times, or places, this man had a Nautilus Bi/Tri machine at his home and asked me if I would like to have it for the gym. I accepted his offer, and that night went to his residence, disassembled the machine, transported it to my gym, and reassembled it on the gym floor for the members to enjoy. That is the type of camaraderie that existed at my club. Everyone was part of something larger and did his or her share to make it a great experience for all.

One of my gym's hard-core members was a guy named Russell Cunningham. Russell was a no-nonsense type, who openly displayed a bullet lodged in his muscular abdomen. In May of 1976, I witnessed him easily win the WBBG Mr. Staten Island competition among a large field of competitors. I remember how awesome he looked standing there onstage with his heavily muscled physique and ripped abs. He looked unbeatable that night and inspired me to train harder and heavier, so I too, one day might win the coveted Staten Island title. Later that year, Russell walked into my gym wearing a short sleeve flannel shirt that exposed his thick forearms and neck. As overpowering as he looked, he was equally nice once you got to know him. Russell was a bodybuilder who trained for the love of it and gave advice willingly to all the up-and-coming muscle builders. One day, while on the way to the gym, he saw a building on fire. Without hesitance for his own safety, he ran into it and saved the lives of those who were trapped inside. The incident made the pages of the *New York Daily News* and brought Russell some much-deserved praise. But to him it was just another day of training.

Another one of my members who was destined to succeed was Dennis McKnight. Although he was not a bodybuilder in the pure sense of the word, Dennis took his training quite seriously and gave it 110% effort. He joined my gym in 1977 while a member of a local high school varsity football team. Dennis pushed and pulled his way in the gym and on the field to earn himself a scholarship to Drake University. He then went on to play eleven successful seasons as an NFL offensive lineman, most of which was for the San Diego Chargers. Dennis was always psyched and flexing in a similar manner as Hulk Hogan. Therefore, it seemed only natural, when after finishing another workout one day, he decided to walk outside of the club and jump on top of someone's parked car while doing his impersonation of the Hulkster. It was funny to watch as onlookers, who were walking and driving by, stare in bewilderment and horror as they tried to understand this massive fellow's odd behavior. To us, it was just Dennis's way of letting the world know he was psyched and ready to meet any challenge that came his way. After his NFL career, Dennis became a football coach for the University of Hawaii's Warriors and for a time, tried his hand as a radio broadcaster in California.

One member in particular, whose physical presence demanded your attention, was the big burly Raymond Irving. Ray was also an avid football player that liked to hit hard and made sure you felt it. In the gym, he was not satisfied unless he racked the entire stack of weights on any exercise he performed. Sometimes it seemed he wanted to lift the machines as well. When Ray trained, the other members kept their distance. He had a deep dark stare that made you wonder what he was thinking. However, once you got to know him you realized that he was a nice guy who would give you the shirt off his back if you needed it.

There was also Rocco Votinelli. Rocco's membership number was 38, the same number as his age when he joined my club during its first month of existence. Rocco was the senior member of the gym and always had some words of wisdom to give the members. He trained consistently hard and turned his frail body into a muscular work of art that matched the colorful battleship tattooed across his entire chest. Whenever there was any gym equipment broken, Rocco would take it to a friend of his to be repaired and never asked for anything in return. For him, the gym was like a happy home he cared about; you could see Rocco's inner joy as he toiled away at the cold steel. After several years of intense training, Rocco brought his son, Al, to the gym and being the good father that he was, helped Al build a massive physique in much the same manner that he had. Like father, like son.

Tom Kirdahy is a gym member that I have personally known for over three decades. Tom joined my gym in the late 70s. Although his goal during the Iron Age was to compete on the physique stage, he also liked to lift heavy and trained like a seasoned powerlifter that had twenty years under his lifting belt. Tom was a teenager during the years he trained at my gym. What he lacked in experience he made up with heart, as he would constantly challenge himself to lift heavier steel with every workout he executed. If a barbell was not bolted down to the floor Tom would lift it with every once of strength he could muster. There wasn't any amount of heavy steel that intimidated him. Because of his heavy training practices, he eventually built a Herculean physique rarely seen on a teenager. Tom's mass monster mentality would bring him a string of physique awards as he became one of the main faces in the close-knit Staten Island bodybuilding community. Fast forward into the 21st century, Tom is still lifting poundage that astonishes onlookers. Occasionally, I train with him for periods of time and always enjoy the gains made in size and strength from our high intensity, heavy-duty workouts. He is one of the few original Island muscle builders that has lasted through the test of time and knowing Tom the way I do, I am sure he will still be pushing and pulling the heavy steel when he is ninety-nine.

One of the most dynamic figures to ever train at the Staten Island Bodybuilding Club was Tony Bartollotta. Tony was one of my gym's original members. From the onset, he demonstrated a great ability to focus intensely on his training and desired goals. When he trained at the gym, it was an all out war as he pushed and pulled the steel with every ounce of strength he had. Tony was and still is a tri-athlete who possesses tremendous stamina and has competed successfully in many endurance competitions. One day in 1976, before his workout, Tony put on a pair of boxing gloves and challenged me to some friendly sparring. Reluctantly, I agreed and we stepped outside my gym's door and into the view of the public at large, we both started to swing away. As the gym's members exited its door to watch the battle take place between the two egomaniacs, both Tony and I continued to swing away as we hit harder with every punch. As the spectacle raged on, it became apparent to the members that they were watching two individuals that did not know the meaning of the word *quit*. However, before things got ugly they jumped in and ended the heated battle. That's the way Tony was and remains. He is not a quitter, but someone that challenges himself each and every day to go a little further on his quest for physical excellence. Today, Tony still trains hard and continues to focus on future endurance competitions. I am sure that twenty years from now, Tony Bartollotta will still be breaking athletic barriers in much the same way he did in the past.

Another member, who also happens to be a long time friend of my family, is John Foti. I have known John since we were kids in high school and remember when he would come to my home to pump iron with my brothers and me. John continued his dedication to lifting heavy steel and occasionally would help me in the gym. One Sunday morning in 1978, after an intense arm workout with John, I got the bright idea to build a small office near my gym's main entrance. Since it was a Sunday, every lumberyard on the Island was closed. After several phones calls, we managed to find one in Brooklyn that was open and sped over the Verrazano Bridge to arrive at the lumberyard as it was closing. Hastily, we ran in, purchased about two dozen boards of sheetrock and paneling, and placed them on the top of John's 1968 Ford International Scout for the ride back to the gym. When I requested some rope to tie the boards down, the lumberyard manager told me he was out of rope and locked the loading area gate behind us as he walked away. John and I looked at each other and said, "What the heck?" As John drove his vehicle with his right arm, he had his left hand on the roof, holding the boards down. I was in the front passenger side of the vehicle and practically hanging out the window as I held the boards down with both hands and fought the winds while traveling over the Verrazano Bridge. Along the way, we had to make several stops to reset the boards, but eventually did make it back to the gym. After that ordeal came the creation of an office that lasted well into the twilight. For hours, we both sawed and hammered our knuckles away to build a wood-paneled office with functional windows and a door. By the time the early morning arrived, the office was complete. This long time friend would later marry my first cousin, Donna. Today, as we reminisce about that day and the many other challenges we overcame because of bodybuilding, we smile and laugh, knowing that we would not have done it any other way.

A bodybuilder by the name of Carl Stair, who came from a family of champion arm wrestlers, was also a member of my gym. Carl's father and grandfather had genetically-gifted forearms that gave them bone-crushing strength and quick speed to takedown any opponent in an arm wrestling match. Carl had the same fire in his genes and was determined to be one of the best in this intense sport. In the gym, Carl regularly performed heavy Barbell Wrist Curls (see page 47) and various other exercises with the goal of creating great forearm strength and speed. Eventually, he succeeded in his quest and became one of the best in his chosen sport.

There were many such members as Russell, Dennis, Ray, Rocco, Tom, Tony, John, and Carl that stand out in my mind. In fact, there were over ten thousand members during my club's history with which I shared some great times and some not so great times. The members of my gym were the furnace that heated up and energized the Staten Island Bodybuilding Club. We all shared one common bond and passion that drove us to excel in our quest for excellence. We were a group of bodybuilders that truly loved the sport of muscle building and we lived our lives for that purpose. It was a unique time for bodybuilding on Staten Island that can never be duplicated. The main faces in the Island's muscle scene gathered at my gym on a daily basis and together they united to create a magical atmosphere that brought them many years of hard-earned achievement. Each of them was dedicated to the core and together we all pained through endless workouts of Guts and Glory. Life seemed to be ours for the taking as we were youthful and had little sense of fear or doubt. The only question was, *How long before we gained another pound of pure, rock hard muscle?* To us, that was all that mattered.

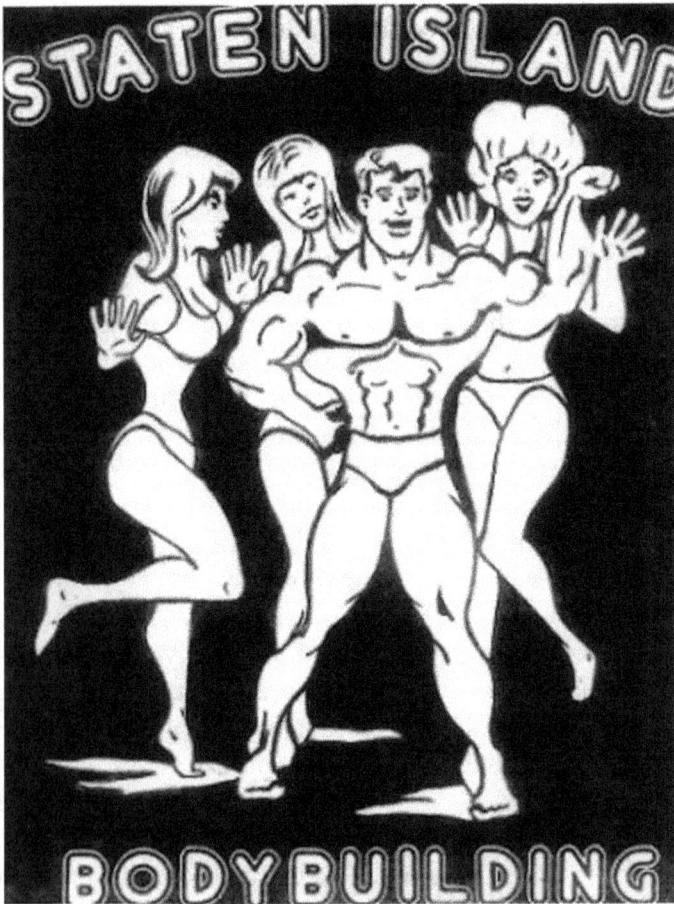

EXTREME EXPLOSION

In January of 1978, I found myself preparing for yet another role to conquer. Dan Lurie had asked me to perform a feat of strength at his upcoming WBBG Eastern American Bodybuilding Championships to be held in New York City in May of that same year. Having never really performed a feat of strength for a large audience, I took the request to heart with a serious determination to entertain and capture the crowd's imagination. However, what would satisfy the muscle savvy New York spectators? After debating several ideas such as tearing phone books, bending spikes, and breaking loose from handcuffs, I recalled seeing Franco Columbu explode a hot water bottle in the bodybuilding documentary *Pumping Iron*. In 1997, I went to the premier of the film and witnessed the awe and amazement of the audience as they watched Franco perform this death-defying feat of strength. Having marveled at pictures of Bill Pearl and Chuck Sipes blowing up hot water bottles earlier in my bodybuilding career, I realized that this was the feat of strength that I was seeking. That was it! I would explode a hot water bottle at Dan Lurie's show and captivate the audience just as Franco Columbu did in the movie.

Little did I know what kind of extraordinary effort it would take to accomplish this colossal task. I soon purchased several hot water bottles and brought them to my Staten Island Bodybuilding Club so I could practice. Before I go any further with this story, let me warn you: DO NOT ATTEMPT TO EXPLODE A HOT WATER BOTTLE! If you do, you run the risk of serious physical injury or even immediate death. Having stated that, let me say that my first attempt at blowing up one not only resulted in failure, but caused tremendous pain throughout my lungs and facial muscles, along with traces of blood in my mouth and on my lips. The exhaled wind pressure necessary to explode one of these babies is tremendous, and after trying this for the first couple of times, you will discover muscles in your face that you never knew existed before. It's not only extremely difficult to blow up a hot water bottle by getting the thick rubber to expand with your lung power, but once you get it to start inflating, it's even more difficult to keep it pressed against your lips so the forced air doesn't escape. Similar to weightlifting, building up the lung stamina and facial muscles necessary to be able to perform this feat of strength takes effort. Already being in great shape at the time, I was able to conquer this dangerous quest in about two weeks time, which led to another surprise. At the moment the rubbery bottle explodes, it gives off a loud bang as it whips pieces of rubber with extreme force against the face and elsewhere. After my first successful attempt, I was left with two giant welt marks on my face from the force of the whipping rubber. The welts lasted several days, causing me not to be too popular with family and friends when they found out what I was up to. To be able to keep on practicing blowing up the bottles without harming myself, I came up with the idea of wearing a ski mask and goggles to protect my face and eyes from the stinging rubber. This worked well and afforded me the ability to practice daily without having to worry about the risk of scarring or going blind in the process.

A couple of weeks before Dan Lurie's WBBG Eastern America Show, I wanted to test it out in front of an audience and gave a demonstration at my Staten Island Bodybuilding Club to some members. As they gathered around, I began to blow up the hot water bottle with tremendous force and will, while continually pressing it against my lips so no air pressure would escape. After expelling eleven breaths into the challenging receptacle some members began to back away for fear that the exploding rubber might injure them. As the hot water bottle continued expanding in size, more members cleared the area until I was left standing alone forcing air into this hellish vacuum of space. 15-16-17-18-19 BOOM! It suddenly exploded with a loud bang that brought a passing NYPD patrol officer into the club to see what was happening. The members were stunned by what had just transpired, for this was the kind of thing you only saw in the muscle magazines or on the big screen and now it happened right there on their home turf of Staten Island. The reaction of my members was one of awe and amazement, which made me excited for my performance at Dan Lurie's big show.

The night of the Eastern American competition was filled with the kind of great excitement that all of Dan Lurie's shows produced. Bodybuilders from all across the land gathered to battle for top honors in front of thousands of screaming muscle fans. I was scheduled to start the second half of the show with a bang and I did not fail to deliver. I also participated as a judge that day and was very busy with little time to contemplate the task before me. As the second half of the show began, I walked behind the curtains to center stage and stood there while waiting for the stagehands to open them. Within a minute or two the show's MC said a few words about Dan Lurie and the WBBG and then began the second half by saying, "Ladies and gentlemen, to start the second half of tonight's show with a bang is last year's Mr. Staten Island winner and *MTI* author Mario Strong, who will perform a death defying feat of strength." With that, the curtains slowly opened, exposing me to a hoard of enthusiastic fans whose cameras sent flashes of blinding lights in my direction. There I was, standing onstage in the thrones of Muscledom and I immediately felt a surge of energy electrify my mind and body as I heard the trumpets from Rocky Balboa's inspirational theme song *Gonna Fly Now* echo loudly throughout the auditorium. I raised the hot water bottle up and sealed it tightly to my mouth by pressing it hard against my lips as I began to force air into its seemingly endless void. As I approached the tenth expelled breath the MC chimed in with the audience by counting loudly with each breath I took. It felt like an eternity and I soaked it all in as I fulfilled my goals to entertain and capture the imagination of my bodybuilding peers. When the hot water bottle exploded, the crowd went into a roar as I threw it into the audience and performed a few Hulk Hogan style poses as I strode mightily off the stage with a feeling of great accomplishment. I had fulfilled Dan Lurie's request to perform and in the months and years ahead found myself performing this same dangerous feat of strength for thousands of spectators everywhere.

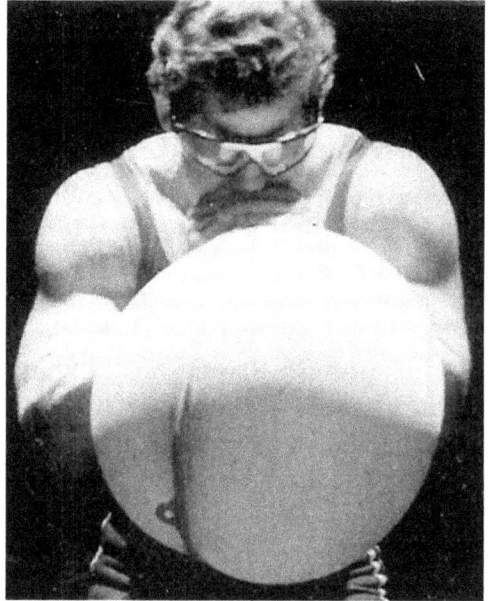

Another important thing that happened that exciting evening was the crowning of a new Mr. Staten Island. A member of my gym by the name of Frank Rapacciulo, who had good symmetry with flowing lines and great persona, was victorious in his quest for the championship. I was glad to hand Frank the 1st place trophy, as I knew how dedicated he had been in his pursuit to win the prestigious title. It was a deserving win that saw the Staten Island Bodybuilding Club rejoice in knowing that one of its own had once again brought home the championship. This day, was another memorable one in Staten Island bodybuilding history.

A BODYBUILDING PRODIGY

As time went on, I lived up to my reputation as a builder of champions and in 1979, I entered about a dozen of my gym's members into the WBBG Mr. Staten Island competition. All of my students trained hard and were ready for the challenge, but one stood out and would shine for years to come. His name was Joe Carrero (see photo).

I first heard about Joe in July of 1978 through a member of my gym. This member bragged about how Joe had great potential and that at only fourteen years of age, was showing muscle quality usually seen on much older bodybuilders. He continued telling me how well built and strong his friend Joe was. From some of the things he was saying I was beginning to think he was a bit crazy. Finally, one day in August of that year, Joe visited my gym and became a member. Well, I took a good look at him and realized that he did have tremendous potential just like his friend said.

Joe Carrero started working out at my gym and immediately began training six days per week. It was the first time that he had trained with a variety of equipment and it was amazing to watch his natural genetics benefit from every exercise he performed. Until that time, he had only trained at home with some free-weights and an adjustable bench that his parents bought for him. Now he was at a hard-core gym, and while other members of my club were making good gains, they were nothing compared to Joe's progress. The kid became stronger day by day. It was amazing to watch him grow, and other members of my gym wanted to know his secrets. If there was any secret for his tremendous gains it was the belief that he had in himself. He was only fourteen and worked out with 260 pounds in full squats, leg pressed 520 pounds, and bench-pressed 210 pounds for 3 sets of 8-10 repetitions. When training at my Staten Island Bodybuilding Club, Joe always expressed a positive outlook towards his workouts and for life in general. He had that look of confidence, that same Schwarzenegger-style attitude, that one day he would be a champion. Time would tell.

In October of 1978, several members of my gym began training for the upcoming WBBG Mr. Staten Island Competition, which was slated for May 1979. The competitive spirit was in the gym and it was suggested by some members that Joe enter the competition to get some experience. Joe asked me about this and I agreed that it would probably be a good idea, because if he planned to go far in bodybuilding it would be necessary to get all the experience possible.

Joe's training intensity picked up at an incredible rate. His bodyweight grew naturally from 155 to 175 pounds in just five quick months. By February of 1979, Joe had turned fifteen and was training like a professional bodybuilder with ten years experience under his lifting belt. In whatever exercise he performed you could see that he felt it within the muscles he worked, as he trained for a deep pure pump in every muscle group. Three weeks before the contest, I checked Joe's leg development and was slightly disappointed. They had mass but lacked some sweep and separation. I put him on a special program emphasizing Front Squats and Heavy Leg Curls. The results spoke volumes. By contest time, Joe's legs had greatly improved, enough so that he earned several votes for the Best Legs Award.

On the day of the contest, the audience was amazed to say the least. Joe weighed in at a ripped 150 pounds. Whether he stood relaxed or tensed, he looked superior next to most of the other competitors, some of whom outweighed him by 40-50 pounds. I will never forget the audience's reaction to his vacuum pose. He actually pulls his abdominal muscles under his diaphragm and behind his chest. It had to be among the best in the world at the time. I have never seen any better since.

At the end of the competition, Staten Island bodybuilder Lou DeBella was declared the overall winner. This was Lou's third try at the title and his winning physique displayed good size and proportions. In fact, good enough for him to win the Best Arms Award among all the other New York City competitors that evening. Joe placed a close second, which was very good considering he beat out Bill Cirelli, who placed third and was a well-known bodybuilder on Staten Island.

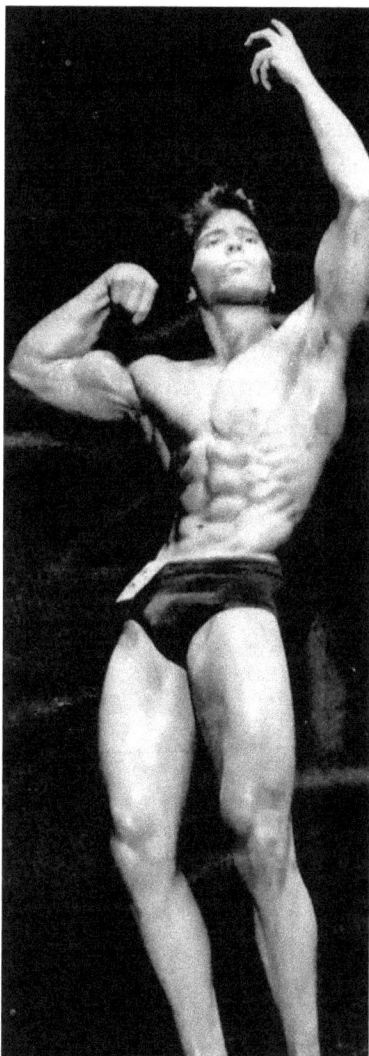

However, Joe's night was just beginning. During the evening's best body parts awards presentation, Joe won trophies for Best Back, Best Abdominals, and for being the Best Poser, beating all other 78 New York City competitors. Such an accomplishment was unheard of for a 15-year-old bodybuilder from Staten Island, but for Joe Carrero, it was just the beginning of the historic journey that would span fourteen years. The future looked bright for Joe. He had all the ingredients to become a national bodybuilding champion...and with time, he did!

THE CLEANING CREW

Every bodybuilding gym has its members who cannot afford to pay their dues. My club was no exception. If anything, it had a surplus of muscle-heads that wanted to train at my facility, but just did not have the funds necessary for their memberships. Since I knew these guys were sincere with their financial dilemmas and that they really wanted to body build, I gave them the option of trading sweat for their time. The deal was they would work for me by helping to keep the gym clean on specified days and times of the week. Most of these members were of high school-age, so each day after school a few would come to the club firstly to workout and secondly to mop or vacuum the floors.

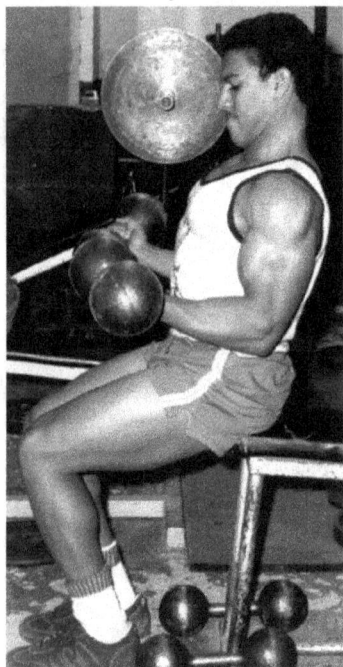

While some cleaned weekdays, others cleaned on the weekends. The weekend crew was an unusual bunch that spent more time laughing than actually cleaning. Everything was amusing to them. That is until I would point to a spot they missed or found something new that needed cleaning. Then they would just frown and struggle along with their assigned duties. The weekend crew was lazy! When working out they would put all their efforts into it. However, when it came to cleaning the gym, they were as slow as box turtles and let any and every little thing distract them from their work. It was more of an effort for me to get them to do the cleaning than for me to do just clean it myself.

One such member of the weekend cleaning crew was a kid named Keith Miguel (see photo). Keith was a promising young bodybuilder with great genetic potential and a true love for the sport. Whenever he posed on a physique stage, he would receive a thunderous applause from the audience, thanks to his great ability to communicate with them through his artful skill. While he was a natural on the stage, he was definitely out of place when it came to performing his assigned duties as a member of my weekend cleaning crew. Keith's sole purpose for being in my gym was to train for size and strength. Anything else was a waste of his energy, and therefore shunned as a detriment to his muscle building lifestyle. Like clockwork, every Saturday morning he would come to my gym for his workout and try to weasel himself out of his agreement with me. I would practically have to plead with him to take out the trash and it wasn't much easier when it came to his other chores. Whenever I would leave him on his own he would head back to the weights and sip a protein drink in between sets to replenish his tired muscles. Perhaps if I had attached a broom's brush to the end of a barbell he would have been more motivated to perform his assigned duties.

HOME OF CHAMPIONS

In the spring of 1979, when Arnold Schwarzenegger was king of the bodybuilders and Sylvester Stallone was fighting his way to the top of the box office, I invited national bodybuilding superstar Ron Teufel to my Staten Island Bodybuilding Club, for what turned out to be a very well-received and momentous seminar. The seminar gave Ron a forum to express his opinionated views on the world of Muscledom through the national coverage it received in a bimonthly feature within the pages of Dan Lurie's *Muscle Training Illustrated.*

I remember the day of the seminar very well. It was a bright sunny day and several hundred members waited outside my gym to see and learn from the man with the legendary "slabs of abs." However, there was one small problem. Ron Teufel was nowhere to be found and the door to my gym remained locked for fear of a riot. As the minutes ticked away, the crowd began to get impatient. After nearly an hour of waiting, they began to get loud and shades of panic began to set into my usual calm self. Against my better judgment, I went outside the gym to answer questions about Ron's whereabouts while hoping to stall for more time. Suddenly I heard the sound of screeching tires coming closer. As I looked up in disbelief, I saw Ron Teufel racing his red Trans Am directly at us with his head and left arm out of the car's window while waving widely. He nearly drove over some of the fans who rushed into the street to greet him as he hit the brakes and slid into a spinning stop. As the fans circled around the Trans Am, Ron exited the car. You could immediately sense the energy and joy that he was feeling as he said hello and signed autographs for every one that came to see him that day. After all the excitement had cooled a bit, Ron entered the Staten Island Bodybuilding Club for the first time to give what was probably one of the most detailed and honest seminars ever given by a nationally recognized bodybuilding champion. The seminar lasted about three hours, but to those in attendance, it seemed much less. There were questions regarding training, nutrition, steroids, and a host of other topics. Ron answered each question to the best of his ability, while adding shades of humor to lighten the intensity of the seminar. The Ron Teufel seminar was a major event for the Island's muscle builders and to this day remains the most widely publicized bodybuilding event in the Island's bodybuilding history. After the seminar, Ron was the guest of honor at a special gala dinner that was attended by the members and staff of my Staten Island Bodybuilding Club. That day was truly one of Ron's happiest occasions as he was in his element, celebrating his joy of bodybuilding with those who shared the same passion. The Ron Teufel seminar was definitely a turning point in the history of my club.

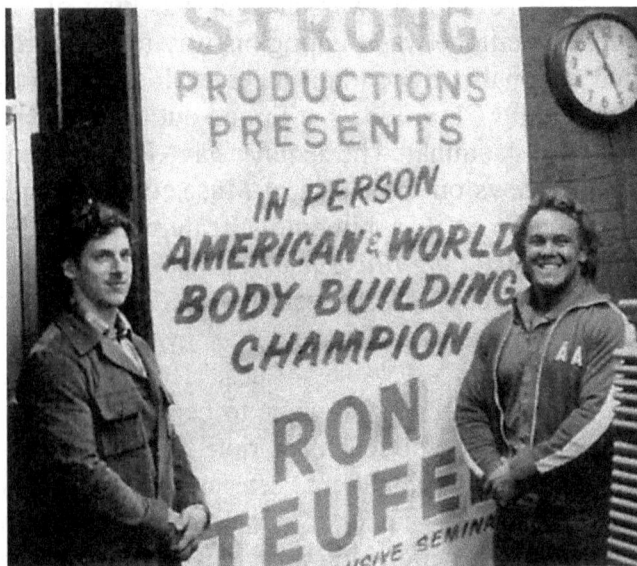

Author Mario Strong, "King of Staten Island Bodybuilding," and Ron Teufel.

Note: For some unknown reason Ron Teufel was never awarded the title of Mr. America. A title he so richly deserved, but was denied; placing runner-up several times. I always felt this was the lever that pushed Ron over the edge. He was so close to realizing his dream but was denied because of politics in the sport he loved. Through the years, I occasionally heard from Ron and always enjoyed his phone calls and ideas about muscle building and the sport in general. One thing he was always passionate about was the topic of politics in bodybuilding. Ron strongly believed he had been wrongfully denied his place in the sport's history. When I got the news of his passing in 2002, I was saddened, but not shocked, for I knew deep inside he felt emptiness in his heart where joy should have been.

The Staten Island Bodybuilding Club had become a nationally recognized muscle building gym and whenever bodybuilders would pick up a physique publication on any newsstand in the country, there was a good chance they would see a picture or read a story with my gym somehow mentioned. The tide was turning towards Staten Island and bigger waves were about to hit its shores.

A month after the Teufel seminar, another legendary figure in the sport walked through my gym's door. It was none other than world champion bodybuilder Robby Robinson, who was nice enough to visit my gym and meet with the local muscle builders. Staten Island legend Leon Brown and Bath Beach Bodybuilding owner John Barberro also accompanied Robby. It was great meeting Robby for the first time. I had followed his career for years and had seen him on the silver screen in the movie *Pumping Iron*, and now here he was in the flesh to say hi to the members of my club. One incident I can still vividly remember about that day was when a couple of my members were performing Barbell Curls incorrectly. These two were nicknamed the Herculoids because they were always trying to lift a ton of steel in every exercise they performed. It did not matter to them if it was the Bench Press or the Dumbbell Wrist Curl. These two guys would always lift as much steel as humanly possible. Robby was gracious enough to walk over to them and demonstrate the proper technique as I cringed, knowing that the Herculoids would never lower the poundage on the barbell for the sake of form. After Robby spent what seemed like an eternity trying to get them to use the proper technique, the Herculoids thanked him. As he walked to the front of the gym, Robby looked back only to witness in horror the Herculoids performing their sloppy form once again. Robby just shrugged it off and after an hour or so he, Leon, and John Barberro said goodbye. When they left the gym, I walked over to the Herculoids to explain once again the importance of proper form in weight training. They both acknowledged my advice but as soon as I walked away, they were back to lifting impossible numbers in their usual manner. Several months later, I got a nice surprise when I picked up a copy of Joe Weider's *Muscle Builder & Power* publication and saw a photo of Robby Robinson wearing a Staten Island Bodybuilding sweatshirt that I gave him on his visit to my gym. It was the first time I had ever seen a world bodybuilding champion wearing one of my shirts in a major muscle magazine and it felt great.

As my gym became more popular, it received greater attention from the media and became a constant hot bed for physique champions to stop by and visit. One day, Bill Pearl, a five time winner of the Mr. Universe title, stopped by to check out the Staten Island Bodybuilding scene. Bill Pearl was, and still is, a much-respected star in this world of muscle and it was truly an honor to have him come to my club. I had first received word that Bill Pearl was headed to my gym only about an hour before his arrival. Luckily, it was on a Saturday morning and I had the cleanup crew working quickly to spruce up the gym for the arrival of this legendary Mr. Universe. I also made about twenty phone calls that morning to alert as many Staten Island bodybuilders as possible that Bill Pearl was paying a rare visit our way and this was their chance to meet him. When Bill Pearl (see photo) arrived it was as if the Holy Lord had just entered my gym. He had an aura about him that glowed with confidence. Even legends looked up to this man. Bill Pearl was bodybuilding royalty and it just did not get any better than that. His physique was world-class and his knowledge of the sport of bodybuilding was unmatched. He was the epitome of what bodybuilding was meant to be, and it was an honor for him to be at my club. In awe, my club's members greeted the champ as he signed autographs for them while happily answering the many questions they asked him. Bill told some great bodybuilding stories to my members as

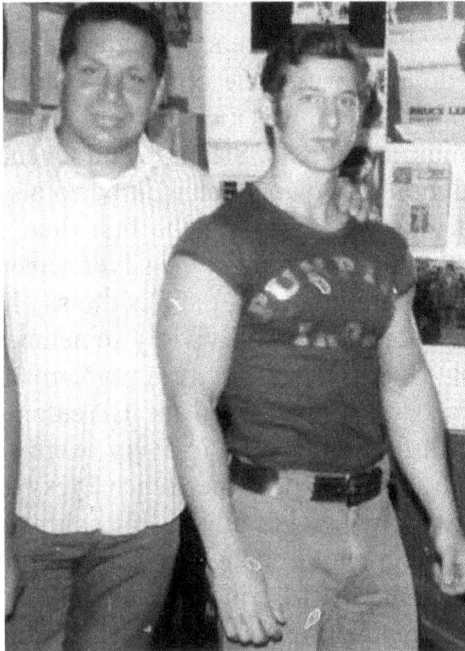

they listened and absorbed his every word. His history in the sport was as vast as the universe itself and his presence at my club seemed to make time stand still. Bill Pearl is a true gentleman in every sense of the word and if more bodybuilders were like him, this sport would be less looked upon with suspicion, and instead, highly respected for what it can offer. The day Bill Pearl came to the Staten Island Bodybuilding Club was one of the most memorable days in my club's ten-year existence. That day, as well as the ones before and the many to come, only served to fuel my member's ambitions even more as they trained harder than ever before and with a keener vision on where they were headed in their quest for muscle. The Staten Island Bodybuilding Club had become an institution that was recognized by some of the biggest names in the sport. On Staten Island, it was the *Home of Champions*, where legends not only visited, but were created as well.

THE BROWN BOMBER

Speaking of bodybuilding champions, none was ever more legendary on Staten Island than the Brown Bomber himself, Leon Brown. As fate would have it, I would meet the Brown Bomber a few years prior to the opening of my club.

In February of 1973, I attended an AAU weightlifting and bodybuilding competition held on Staten Island with my brothers, Johnny and Domenic. It was my first ever attendance at an iron and physique competition, so my expectations were high. While there, I heard a rumor that Leon Brown would be at the show sometime late in the afternoon. I never met Leon before, but knew much about him since he was somewhat of a legendary bodybuilding figure in the metropolitan area as well as a constant feature in the muscle magazines. Around 4 PM that afternoon, while watching the weightlifting portion of the competition, I noticed people in the audience turning around and gazing towards the back of the auditorium. Naturally, I also looked back and could not believe what I saw. Larger than life, there he stood, grinning and shaking hands with all that greeted him. Big, bad Leon Brown was in the house and the competition practically came to a halt as the Brown Bomber's presence nearly stole the show. There he was, this legendary muscle figure from Staten Island, wearing fitted corduroy pants with a dark purple knitted muscle shirt, which revealed a Herculean physique that glowed transparently through. The crowd just stood and studied this celebrated national physique champion. Then one fellow yelled out "Look, it's Leon Brown," Leon, always the master of comic relief, answered back in the Terminator-style dialect, "No, you are wrong, it's Leon Purple," sending the crowd into a laugh as they gathered around to welcome their local muscle hero. My brothers and I introduced ourselves and were instantly psyched by this legendary champion, who on this day, possessed a muscular structure rarely seen on Staten Island before.

Three years later, during the Staten Island Bodybuilding Club's first week of existence, the Brown Bomber walked through its door for the first time. When Leon entered my gym, his electrifying persona completely captivated its members. Immediately, upon seeing this legend, the Island bodybuilders bombarded him with questions ranging from training and nutrition to posing and muscle folklore.

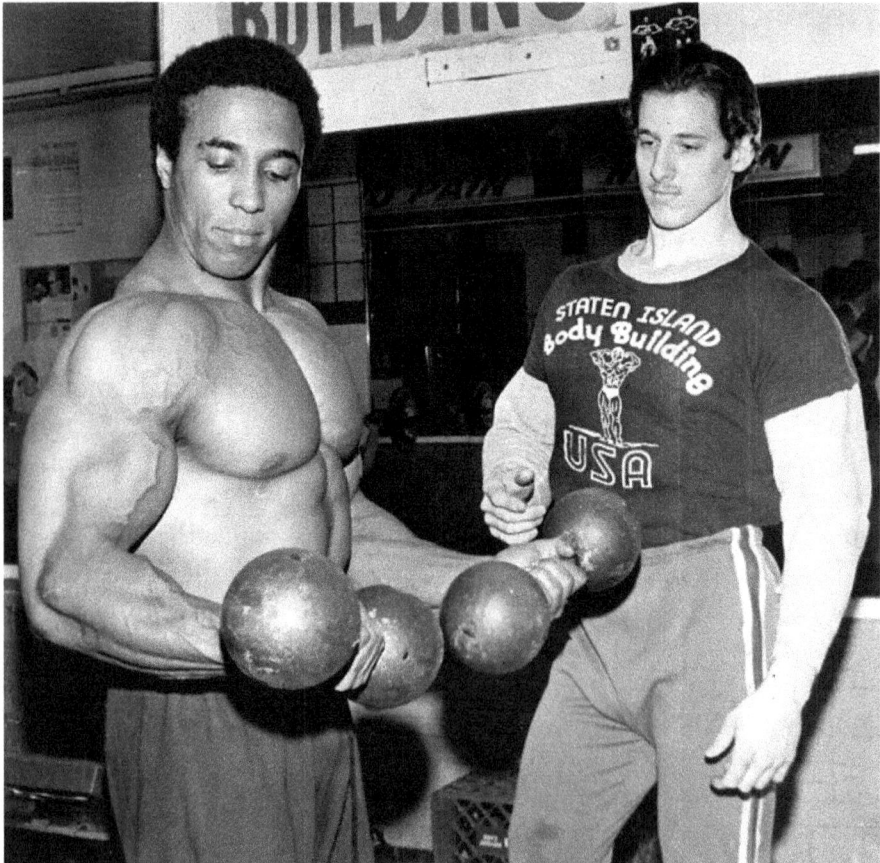

Mario Strong watches bodybuilding legend Leon Brown train – 1979

Leon just stood there, happily and patiently answering all the questions, while adding a few of his own stories about the Golden Days of Bodybuilding. After an hour or so, I managed to get Leon's attention and welcomed him to the club by giving him an honorary lifetime membership to the Staten Island Bodybuilding Club. I have been good friends with Leon since those early times in our history, and throughout all the years I have known him, I have never met anyone who had a greater love for the sport. That love comes from the passion Leon has for bodybuilding, as the sport burns deep within his heart. Leon Brown is a bodybuilder from the sport's Iron Age. A time when Guts and Glory ruled the day, and champions such as he, basked in the warm light of their fans and peers. Today, the Brown Bomber is well into his sixties, and to him age is just a number. He is the living legend that defies time as he continues to train with the same fire and drive that once led him to the top of the muscle world.

Leon Brown is an old school bodybuilder. He trained with and competed against some of the greats in bodybuilding. His history in the sport is rich as evidenced in the bodybuilding documentary *Pumping Iron*, in which photos of the Brown Bomber are spread throughout the book's pages alongside legendary muscle icons such as Arnold Schwarzenegger, Franco Columbu, Frank Zane, and Lou Ferrigno, to name a few. He was also the first bodybuilder ever featured in *Sports Illustrated* and in many ways is responsible for helping to open the doors of the public to bodybuilding in an era that witnessed the emergence of Arnold Schwarzenegger.

In 2007, Leon Brown was inducted into the WBBG Hall of Fame. As a plaque was presented to Leon for his endless dedication to bodybuilding, a video of his history in the sport was played on a giant screen while the film's moderator spoke the following words: "Leon Brown, a Staten Island bodybuilder who became a national treasure. In 1972, Leon Brown was the first bodybuilder ever featured in Sports Illustrated. He has trained with the champions of the sports Golden Era and has beat many of the great legends in bodybuilding. Leon Brown is the last true bodybuilding warrior. He is beyond a legend. He is a bodybuilding icon who has trained and competed with pride for five decades. Leon Brown loves to train and loves to compete; if he lives to be 100 years old, the man will still be onstage. That is Leon Brown, a bodybuilder from the Iron Age on his journey into the future. Leon Brown, a true bodybuilder throughout the ages."

A WASTED GIFT

The late 1970s saw the emergence of a member to my gym whose physique had the potential to be one of the best in the world. I first met Jake during the summer of 1976, when he, along with his younger brother and father, visited my neighborhood garage gym. Before I opened the Staten Island Bodybuilding Club, I was training local Islanders and Jake was one of many who entered my neighborhood gym. I put him and his brother through a trial workout and did not see them again until they joined my club in 1978. Jake showed enormous potential, as he seemingly grew larger and became stronger with each day that passed. He was dedicated to his training and it was amazing to watch as he progressed at a fantastic pace. He was also a practical joker, who one day entered my gym and dropped a live six foot snake on me while I was relaxing on my office recliner, thus sending me soaring into the air and heading for the door.

Jake was very popular on the Island and one year decided to enter the Mr. Staten Island competition. The show was held in a small building that had an auditorium surrounded by balconies. Jake's entry in the show made it an instant sellout. When his name was called to pose at the evening portion of the event the crowd went wild as they shouted his name repeatedly. It was one of those moments in Staten Island bodybuilding folklore that would snowball into a storm, as Jake easily won the overall title and began to look ahead. As he continued to train, his physique grew into Herculean proportions. Jake's physique was huge and got the attention of a certain member of the bodybuilding community, who unfortunately introduced him to steroids. As his pictures and stories began to appear in the physique publications, Jake began to follow a philosophy towards bodybuilding that I strongly condemn. He wanted to be a pro and was very much on his way until he took another wrong turn on life's path, a turn that brought his competitive career to a screeching halt. His was the genetics of champions never to be realized because of bad choices. He soon got involved with the wrong crowd and began selling both recreational and muscle building drugs, while also running weapons to make some easy cash. Eventually, he found himself in trouble with the law and was sent to prison for his wrongful actions. While behind bars, Jake turned states evidence against the mob and left New York before revenge could be taken against him. However, before he left town forever, he swindled thousands of dollars from his fellow Island bodybuilders by falsely promising them a truckload of steroids.

Unfortunately, I have witnessed this type of scenario all too often. When young minds get a little muscle and some attention, their egos go unchecked and they begin to think of themselves as invincible. This is acceptable when applied in a positive way, but every now and then a muscle builder gets to full of himself and uses his gains for wrongdoing. Over the years, I have heard of several bodybuilders who were killed because of their involvement with the wrong crowd and of many others who have done years in a cellblock for breaking the law. Like the saying goes, "Life is wasted on the young," and at times, so too, is the sport of bodybuilding.

FLEX APPEAL

The year 1979 saw the arrival of women bodybuilders to the Staten Island Bodybuilding Club. Well, they were not exactly bodybuilders but I needed some girls who looked the part, immediately. Early one summer day, I received a phone call from a *Staten Island Advance* reporter. The newspaper was doing a story on the growth of women's bodybuilding in America and wanted to know if I had any women bodybuilders training at my gym. I said, "Of course, I do." Before I could take back my words, an interview was slated for later that evening at my gym, and was to include several women bodybuilders and myself. Up until this time, it was hard to find women who weight trained anywhere in New York, let alone on Staten Island. Nevertheless, I had committed myself to an interview and needed to find some fast.

Luckily, my then-girlfriend, Denise, trained with weights and looked fit for the part. But that's all I had, so I got the bright idea to draft my sister, Patricia, and cousins Lisa, Sally Ann, and Nancy who were free that evening. When the gals arrived, they didn't look much like muscle builders, but after a few alterations in sportswear and some coaching on how to act the part I was confident enough that the interview would go over well. After all, outside of the narrow sub-culture of bodybuilding, who in 1979 really knew what women bodybuilders were suppose to look like? The sport was still in its infancy, so it wasn't too hard to satisfy the reporter as the ladies and I answered every question asked of us. As the interview was taking place, a photographer shot photos of the women working out with weights. About a week later, the story on women bodybuilders training on Staten Island hit the newsstands and all hell broke loose at my gym.

Suddenly, I found myself swamped with women wanting to join my club and look like the girls in the newspaper story. This did not go well with the gym's all-male membership, who came to train without the distractions of ladies getting in their way. However, the women wanted to weight train and since I am a firm believer that bodybuilding was for everyone I let them join; thus, women's bodybuilding had become a reality on Staten Island. Because of this, some of my male members actually left the gym in protest and joined other local gyms. However, they were to return a few months later as the other Island muscle gyms also began to enroll the gals. The beginning of a muscle revolution had arrived on Staten Island. At the annual Staten Island Bodybuilding Championships, a women's division was created, which allowed the ladies to compete in a similar manner to their male counterparts. At first, only one or two female competitors entered the new competitive division. As the acceptance of women's bodybuilding grew throughout America, it also grew on the Staten Island physique stage. Before you knew it, not only were the women's divisions seeing lots of competitors, but an even newer division was created for couples, which allowed males and females to pair and compete in harmonic fashion as they flexed for the approval of the judges and audience. What began as a newspaper story flourished into a way of life for thousands of Staten Island women. Today, no matter what hour of the day it might be, you can always find women training with free-weights at most gyms on the Island. Looking back at it now it is hard to fathom a time when women did not train with weights for improved health, sports enhancement, and figure. However, that is the way it really was on Staten Island a long, long time ago.

MARIO STRONG MULTI VITAMINS

It was also around this time that I ventured into the supplement business by selling my own line of nutritional products at my Staten Island Bodybuilding Club. The club was humming with hundreds of members entering through its door each and every day. My members trained hard and supplemented their diets to help insure their gains. They were constantly asking me to stock my shelves with some nutritional products as a convenience for them. The problem was that even though I knew that some supplements worked to a degree, I believed in natural nutrition to achieve maximum benefits. I myself had not taken any form of supplementation since my high school days and found it hard to recommend such products to those that trained at my establishment. Nevertheless, reality won over and I decided to make the supplements available in a limited degree. After researching several possible brand names to sell at my gym, I decided to go with a laboratory whose products had the least amount of artificial ingredients, yet supplied the most in nutrients. I also had my own label designed and placed on every bottle I ordered and sold.

The supplements were a big hit. Not only were my members emptying my shelves on a daily basis but visitors were also stopping by the club to purchase products to fill their own needs. Every day shipments would arrive from the lab to fill my shelves and every day I would be sold out. I offered just several items for sale. They were vitamins A, B-Complex, C, D, E, desiccated liver, calcium, and a multi-vitamin/mineral supplement. I also sold fruit juices and was one of the first to sell Snapple (when it had fewer ingredients than today). There were many more types of designer supplements that I could have sold, but to me they were more about making a buck and less about health and strength. In my mind, the supplements I offered were sufficient for any normal trainee and if anyone wanted more, they could go to the local health food store down the road and help themselves to whatever they desired.

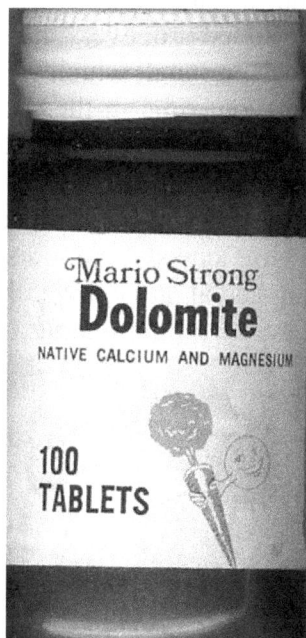

Mario Strong
Dolomite
NATIVE CALCIUM AND MAGNESIUM

100
TABLETS

THE ISLAND OF MARIO'S MONSTERS

By the 1980s, the popularity of the Staten Island Bodybuilding Club had grown tremendously. Every local bodybuilder who had a competitive edge to his training was at my gym pumping daily in hopes of bringing home a championship title to the club. Such was the influence of my Staten Island bodybuilders on the metropolitan area that *MTI* editor Denie coined the phrase "The Island of Mario's Monsters" in an article he penned for *Muscle Training Illustrated*. When my gym's bodybuilders entered a competition, they were supported by its members who traveled by the busload to cheer on their favorite local muscle builders. The Staten Island bodybuilding community was a close-knit group of guys and gals that shared the same goals and passions while making their mark on the competitive trail.

My club was unique in many ways. Not only was it the first bodybuilding gym on Staten Island, it was also the Island's bodybuilding epicenter, where the top local muscle builders of the era would train side by side to create a unique atmosphere. There was a strong camaraderie among its members that translated into friendships that would last a lifetime. It did not matter if you were a beginner or a seasoned pro, everyone trained together in harmony and with the same goals in mind, which were to get big and strong. If you were willing to put your time in the gym and pour enough sweat onto a barbell, you were all but guaranteed to build a physique worthy enough to step onto a bodybuilding stage. My members built muscles they never knew they had and lived for more. When you entered my gym, the realities of life stayed outside its door. This was a place for results. It was not for social gatherings. It was a place for pain beyond imagination. There were no phones, no TVs, no magazines, and especially no idle

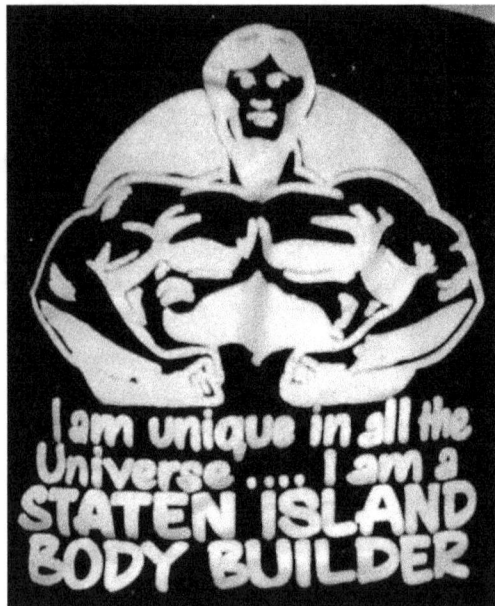

I am unique in all the Universe .... I am a STATEN ISLAND BODY BUILDER

chatter. What the gym did have was screams that would horrify the curious. It had huge mirrors filled with moving images of raw muscle. It had tons of cold steel to lift and big gains to be realized. It had bodybuilders whose sole purpose for being alive was to train in order to reach ultimate strength and muscle power. The Staten Island Bodybuilding Club had an energetic and empowering atmosphere that would last for years!

Champions were created and perfected at the Staten Island Bodybuilding Club! The right combination of genetics, desire, application, and knowledge helped me build some of the greatest natural physiques ever to walk the Island's streets. In 1976, I opened my gym because I had a burning desire to teach bodybuilding. I was a living library of muscle building know how. I trained using the principles I had mastered over a lifetime and wanted to share my expertise with those willing to listen. Throughout the club's ten-year history, I personally trained thousands of men and women. Long before the term *personal trainer* ever existed, I was designing personalized bodybuilding programs for each one of my members. It didn't matter if they wanted to gain 50 pounds of solid muscle or lose 100 pounds of unwanted body fat; I was there every step of the way to help guide them towards their desired goals.

Some of my members were gifted with extraordinary genetics. Their physiques had long muscle bellies and symmetrical structures that were proportioned with fibrous tissue designed for bodybuilding. When I gave advice to my members, they eagerly listened. I had the ability to see the potential in everyone I trained and brought out the best in those genetically gifted for success. The Staten Island Bodybuilding Club was known for pumping out winners and its reputation as the Home of Champions was well respected. Throughout my gym's history, many champions emerged from its deep core. It was a place to focus on one's individual goals, and many dreams that began there became future realities.

THE SHOW MUST GO ON

In 1980, I unexpectedly found myself in the role of show promoter. Early in May of that year, my students as well as other bodybuilders throughout Staten Island were training hard to be in competitive condition for the WBBG Mr. Staten Island competition, which was about ten days away. Regrettably, the WBBG suddenly cancelled its big New York City show, which consisted of all five boroughs, including the Mr. Staten Island competition. It was left up to me to find another venue for the Island's big bodybuilding event. On such short notice, it was impossible to find an auditorium to hold the competition. Since most athletes were nearing peak condition, it was not practical to reschedule the event, so the only choice I had was to hold the competition inside my Staten Island Bodybuilding Club.

Through some fast footwork and ads in the local newspapers, I was able to get a good field of 18 competitors. On the day of the show, a section of the gym, which was approximately 1000 square feet, was used to hold the event. After several exercise machines were moved and two hundred chairs put in their place, we were ready for some muscle flexing. It actually worked out fairly well. Before posing, the bodybuilders were able to pump their physiques with the free-weights in the gym's lower level, then just walk up the stairs and step onto the posing dais to do their thing. The only big problem I had was with Mother Nature. The day of the competition was extremely hot and humid. To make matters worse, my gym's air-conditioning system was not designed to service such a large crowd. The place was packed and my stock of bottled fruit juices and spring water sold out within the first hour. Nevertheless, the show went on and all the competitors had their chance to pose. The crowd was even treated to special posing performances by Russell Cunningham and Leon Brown.

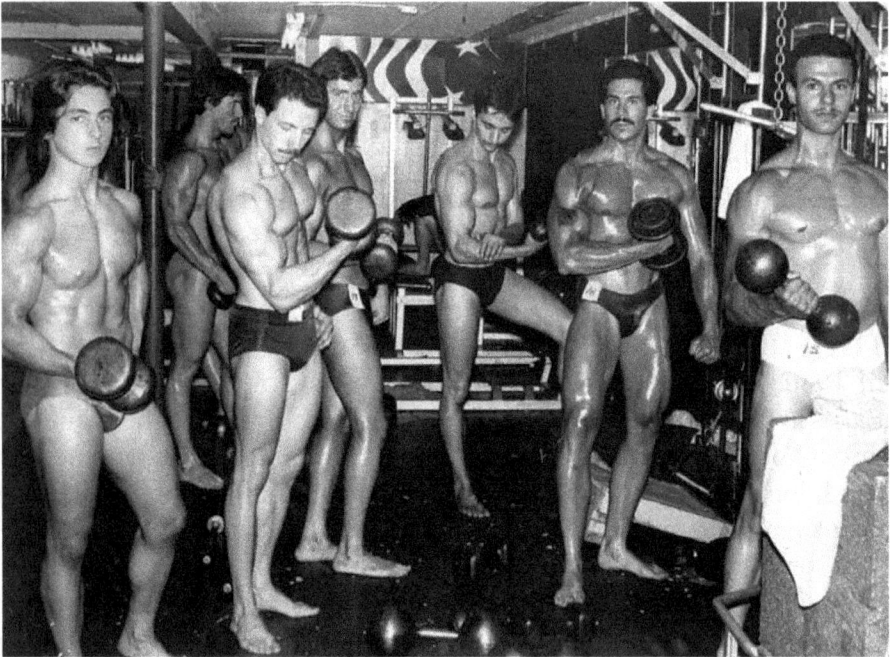

Mr. Staten Island competitors prepare for battle in the Animal Room – 1980

To say it was not comfortable would be an understatement. However, the crowd was orderly until tempers flared towards the end of the evening when the awards presentation commenced. After the top five place winners were announced, a couple of spectators took it upon themselves to stand up and start yelling at the judges when their favorite bodybuilder did not place. In a steamy room, sitting shoulder to shoulder, it did not take much for a near riot to happen. One of the judges was Russell Cunningham. Russell was a former Mr. Staten Island winner and was someone you did not shout expletives at. Along with the other judges, he stood up firmly and angrily questioned the shouting duo. When reason did not suffice, Russell quickly rushed towards the complaining duo as they cowardly jumped off their seats and headed straight for the exit door, while knocking others from their chairs. As the audience returned to their seats, I stepped onto the posing dais and ended the show with a real bang by exploding a hot water bottle for the upset crowd. It was another first in the history of the Staten Island Bodybuilding Club and for me the first of what would be many physique competitions I would promote.

THOU SHALL

Bodybuilding clubs throughout America are notorious for having poor gym etiquette. These hard-core muscle-head gyms are full of foul language, dirty locker rooms, and weight-plates that are never returned to the racks where they belong. It is amazing how some of these places even survive. At the Staten Island Bodybuilding Club, I faced a similar situation early in its history and came up with a solution to the problem. It hung as a reminder and was used only once. In today's politically-charged environment, where everything seems to be misconstrued and negatively slanted, it would never be allowed. However, in the days of Guts and Glory, it served its purpose without question, while symbolizing the law of the gym. It was a cowboy style noose that hung high from the ceiling, and was placed there to discourage unruly members who did not want to follow the gym's three commandments:

Thou shall not crash thy weights on thy gym floor.
Thou shall put thy weights back on thy rack after thy use.
Thou shall pay thy gym dues to thy gym owner on thy due time.

On occasion, I would have to point to the noose as a friendly reminder for some members to follow the commandments. Nevertheless, I had a problem with one individual who just did not get it. He was a big and strong guy that did not respect the gym or its members. Finally, after three months into his membership and after giving him enough warnings, I had enough of his bull and decided to put an end to this jerk's bad behavior. To give him a good lesson I had one of my members get a painter's ladder from the storage closet and place it under the noose while I walked over to this wise guy and gave him an ultimatum. Upon giving him a friendly warning, he stupidly gave me a little lip and my temper hit 1000 degrees. In anger, I, along with a couple of members dragged his sorry ass towards the ladder and yanked him up the steps as he struggled to get free. Although we had no actual intentions of hanging him, it was somewhat funny watching him squirm in fear, as he believed we were going to do so. Suddenly his behavior changed and he began to plead for mercy by apologizing profusely for his actions in the gym. I warned him once again and he nodded in acceptance. I then let him loose and watched as he crashed to the gym floor and ran out of the building. Twenty years later, I would meet this same individual as he was shopping in the Staten Island Mall with his two children. He recalled the incident laughingly and thanked me for my actions, saying that it had made him a better person in life. I told him it was my pleasure and anytime he needed further assistance to look me up.

A CHANGE OF COURSE

From 1976 through 1979, my club was primarily the only bodybuilding gym on Staten Island. There were a couple of small garage gyms and a Nautilus fitness center on the Island but that was it. The Staten Island Bodybuilding Club was the place to be. It was the epicenter for Island muscle builders and remained so throughout its history. In 1979, a fellow by the name of Mike Cassaro opened the second bodybuilding gym on Staten Island. The gym was appropriately named "Mike's Gym," and was equipped with exercise machines that Mike designed and welded himself. Mike's Gym was spacious and had a good group of members that trained hard on the equipment he built for them. He was someone who loved bodybuilding and helped promote the sport in a positive way.

In 1980, the Staten Island Bodybuilding Club's membership roster was soaring. The club was well-known throughout the city and appealed to those seeking championship physiques. Mike's Gym was on the opposite side of the Island and his gym was also producing great bodybuilders. My gym had many dedicated members that had been with me for years. A couple of those members were guys named Dennis and Ernie. Both were dedicated to their training and always worked out on their scheduled days. They were like the rest of the members in that they desired more mass and strength. However, their action caught me off-guard one day when I found out that they were secretly opening a bodybuilding gym just two blocks from mine. Now I know America has a free enterprise system and it is the land of opportunity, but to open a club in the same neighborhood as mine was betrayal in my eyes. At the time, there just wasn't enough business on Staten Island for two clubs so close together to function successfully and there still isn't. To me, it really felt like a stab in the back as I felt they were trying to steal what I had created.

Human nature being what it is caused me to lose about half of my membership to those seeking something new while the rest of my students remained loyal. I began to look towards the future and decided to take my club in a slightly different direction. I wanted to tone down the hard-core aspect of my club so it would seem more appealing to the general public. At the same time, I did not want to deter from the true reason I opened the gym in the first place. After several months of studying my options, I decided to equip the Staten Island Bodybuilding Club with the widely-popular Nautilus Time Machines. Nautilus was a well-respected name in the industry and their equipment was built to last. More importantly, the original Nautilus Time Machines were engineered to produce results. They were popular in the NFL and sought after by strength coaches everywhere. Besides, I had trained on several Nautilus machines in the past and knew of their muscle-building potential when used correctly. After very careful consideration, I went ahead and purchased twenty new Nautilus Time Machines for my gym.

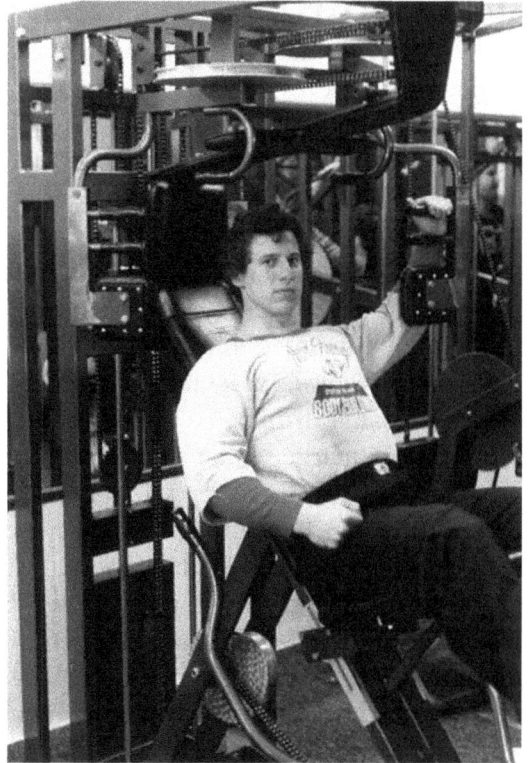

And with that move, a new era on the Island of Mario's Monsters had begun!

My club already had a large clientele of muscle builders and now I wanted to increase its membership with a greater diversity of people from the Island's population. The Nautilus machines were the answer. They attracted thousands of members to my club, many of whom were more into sports and fitness than just pure muscle building. Unlike the other Nautilus gyms on the Island, my club also offered a full line of weight training equipment – plus unlimited use of the Nautilus machines as opposed to the twice weekly, one-set-per-exercise rule the other clubs were following. In a way, Dennis and Ernie actually did me a big favor by forcing me to open my club's door to a wider range of students. Because of the club's transition, I was also able to rid it of the "gym-rats" that practically lived there, and the couple of steroid users it had. Once again, I looked forward to teaching health and fitness to the many ears that were willing to listen. I had the best of both worlds and my club's cash register never rang so cheerfully!

MR. ANATOMY

In 1981, I was dating a girl who was studying to be a nurse at the College of Staten Island. Occasionally, I attended class with her. One day, during an anatomy lesson, the class professor asked me how developed my physique was. As my then-girlfriend watched, the professor placed her hands on my chest and biceps while asking me if I would like to model for her class. She explained that every semester she would have a muscular male demonstrate the actions of the muscles for her students and stated that I would be perfect for the part. Being the egomaniac that I was (am), I said, "Sure." I found myself in her class a week later, standing on top of a desk and wearing nothing but my posing trunks. While gasping in awe of my physique the professor remarked that my body was the most muscular and proportioned she had ever seen. This only fed into my ego more as I flexed away on her demand and watched as the nurses came over to study my anatomy more closely. One by one, I flexed each muscle group as the professor demonstrated its action. On her command I extended, twisted, and turned my physique as I displayed my muscularity. I served her class well. After completing my demonstration, I received a nice applause from the students and was asked by the professor if I would like to pose for future classes. I said,

"Sure," and returned for several semesters to do my thing while also gaining an occasional new member to join my club. Such is the life of a bodybuilder.

THE LAST LAUGH

At the Staten Island Bodybuilding Club, my members were always playing practical jokes on me and having a good laugh at my expense. One day during the fall of 1981, I came up with a scheme to get them all back at once. I needed to set them up for something big and to catch them totally off-guard. At the time, I was training hard and was in good competitive condition. Knowing that one of my staff members could not keep a secret, I purposely told her that I was getting ready for a national level show. I said I would be out of town sometime in the near future. Sure enough, by the end of the day the rumor of my return to the physique stage was circulated throughout my club.

As the days passed, my members bombarded me with questions about what show I was preparing for. Every time I was questioned, I laughed to myself more and more, knowing that they were all falling for it. I continued to train hard and dieted to help lose some excess body fat to further raise the bar of suspicion. About a month into the joke, I took some time off from the gym and advised my staff that I was going to Ohio to see the Mr. International physique championships. I totally disappeared from the Staten Island bodybuilding scene. On the Saturday night of the Mr. International show, I had a couple of friends visit the *Staten Island Advance* to report that I had competed in the show and won the big title. Sure enough, the story hit the newsstands that Sunday morning. In the sports section of the newspaper was the bold headline: MARIO STRONG WINS MR. INTERNATIONAL. The story detailed my victory in Ohio and how I defeated seventy-two national level competitors. It went on to state that I was now training hard in hopes of winning the Mr. Universe competition in Paris the following month.

My members were completely duped by the story. Continuous phone inquires to my gym went unanswered. It seemed that every one of the newspaper's subscribers read the story and wanted to know more about my victory. However, I was nowhere to be found. My scheme had worked perfectly. My members took the bait and began calling each other to see if anyone had an update. I was having a good laugh at my upstate cabin while receiving messages from my family and staff as to what was transpiring on the Island. The joke seemed flawless until some gym patrons started visiting my parent's home. They caused my father to get extremely irritated with their knocks on the door. After a few hours, I decided I had enough of a laugh and called my staff, telling them to let everyone know the joke was on them. The next day I returned to my gym and received a call from the *Staten Island Advance* threatening me with a lawsuit for filing a false story. The call worried me for a few days until one of my members admitted he was the prankster. He said with a big smile, "Ha! I got the last laugh."

A SECOND PASSION

I have always enjoyed watching the martial arts films on the big screen. As a teenager, I would go to the movies with my brothers, Johnny and Domenic, to see Bruce Lee take on what seemed to be impossible odds. The smooth form and focus that Bruce Lee displayed as he fought villains motivated me to try my hand at the sport. The martial arts seemed to come natural for me. During my high school days, I spent several years learning the art of Vada Kempo from a schoolmate named Jackie Aversa. He was a master in this style. Jackie's karate school was in the basement of a clothing store on New Dorp Lane in Staten Island. The basement was well lit and had a couple of sand bags that hung from a steel beam over a concrete floor. In a twist of fate, it would be in that very building – basement and all – that I would open the Staten Island Bodybuilding Club several years later. Before I would ever drop an ounce of sweat at my bodybuilding club, I would first pour blood onto the same floor, as I punched and kicked my way in a building that would witness many years of my own pain. Sadly, Aversa's school closed after a few years of operation and I was left to train on my own.

In 1982, I joined my then workout partner, Myke Decembre's karate studio to learn the style of Go Ju. This style was more suitable for my frame as I enjoyed the close hand-to-hand combat. For me, it was a more practical style for the street and after several years of painful stretching and heavy-hitting, I found myself about six months away from taking an exam for my black belt. Once again, my training in the martial arts would be derailed as Decembre's karate studio eventually closed and forced me to practice what I had learned on my own. Although I continue to practice the basics of martial arts today, I look forward to the day when I will have the extra time needed to return to the mat in a class setting. It is a goal that I have waited decades to accomplish. I will once again take up where I left off in my quest of that elusive black belt.

A LOST FRIEND

March 10, 1983 was a sad day for Staten Island bodybuilders. A long time member of my gym and one of the most well-liked and respected bodybuilders passed away after battling cancer. His name was Jerry Valente (see photo).

I first met Jerry in the summer of 1976, after reading an ad about some exercise equipment in the *Staten Island Advance*. I was preparing to open my club and was looking for several pieces of gym equipment. Jerry had a Dan Lurie Moon Bench for sale and I took a ride to his house to see it. When I drove into his driveway Jerry was there waiting for me with the bench.

Jerry was a big strong guy who had an easy smile and friendly personality. He was also a former training partner of Lou Ferrigno. The two bodybuilders use to train together at the original R&J Bodybuilding Studio on Avenue U in Brooklyn. Photos of Jerry appeared in physique publications nationwide from time to time. He was a well-known bodybuilder that had competed against some of the greats in the sport including three time Mr. Olympia, Frank Zane. After talking to Jerry for a while he showed me his well-equipped home gym and I was amazed at all the exercise equipment he

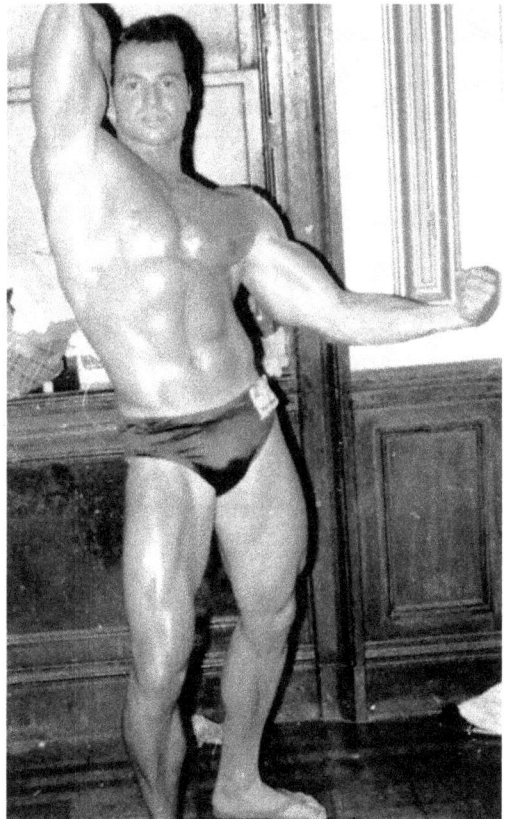

housed in his spacious basement. He had everything imaginable and was replacing the Moon Bench with a new piece of equipment. After the tour, I purchased the bench and invited Jerry to stop and train at my club any time he liked. About a month after my club opened, Jerry stopped by to see what it was all about and started to lift weights alongside the members. He was an inspiration to watch because he performed his exercises in perfect form. Not before long, Jerry became a staple at the gym and was always happy to give training advice to my club's members. That is what Jerry was about. He loved bodybuilding and was always there to lend a hand.

When I was training for the WBBG Mr. Staten Island competition in 1977, Jerry was there for me, as he had been so many times before. He constantly monitored my progress and even brought a dais to my gym to help me with my posing. At the premier of the film *Pumping Iron*, Jerry introduced me to his old training partner Lou Ferrigno. The two had been out of touch for several years, since the time Jerry was nearly killed in a job-related accident that left him partially deaf. Lou hugged his old friend and took Jerry backstage to get reacquainted. Everyone liked Jerry! He was a positive person who gave it his best.

In 1982, he was training for a physique competition when he became ill. Jerry fought against all the odds as he sought the medical attention needed to rid himself of this terminal illness. Sadly, Jerry lost his battle the following year, and to this day is remembered fondly by all those that knew him.

TRAINING WITH ARNOLD

In the summer of 1983, I flew to California for a few weeks of muscle pumping at the new Gold's Gym and original World Gym in Venice. For years, I had read about the champions in the physique publications and had met a few throughout my bodybuilding career but never had the opportunity to train with them. While in Venice that all changed. I was training twice a day. Between workouts, I tanned at the beach with other male and female muscle builders that shared my same passion. I was in muscle heaven and living the bodybuilding lifestyle alongside the champions. Every morning I arrived at World Gym at 7 AM. Already training at that early hour were Arnold Schwarzenegger, Franco Columbu, Frank Zane, and a host of other well-known bodybuilding legends. It was a great environment to train in and I gave it my all to make the most of my time there.

I had the pleasure to workout with Arnold. One thing about Arnold that stood out was his ability to focus intensely on each and every exercise he performed. Watching him train you could see the fullness of his muscular structure change as he pulled and pushed the steel with perfect form. When I trained with Arnold, I performed the same exercises and techniques. We both trained with moderate weights and rested little between sets. Every single repetition we pained through was performed using a full range of motion and unique style. It was a great experience for me to workout with the Austrian Oak. I not only learned how the Muscle Beach bodybuilders trained but also witnessed my physique respond well to Schwarzenegger's bomb and blitz routines.

Arnold liked to joke between sets. He'd banter with Franco across the gym just to get him going. Franco also had a great sense of humor and would always swipe back at Schwarzenegger, sending the gym's members into an uproar. Bodybuilding to Arnold seemed like a celebration of life! He always looked happy while he trained and seemed fulfilled with his efforts. For me, training with the Austrian Oak proved to be a once in a lifetime experience. Not only for the workouts we shared together, but also because of the positive attitude he exuded throughout the gym.

In contrast to World Gym, Gold's Gym was huge and filled an entire warehouse size building with every piece of exercise equipment imaginable within its walls. While training at Gold's Gym in the evenings, I had the opportunity to workout with many well-known physique champions of the era.

One evening I had the pleasure of bombing my thighs with bodybuilding champion Tom Platz. Tom was an extremely intense bodybuilder to train with. One exercise I remember was the Hack Squat. Together we worked up to several hundred pounds in the exercise and what was truly amazing was not the heavy weight used by Platz but the way he performed the movement. While performing Hack Squats, he would put both feet close together with toes pointed out and placed near the bottom of the Hack machine's footboard. From the top starting position, he would crash down in an exaggerated motion while stretching his quads forward for maximum stimulation. From there I would slightly assist him back to the top where he would immediately repeat the same crashing motion. How his knees didn't explode, I don't know. Nevertheless, this is the manner in which Platz performed all of his thigh exercises – with lots of explosive force and extreme intensity. I can still remember the pain I felt in my thighs in the following days. I also remember how great it felt to be in California during that era when bodybuilding was still a close-knit community. So much has changed!

It came as no surprise to the bodybuilding community that Arnold achieved his lofty goals. Arnold is a conqueror! After he dominated the bodybuilding and film industries, he set his deep grey Austrian eyes on his long time political aspirations. For years, we all talked about him becoming the governor of California and when the opportunity arrived, he threw his hat into the political ring to win the job. In a way Arnold is much like that of the character Conan that he portrayed on the silver screen. He knows deep in his heart that his is a life that will lead many. He has a purpose for being here. He must never rest until all his goals are realized. The only thing stopping Arnold from becoming a future U. S. president are the words within our Constitution that state one must be born in this country to serve as Commander-in-Chief. Too bad, I believe Arnold would really try hard to be a good leader of the free world.

THE ANIMAL ROOM

If there ever was a hell on earth for mortal man, then it was my gym's Animal Room. Located in the dungeon of the Staten Island Bodybuilding Club, the Animal Room was a training section of my gym. This is where my members went to lift enormous amounts of steel while bellowing horrifying screams that could be heard on street level. While my gym's upper level featured wall-to-wall carpeting, wood paneled walls, and bright lighting; the Animal Room in contrast was dimly lit, had sweat soaked mirrors, and drawings of Herculean figures painted on its red, white, and blue concrete walls. Only those brave enough dared venture into its cavernous chambers, where the air remained stagnant and the training equipment barbaric in nature. When you entered the Animal Room, it was as if time stood still. There was only one purpose for being there and that was to put your life on the line while lifting as much steel as super-humanly possible. Today, in the many multi-purpose fitness centers, such a training environment would never be tolerated. However, back in the days of Guts and Glory, it was welcomed by the few that understood what it took to create giant muscle and raw power.

As the theme from *Rocky* constantly blared off the Animal Room's walls, the echoes of clanging and crashing from the iron being lifted and dropped, fell in tune with the trumpets of *Gonna Fly Now* and the drumming beat of *Eye of the Tiger*. The Animal Room had a vibe that exuded results. Its very environment created a magical atmosphere by those that poured their blood onto the rusty barbells. It was a no-holds-bar, winner takes all mentality, which saw some of the greatest workouts in the most primitive conditions ever to take place on the Island. As you walked down my gym's staircase, the words ANIMAL ROOM boldly greeted you. Looking across the training area you saw the words TRAIN WITH THE INSANE painted across one of its long walls. That pretty much summed up the attitude that was needed to survive in such a hellish environment.

It was a remarkable sight! The Animal room was filled with huge 100 pound and 75 pound weight-plates on its machines and racks. The dumbbells, large round balls of black steel, had thick handles. They endured endless gripping by those strong enough to lift them. Its angle iron benches were held together by welds that strained under the force put upon them while their vinyl coverings stretched and shredded from the muscles that dug deep into the fabric. What was hell for others was heaven on earth for the hard-core muscle maniacs of the Staten Island Bodybuilding Club. They lived and dreamed for such torturous days of iron pumping madness and big gains. Training in the Animal Room was an experience that relatively few ever had the pleasure to enjoy. To this day, I can still feel the enthusiasm and taste the pain I shared with the members of my gym as we met and conquered the many challenges that dared come our way. It is the fond memory and the strength that stays with me as I continue to push forward with this thing called bodybuilding.

HE FINALLY GOT RESPECT

In the summer of 1983, I received a phone call from someone claiming to be a location scout for a movie being filmed on Staten Island. The caller stated that the movie starred Rodney Dangerfield and asked me if I would be interested in having a few scenes shot at my club. Not knowing if this was a legit or prank phone call I said, "Sure," and let it go at that. A couple of weeks later, a man and woman entered my gym and said they were location scouts for the film, *Easy Money* starring Rodney Dangerfield. With curiosity, I gave them a tour of my club, and watched as they snapped photos and drew sketches of its layout. The scouts said that with some slight modifications the club would be perfect for the film. They also mentioned that they would need three days to do the shoot. With some hesitance, I said, "Okay," and received a generous financial proposal for the use of my facility.

Several months later, while the gym was in full swing, none other than Rodney Dangerfield and a woman came for a visit. They introduced themselves and told me about the film as I gave them the tour of the club. As we walked towards the back of the gym, Rodney heard loud screams coming from the Animal Room below. Without pause, he ventured down the stairs and gazed up at a large poster of Arnold Schwarzenegger that hung high on the room's musty wall. Jokingly, Rodney said, "He thinks he's big, I'll show him," as he walked over to a power-rack and tried to lift what seemed to be 400 pounds on the bar. As his eyes bulged, he looked around to see if anyone noticed. Unfortunately, the members were too busy doing their own thing and paid no attention to Rodney's hilarious efforts. Sadly, he then walked over to me and said, "You see, even here I get no respect." With that, he shook my hand and said his team would be in touch.

Later that year, I had heard that *Easy Money* was being filmed on Staten Island, so I took a ride and visited Rodney on a movie set in Grant City. While there, I was disappointed to learn that the gym scene had been cut from the movie. After a few minutes of watching the filming, Rodney walked over to me and flexed his right bicep. Amazingly, he displayed a nice peak and I told him that Arnold was lucky he retired from competition when he did. This caused Rodney to laugh loudly and say, "Finally, I got some respect."

THE WRONG KIND OF PAIN

Bodybuilding gyms can sometimes be dangerous places to be. Besides the residual pain felt from training with the iron, the heavy weights can lead to unfortunate accidents. On any given day, every bodybuilding gym has its share of heavy lifters pushing and pulling the steel to their very limits. A good way to experience some real pain is to stand in front of a big boy when he is performing the Overhead Dumbbell Press and block his vision to the mirror. I've seen plenty of dumbbells fly like "smart bombs" in the direction of feet that weren't suppose to be there. It is amazing how instinctively accurate some of these big boys can be. Another way to experience some real pain is not to focus on what you are doing. There's been more than one time in my life when I've found myself leaping into the air after a 45-pound weight-plate fell off a weight-rack and onto my foot, all because I was looking at some hot babe and not paying attention to the task at hand.

I remember one unfortunate incident when a member brought some friends to my gym for a visit. After they were there for about five minutes, I heard a loud commotion coming from the back of the gym. One of the visitors had put his hand where it did not belong and his index finger was chopped off as one of his friends unknowingly lowered 500 pounds onto it while performing the Leg Press movement. Needless to say, the victim ran out of my gym with his detached finger in his other hand in hopes of having it reattached at a local hospital.

In the 1980s, most overhead pull-down machines had pulleys that used steel cables and S-hooks to hold the pull-down bar in place. The steel cables were plastic coated and occasionally would snap, sending a bar crashing down on a victim as he or she tugged on a heavy set of pull-downs. One day, a member of my gym had a painful experience while performing Behind the Neck Pull-downs. As he yanked the bar downwards, the cable suddenly snapped and released the bar in the direction of his skull. It was amazing to watch the blood squirt out of the top of his head like a volcanic eruption. The pulling force on the bar had cracked his skull on impact and sent him immediately to the ER for some much-needed stitches. That same pull-down machine sent my then-girlfriend to the hospital one day when she was hit by the pull-down bar after it whipped off the cable's S-hook and landed squarely on her face. After being interrogated by the local authorities for possible abuse, I was free to take her home to her parents with a swollen nose, two black raccoon eyes, and an icepack over her face. Trying to explain to the parents what had happened to their daughter was also another uncomfortable and awkward experience.

Because of the nature of bodybuilding gyms, with members training hard and moving in many different directions, injuries happen more often than not. It is because of this potential for disaster that I had a notice created for all members and visitors to my gym to read and sign before they were ever allowed to step onto the training floor. The top of the notice read: DEATH NOTICE (with a skull and cross-bones under the heading). It was several paragraphs long and detailed the potential dangers that existed within my gym. After members read it, they were required to give their signature with the understanding that they were entering and training at my facility at their own risk. I am not sure of the legality of the notice but everyone that trained in my gym signed on the dotted line. After accumulating thousands of them over a decade that saw plenty of mishaps, no one ever attempted to sue me for some bodily injury or painful experience they suffered while at my club. I guess it worked!

MERRY FITNESS

The holiday season was always a joyous time for me. As the fall leaves blew away, the winter's cold would usher in mountains of snow and new hopes for increased size and strength in the upcoming year. For me, Christmas and New Year's Eve were not only a time for gifts and parties, they also marked the beginning of my bulk and power season. Most Christmas Days were the same. After my family and friends finished feasting on their elaborate holiday meal, I would take a ride to my gym and pump iron while listening to tunes of *White Christmas* and *Jingle Bell Rock*. Occasionally, my three brothers: Johnny, Domenic, and Philip, would join me in the true celebration of life. There was always some magic on Christmas. The holiday itself was one of hope and spirit; it brought a positive light that shined into the coming year. New Year's Day was quiet in contrast to Christmas, as the holiday was one of remembrance of times past and hopes for better tomorrows to come. Every January 1st was the same. While the hard partiers were recovering from their hangovers, I was curling and squatting to *Auld Lang Syne*. As resolutions were being broken, I was laying out the framework for my training for the days, weeks, and months to come. For me, every year was a continuation of the previous one. It was a time to review my progress and fine-tune my strategy towards larger muscles and more explosive power for the coming year. Bodybuilding was my way of life and its demanding needs were with me every minute of every day. For me, the holidays were always a time to experience the joy of the season and to be thankful for the ability to keep training healthily and to reach my goals.

BACK ON THE POSING DAIS

In the spring of 1985, I decided to compete one last time in a physique competition. I knew I was about to cross a turning point in my life and I wanted one last hurrah before I got there. The show I chose to compete in was Bob Boham's 1st Annual AAU Eastern Classic. I had heard good things about Bob Boham through members that trained at his Strong and Shapely Gym in Rutherford, New Jersey, and I felt that he was someone who would run a good competition. The show was promoted as an all-natural event and was slated for the second week of September that year. When I made the decision to *Go For It* in May of 1985, my bodyweight was a solid 220 pounds. After a careful calculation, I decided to target the middleweight class and compete at a bodyweight of less than 175 pounds. My thinking was that since I already carried a lot of muscular mass at 220 pounds I would easily out muscle everyone as a middleweight. I wasn't far from wrong!

Preparing for a physique competition is an exact science! After years of pouring sweat in the gym, the time comes for some of us to put on our posing trunks and flex our stuff on the big stage before the judges and audience alike. It is a unique experience to be up there on a physique stage. You stand, side-by-side with other muscle artists, being compared and critiqued by judges, family, friends, and peers within your sport. It is an experience that only the true goal-oriented bodybuilder should dare venture. It takes time, sacrifice, sweat, pain, hunger, and determination to sculpt hard-earned muscle into Herculean form but once you step onto the stage its well worth the effort. When preparing for the Eastern Classic, I lost nearly 50 pounds of bodyweight to make the middleweight class. Looking back, I could have been just as ripped without the loss of twenty pounds of extra muscle tissue if I would have competed in the light-heavyweight class instead.

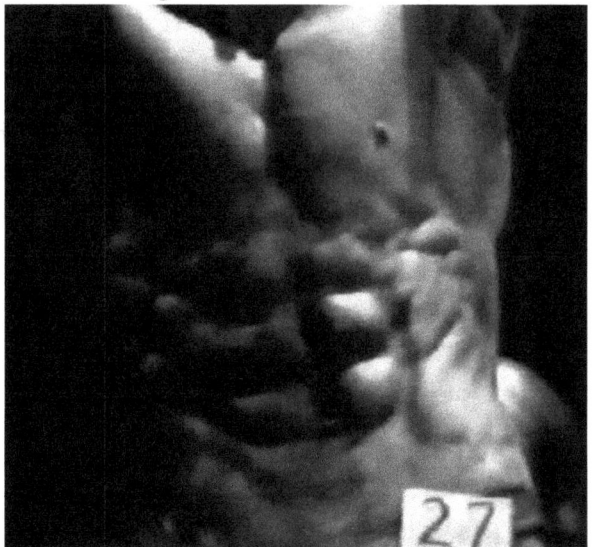

However, my goal was the middleweight class and that is what I trained to compete in. Once again, I became obsessed in my training as I increased my workouts to seven days a week and began to fine-tune my diet. Although my diet was based on all natural single ingredient foods, it was high in calories and complex carbohydrates. As the show neared, I cut my calorie and carbohydrate intake steadily as I brought my bodyweight down to make the middleweight class. The week before the competition, my face looked drawn and my head pained from the carbohydrate withdrawal as I continued towards my goal of being massively ripped for the show. Forty-eight hours before prejudging I eliminated all liquid and fruits from my diet and found myself losing fluids as my body dehydrated to give me that thin, paper skin, polished look. I was ready!

On the day of the competition, I weighed a bit less than 174 pounds and was ripped to the bone. The middleweight class consisted of 28 competitors from all over the eastern seaboard. The class was so large that it took three rows of competitors just to get all the athletes onstage at one time during the pre-judging. Each and every muscle builder looked great as it became apparent to everyone that this was going to be a grueling competition, both for the competitors as well as the judges. The morning's comparisons took about forty minutes as we constantly changed and positioned our Herculean physiques to the demand of the judges. Each posing round was long and torturous as sweat poured from our physiques under the hot overhead spotlights that highlighted our muscular bodies. I felt confident that morning in knowing that I would place in the top five. I was carrying a lot of dense muscle at such a low bodyweight for me that my seratis and intercostals looked liked slabs of jagged steel that had been welded to my sides. I came to win and I would be hard to beat.

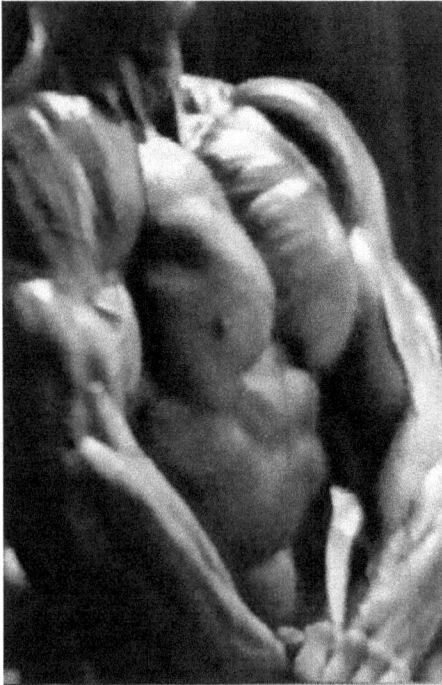

Also competing on this day was my brother, Philip, who entered the teenage division, and my then-girlfriend, Lina, who entered the women's division. After the pre-judging, all the competitors gathered at a local restaurant in anticipation of the evening event.

The evening show saw a standing-room-only crowd. The auditorium was packed to capacity as the show had been sold out weeks earlier. This was a well-promoted competition, with friends and family members present to support their favorite bodybuilders. An hour into the show my class was called and each competitor took their turn flexing their stuff for the muscle hungry crowd. As I stepped onto the stage, I got a rush of exhilaration as the MC announced my name and the crowd of over a thousand applauded wildly. Here I was again, eight years since I first competed in a physique show at the Mr. Staten Island competition, and instantly the magic was back in my veins. As I approached center stage the theater's sound system played loudly with my selected song, which was, "Fanfare for the Common Man." It was a dramatic moment for me, as I knew deep inside my heart that I would never set foot on a physique stage as a competitor again. As the song's trumpets and drums flared, I flowed from one pose into another with the grace of a professional that came from the many hours I practiced my routine. I was back in my element and savored this moment in my bodybuilding history as cameras flashed and rows of fans cheered.

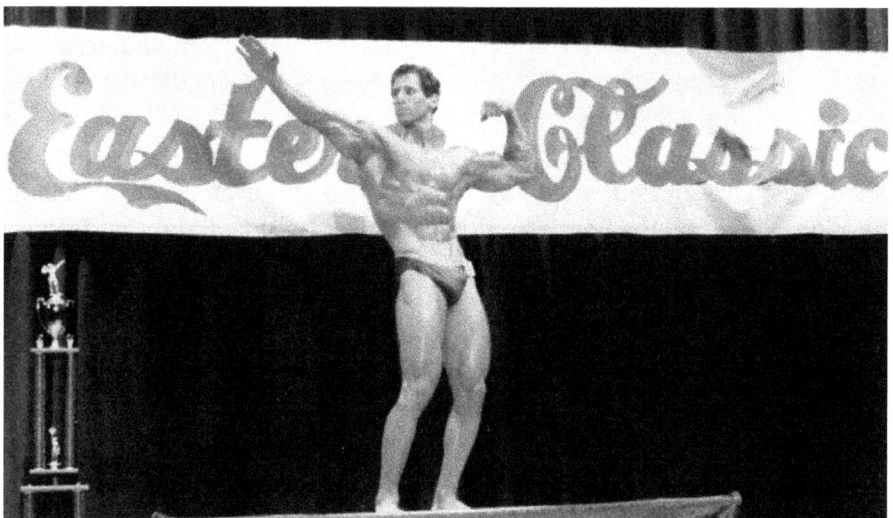

Mario Strong posing at the 1985 AAU Eastern Bodybuilding Classic

After all the athletes in the middleweight class finished their individual posing routines, the top five place winners were called onto the stage for their individual placing. One by one, the athlete's names were called until there were just two remaining, a fellow natural bodybuilder named Rick Trimarco and mine. Rick was a nationally recognized competitor who also owned a gym and came to the contest in extremely good condition. The crowd was in a near frenzy as the both of us posed-down while waiting the much-anticipated results. In the end Rick was the winner, and deservedly so. I congratulated him, knowing that I gave it my best and that either of us could have won that evening. Having fought such an intense battle on stage with him gave me a sense of satisfaction in confirming that I was one of the best natural bodybuilders on the east coast. I had trained long and hard for the Eastern Classic and had accomplished much of my goals. Now for me, the time had come to retire my posing suit.

Lina would go on to take her class in the women's division but lost the overall title in a very controversial decision that rocked the stage with thunderous boos from the audience. My brother, Philip, who came to the show very muscular and posed magnificently, narrowly missed placing in a very competitive teenage division. At the end of the competition, we all left smiling as another chapter in Strong History had been completed, or so I thought.

After the show, my group left to return to Staten Island in separate cars. While driving south on the New Jersey Turnpike I tried to enter the middle lane while another car from the opposite lane tried to do the same. We nearly collided as I pushed down on the accelerator and took the lead. That should have been it. But the fellow in the other car wasn't happy that I took the lane. He decided to tailgate my car with his bright-lights on as we traveled at speeds in access of seventy-five miles per hour. I continually changed lanes to avoid a confrontation with this jerk but after ten minutes of speeding and high tension, enough was enough. In the middle of the turnpike, I slammed on my brakes and sent it into a screeching halt that stopped all traffic on the highway as cars swerved to miss crashing into the both of us. Wearing just shorts and a tank top, I got out of my vehicle and ran over to the other car. In it were a man and woman in their mid-forties. The man was arrogant but seemed horrified as he looked at my tanned, chiseled physique in bewilderment. I yelled to him several times "Let it go, just let it go," and started to walk back to my car. Before I even took two steps, the jerk yelled some obscenities at me while closing his driver-side window. In an unfortunate moment of rage, I returned to his car and as I stood by the driver's window, I made a fist. I then looked the jerk in the eye and with explosive power punched his driver-side window. The window shattered into a thousand pieces as glass flew all over him and the now frantically screaming female passenger. Once more, I warned him to "Let it go." I returned to my car and left the scene, as did my brother, Philip, and the rest of the people who got out of their cars to witness the incident. About a month later, Lina received a call from the New Jersey State Police wanting to know who the man in the car with her was that night. Although she did not state my name, she did advise the police officer of the actions of the other driver. Upon hearing our side of the story, the police officer asked for reimbursement for the window to end the case. She agreed and I sent a money order for the window and closed the book on that ordeal.

On the day after the Eastern Classic, my family celebrated three birthdays. That past week had seen my brothers, Johnny and Philip, as well as myself, get a year older. At my mother's house we had a large ice-cream cake (which I did not taste) to mark the occasion and took several pictures while blowing the candles out. When the pictures were developed, I looked at them in disbelief as I saw how emaciated my face had become from all the dieting and training. I had lost nearly 50 pounds of bodyweight for the competition and looked like I had just come out of a concentration camp with every ounce of fat ripped from my body. The battle had taken a toll on me. I fought hard in the gym and followed a restricted nutritional program in preparation for the muscle war onstage. Now it was time to lay down the arms and look forward to my life to come.

THE END OF AN ERA

The time had finally come for me to close my gym and move forward with my life. The Staten Island Bodybuilding Club had lasted nearly a decade and it was a great experience. From its beginning days as an isolated Island gym, to becoming a major player within the East Coast bodybuilding scene, the gym had finally run its course. My primary reasons for opening the club no longer existed. I had fulfilled most of my goals in teaching bodybuilding and promoting health and vitality. I had trained thousands of students and became an expert and well-known national fitness author. I had championed the bodybuilding stage and had judged those who had judged me. I had come full circle and my heart was no longer in it. It was time to move on.

In 1976, I opened the Staten Island Bodybuilding Club because I believed in bodybuilding, health, and life. I believed I could make a difference with the many, but in reality, it was only with a few. For nearly a decade, I preached the benefits of natural bodybuilding to the thousands of members who had joined my gym. In early 1986, I realized my time would be better spent following a different course in life. So later that year, I sadly locked my gym's door forever. No longer would I hear the clanging of the weight-plates on the barbells or the sounds of *Gonna Fly Now* blasting from my gym's sound system. No longer would I answer the many questions of my students or preach to them about the benefits of physical culture. No longer would I see the smiling faces of my staff or hear the hellos of my gym's neighbors. There was so much to give up and leave behind. It was a difficult decision to make but was something that had to be done. I knew that my destiny lied elsewhere.

Where once my club stood as the only bodybuilding gym on the Island, twenty or so such entities now joined it, some just a few blocks away from my establishment. Financially, it no longer made sense to keep the club's door open for business. Although the membership was sufficient to cover all the gym's bills and expenses, it nevertheless, could not change the predicament of my club. The twenty-plus gyms had thinned my club's membership levels and cut into its profits. Even though my hard-core muscle maniacs were still with me, they were not going to be enough in financial terms to secure a future for me. Like myself, my gym was hard-core to the bone. Similar to the original Pearl's or Vince's gyms in nature, expanding it would have diluted its true purpose. The personal touch would have been gone and it would have become just another fitness center. Although I had the financial means to expand the Staten Island Bodybuilding Club into a major fitness center on the Island, it was not what I wanted to do at the time. Doing so would have been selling out and was not what I had spent the last ten years of my life trying to accomplish. Therefore, after several months of agonizing over this crossroad in both my life and the gym's history, I decided to call it a day and changed the course of my future.

I advised my staff and students of my decision and they stood by me to the end. It was surreal that last day as reality stood before me. The gym was my baby. I had raised and natured it into maturity and now it was time to say goodbye. One by one, the members left giving me their best wishes. One member, named John "The Viking" Delin, had trained at my gym from the beginning. On this last day, he brought in a large poster and hung it high on a gym mirror for all to see. The poster read, "The End Of An Era, The Beginning Of A Legend, Strong Will Return." That poster was symbolic of the closeness I shared with those I had come to know. In a way, it was just as hard for them as it was for me to see the gym close and say goodbye. I will always remember the joy that the Staten Island Bodybuilding Club brought to my life and to those who were a part of it. It was a time that saw me grow into an adult and a time where goals were met and new ones created. I had come full circle in bodybuilding and now it was time for a new direction in my life.

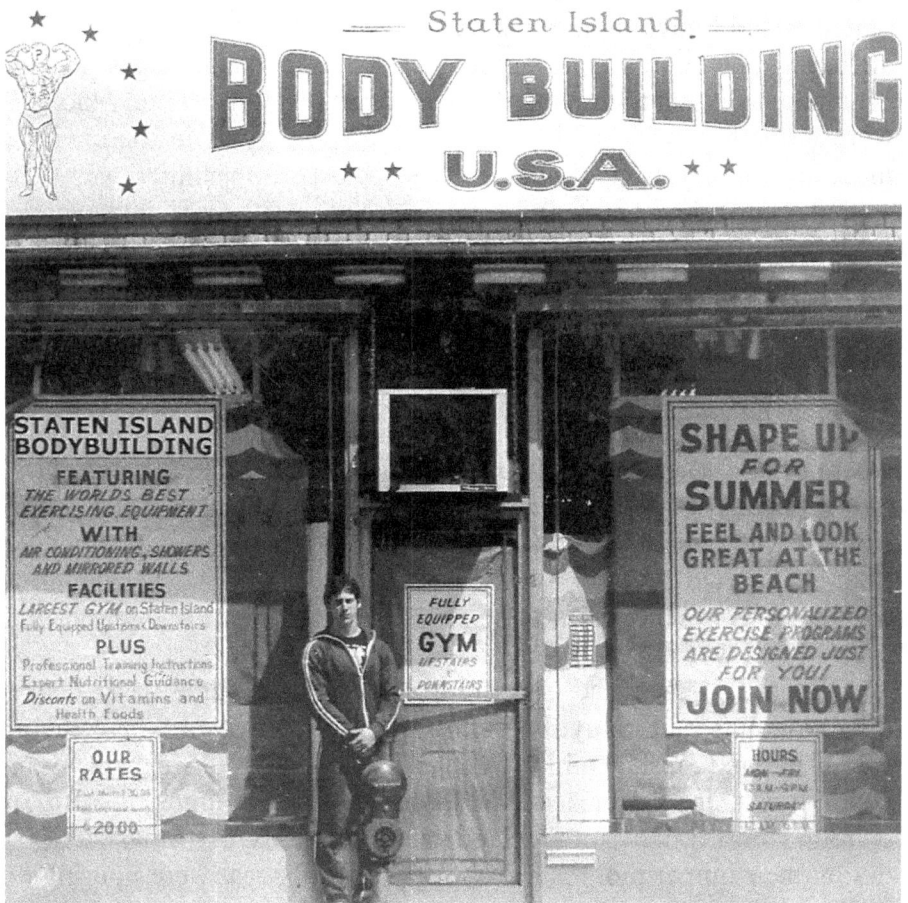

Mario Strong stands in front of Staten Island's first bodybuilding club – 1977

WHAT TO DO

When my gym closed, I had to decide what to do with tons of exercise machinery whose value was equivalent to a new pair of matching Chevy Corvettes. Back in 1986, that was a lot of equipment for a hard-core bodybuilding club and now I needed to find a home for all of my gym's benches, barbells, and tons of free-weights. In addition, I also had twenty Nautilus Time Machines and other pieces of selectorized equipment that still had many good years of use. There was no time for a planned auction so I rented a large truck and removed every item from the club with the help of some of my former members. The tons of iron and machinery that had witnessed the impossible become reality were now leaving the gym forever. They had created champions with their ruggedness and had lasted through the gym's existence. Now it was time to say good-bye to the home they had long known. With some sentimental feelings, I gently placed these pieces of Staten Island bodybuilding history onto the truck. For several months afterwards, I stored the equipment in my home's garage and contemplated what to do with them. Since the Nautilus Time Machines were virtually new, I sold them to a couple of gyms in the area and made my money back. Some other selectorized machines were also sold at a fair price. This left the free-weights and their related exercise equipment. I decided to keep all the dumbbells, weights, barbells, and racks, as well as one piece each of plate-loading machinery and benches. The rest was given to friends and family members that I knew would use the equipment wisely, and not let them collect dust in some damp corner.

I transported the exercise equipment I kept to my upstate home where I had a large barn. The barn's loft was huge and was originally built in the early 1970s as an area to store bales of hay. It had a high ceiling, where wild bats made their home, and reinforced plywood floors supported by thick wooden beams that were strong enough to hold the tons of equipment to be placed there. It made a great place to train when I was not on Staten Island.

When upstate, I had everything I needed for some basic heavy-duty workouts and enjoyed training in an environment where the air was clean and fresh. Unlike commercial gyms, the barn had no air-conditioning or heating system. I found myself training in difficult extremes during the summer and winter seasons. At times, training during the summer months felt as if gallons of sweat were pouring off my body. As the rays from the sun beat down onto the roof of the barn, its interior temperatures would rise in excess of one hundred degrees. Training in those conditions makes it more of a survival thing, than to build muscle. Winters were the opposite. The Catskill Mountains are known for their bitter cold days. When training in my barn during those frigid seasons, I had to wear several layers of clothing just to keep my body heat from escaping. My hands would constantly stick to the icy barbells as hot steam rose off my body and froze onto the loft's paned glass windows. Training in my barn was always an experience that made me not only physically stronger but more mentally capable as well. It also afforded me the opportunity to continue using the same free-weights and machines that had developed my muscle and power over the past twenty-plus years at my gym and home.

IT'S NOT THE SIZE OF THE DOG IN A FIGHT THAT MATTERS, BUT RATHER THE SIZE OF THE FIGHT IN THE DOG

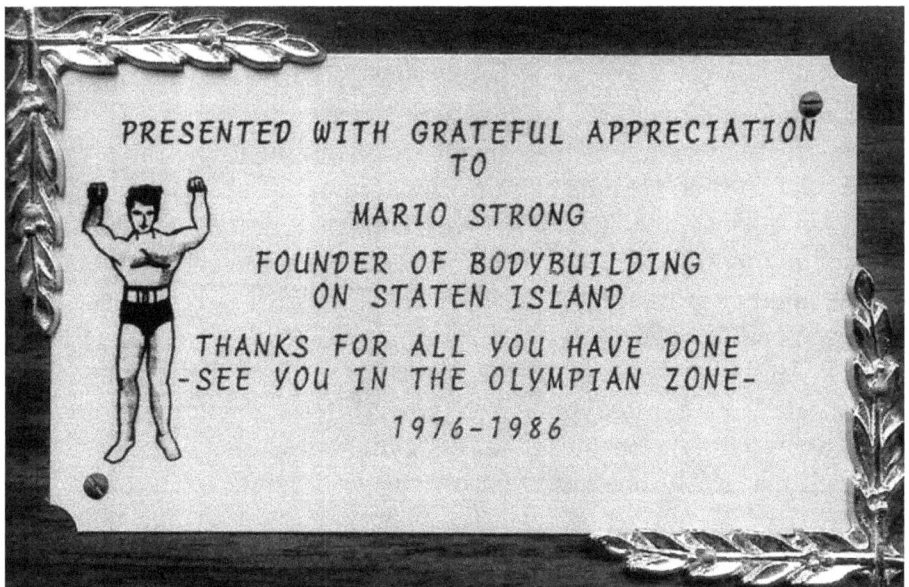

PRESENTED WITH GRATEFUL APPRECIATION
TO

MARIO STRONG

FOUNDER OF BODYBUILDING
ON STATEN ISLAND

THANKS FOR ALL YOU HAVE DONE
-SEE YOU IN THE OLYMPIAN ZONE-

1976-1986

Plaque given to Mario Strong by one of his gym's members

LIFE MARCHES ON

AFTER THE GYM

After the closure of my gym, I realized I needed to wean myself from the Staten Island bodybuilding scene. I trained primarily in Brooklyn for two years. For over a decade, I had been a main face on the Island's muscle scene and needed to step back and reflect on the past as I planned for the future. I literally vanished off the Island's radar as I continued to train like there was no tomorrow at Charlie Corrolo's 5th Ave. Bodybuilding Gym in Brooklyn. I had known Charlie Corrolo through the bodybuilding circles during my reign on Staten Island and was glad that his gym was within close proximity of my Staten Island home. Charlie was also a promoter of natural bodybuilding shows and his club was filled with competitive bodybuilders who trained hard and looked great. The 5th Ave. Bodybuilding Gym was a hard-core club that had plenty of iron to lift and a motivating atmosphere that gave a reason for being there. It was the perfect environment for someone like myself to continue making gains as I let time heal the emptiness within my heart.

As 1988 approached, I felt that enough time had lapsed since I closed my gym. I decided to return to the Staten Island bodybuilding scene and began training at a club named The Palms. A fellow named Vinny Venditti owned the Palms. Vinny was well-known on the Island and in Brooklyn because of the many hair salons that displayed his name. He wasn't a bodybuilder or powerlifter and I am not sure why he was in the gym business, but his gym was well-equipped and that was all that really mattered. During my first couple of weeks at The Palms, I probably did more in the way of answering questions than training with the weights. Many of my former gym's members as well as other Island muscle builders were also members there and they were very curious (to say the least) as to where and what I had been up to for the last couple of years. It had been good to see old friends again and before you knew it, I was helping everyone with their training and nutritional needs, just like the old days.

One member of The Palms worth mentioning was a bodybuilder named Patrick DeLuca (see photo). Patrick was huge and had enormous muscular power with a matching symmetrical frame. He was a former Mr. Florida winner that trained heavy. It made you wonder how the barbells he lifted did not snap from the stress he placed on them. Occasionally, I had the pleasure of training with Patrick. Our workouts together were always competitive. Between the two of us, we dared not show any limits and lifted steel we never thought possible. Patrick motivated newbie muscle builders to higher levels. He was well-liked by everybody that knew him and seemed invincible.

One day in 1991, while training alone at The Palms, I got the shocking news that Patrick DeLuca was killed in a boating accident in Florida. He was only in his early thirties and had a long, bright future ahead of him. It was hard to phantom how such a powerhouse of energy and life could no longer be with us because of an accident. Something wasn't right. If Patrick was vulnerable, then we all were. However, not even death could end Patrick's popularity, as hundreds of people came to his wake to mourn for him and his family. The funeral home had opened three rooms to accommodate those paying their respects to Patrick and his family and it was not enough space. The lines of mourners stretched out of the funeral home and into the street. While kneeling by his casket, I couldn't help but notice that Patrick, in his unfortunate present state, still looked bigger and better than everyone else in the room. Knowing Patrick the way I did, I just laughed to myself because I knew that he wouldn't have had it any other way. He always had to be the best!

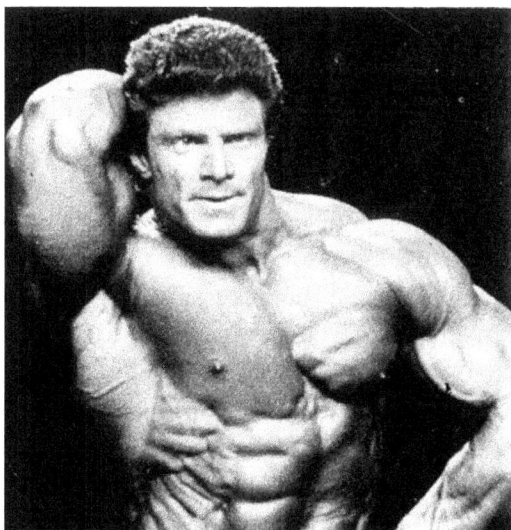

In 1992, The Palms begin to deteriorate as broken equipment remained unusable and bent barbells were not replaced. It was time for me to move on. A couple of friends who had bought Mike's Gym in the 1980s had transformed it into a World Gym. It was well-equipped and had the muscle-building atmosphere so conducive for progress. Ed and Kenny Spencer were brothers who collaborated together to create a gym that attracted the best bodybuilders on the Island. The body-men at World Gym trained hard and were serious about making gains. I enjoyed my workouts there and stayed with the club for several years. Eventually the Spencer brothers opened a second World Gym on the Island and remained in the fitness industry until the mid-1990s.

While still a member at World Gym, I also trained at a newly opened Gold's Gym on Staten Island. It was located in the former Courts of Appeal building, which was a racquetball and fitness center. The Courts of Appeal had a second gym; it was located in Brooklyn and was also transformed into Gold's Gym. My sister, Carmela, began weight training at this time. Several days a week, she joined me at the gyms so I could train her. I also monitored her progress in both physique and strength. We trained mostly on the Island but sometimes took the ride over the Verrazano Bridge to train at the Brooklyn location. Both gyms were well-equipped and professionally managed, which suited me fine until I could no longer take the traffic jams on the Staten Island Expressway. For me to sit in heavy traffic when I was psyched and ready to bomb and blitz, was a test of my patience that nearly drove me insane and caused me to "hulk-out" on occasion.

By the time 1997 arrived, I had finally run out of patience with the highway and joined a new Dolphin Fitness Center near my home. This was the first of several such clubs that would come to the Island. My gains continued as both my sister and I enjoyed training there.

Fate works in mysterious ways. One day in 1998 while training at the gym, I spotted the aerobic section and saw an old friend peddling away on a stationary bicycle. Her name was Aida. I had known Aida from my high school days in the 1970s and it was good to see her smiling face. When she saw I was looking at her she smiled back and waved hello. When I finished my training, I went up to her to chat and before you knew it, I had her pumping iron for the first time. Eventually, our friendship blossomed into a relationship that continues to this day. There is an old Strong saying: "The couple that trains together stays together." Since 1998, that is exactly what we've been doing several times a week and I guess the proverb is true.

While continuing to be members of the Dolphin Fitness Center we've also been members of several other Staten Island gyms over the years including Johnny Lats, Evolution Fitness, and LA Fitness. Johnny Lats and Evolution Fitness have since closed their doors.

We still continue to enjoy both the Dolphin and LA Fitness centers as our favorite places to blast the muscles. I'm not sure where I will be training in the long term future but one thing is certain, you can bet your last dollar that I will be giving it my all as I continue to live long and be strong...naturally!

YOU CAN BRING A HORSE TO THE WATER BUT

In the early 1990s, I was dating a model that not only possessed facial beauty but also had a very symmetrical and proportioned physique. At the time, Dawn was in her early thirties and had never before weight trained. She demonstrated a burning interest in what bodybuilding could do for her. After being convinced of her strong desire to body build, I helped Dawn with her muscle-building regimen and designed an exercise and nutrition program for her. She responded quickly to the training and soon began to see new lines in her physique. She was a natural for bodybuilding and after a couple of years of hard-core training, was Leg Pressing in the neighborhood of 700 pounds and performing the Incline Press with 50-pound dumbbells. Her physique transformed into a work of art and she began competing in natural shows. She did quite well. The seeds of health and strength I planted in her had blossomed into championship form. Her physique remained feminine yet looked mighty while on the posing platform.

Eventually I lost touch with Dawn and was disturbed a couple of years later to learn from a mutual acquaintance that said Dawn had been rushed to a local hospital. Our friend said that while Dawn was training at the gym, her entire body went into a massive spasm. This was the result of diuretics Dawn was using in an effort to lose water for an upcoming physique competition. He also stated that when the EMS crew arrived on the scene they had to strap Dawn to an exercise bench and carry her into the ambulance. When I heard what had happened I went into a tirade and yelled at our friend for not keeping me advised of Dawn's previous actions. Later that evening I visited Dawn in the hospital and saw several intravenous lines attached to her in hopes her electrolytes would return to proper levels. She seemed in pain and when she saw me started to cry and apologized for what she had done to herself. I was both mad and sad for her at the same time. I had spent several years training and coaching her about the benefits of natural bodybuilding and to me this was a form of betrayal. She had been swayed by the advice of some muscle-heads and it nearly destroyed her life. Why had she not known better?

Sadly, this was not the first time I had trained someone into championship form only to watch him or her go the way of the dark side once their egos took over. I have seen many similar occurrences over the years, as bodybuilders would resort to drugs once their biceps became bigger than their brains. How does the saying go?

"You can bring a horse to the water but you can't make him drink it." It is the same story with bodybuilding. As much as I preach to individuals about the benefits of natural bodybuilding and of the dangers of anabolic steroids, my words go in one ear and out the other. If there is one thing that I've learned in my life it's that the individual is going to do what she or he wants, no matter how dire the consequences may potentially be. It is just an unpleasant fact and sometimes lives have to be lost in order for others to smarten up and do the right thing. After Dawn's incident, she lost all desire to return to a hard-core bodybuilding gym and took up exercising in a women's health spa. The atmosphere there was a little saner and conducive to her health and longevity.

NO PAIN NO GAIN

I have suffered many injuries and narrow escapes throughout the decades. In 1973, during my senior year of high school, I was performing handstands on the parallel bars during gym class. I had performed this movement plenty of times before and for me it seemed routine, or so I thought. I had a spotter as required but no mats on the floor to cushion my fall. For some reason, while on the bars with my feet in an upright position over my body, my hands suddenly slipped and I found myself falling quickly towards the hard floor. Instead of breaking my fall, the person spotting me quickly jumped out of the way. There was nothing to stop my momentum and I crashed to the floor with a loud bang as I landed headfirst. What should have brought me serious injuries resulted only in a large head bump and a lesson learned!

Several years later, while riding my horse, Galaxy, on my upstate farm, I got a little bored. To spice things up a bit I got the bright idea of doing some wild bronco riding, but needed a way to make Galaxy start jumping. I found a can of horsefly repellant in the barn and sprayed it on Galaxy's upper tail area. This created a burning sensation on my horse's rear-end and sent him jumping wildly to my delight. After a minute of violent galloping in circles, Galaxy calmed down, but I wasn't satisfied with such a short thrill. So once more, I sprayed the horsefly repellent on Galaxy's upper tail area and again he started jumping wildly. This time he got annoyed with my antics and kicked his back legs higher and higher in an effort to throw me off. Finally, he succeeded in his crazed effort, by whipping me off the saddle and over his backside as I crashed head first into a pile of horse manure. Again, what should have paralyzed me only resulted in my head splattered in what I deserved and another hard lesson learned.

One day I was training in my home gym and banging out Half Squats with a couple of spotters on both sides of the barbell. I worked up to a respectable 365 pounds, which wasn't too shabby for a seventeen-year-old bodybuilder. As I took the weight off the freestanding barbell racks, I stepped back next to a bench and began to squat until my buttocks hit the bench. For some reason on my tenth rep, I found myself unable to lockout and began to fall forward with the weight. As I yelled for the spotters to grab the heavy weight from me its resistance quickly pushed down on my neck and I suddenly saw the floor coming at me fast. With instinct, I somehow somersaulted in midair by using the heavy barbell's pull to swing my body around it as I held my breath and heard the heavy steel crash loudly onto the floor, with me landing on top of it. My spotters didn't know if I had snapped my neck, or was seriously injured as I lay on the floor waiting for some major pain to strike me. After a minute or so, I realized I had dodged another bullet and opened my eyes while smiling to my friends. It was an extremely close call that I would never repeat again. The following day I ordered a power-rack from the York Barbell Company. Since that day, whenever I perform squats I make sure to use some type of safety rack. Another lesson learned!

However, as lucky as I was at times, I have had plenty of real injuries to contend with from my years of karate, running, and weight training. Some of the worst injuries have knocked me out of training for weeks and months at a time. I have suffered through strains and sprains, muscle tears and spasms, both herniated and ruptured disks, and just about anything else you can think of. That is what happens when you constantly train to the max.

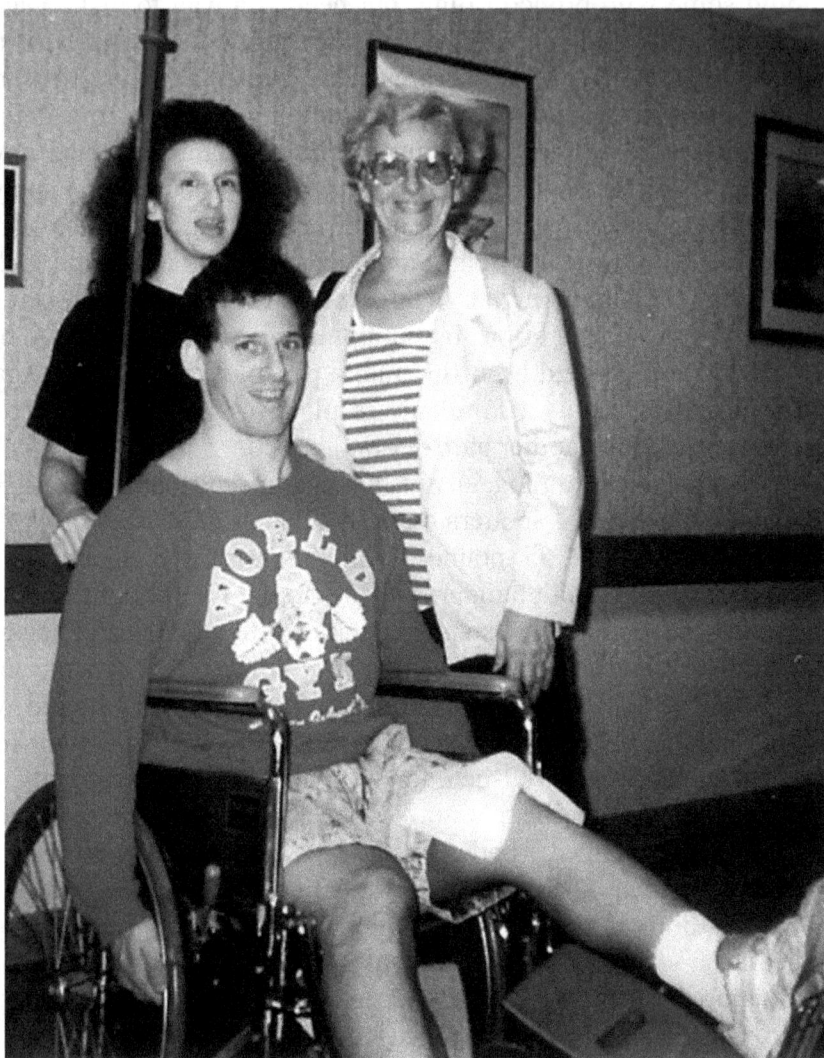

Down but not out! Mario with his sister and mother in the ER - 1987

Every now and then, we all get knocked down. Nevertheless, that is simply a time to re-evaluate your efforts and come back stronger. The important thing is not to repeat the same mistakes again. Remember the phrase "No Pain No Gain." It is so true in this sport. At my Staten Island Bodybuilding Club, I had a forty-foot long red, white, and blue banner with those exact words that boldly hung high as a reminder of what it took to achieve one's goals. It was part of the iron game that we all experienced and accepted without complaint; we always came back hungrier, to train hard for bigger and better gains.

One near catastrophe that I experienced was in 2000 while training at a Dolphin Fitness Center on Staten Island. What was unusual about this injury was that it occurred while I was resting between sets. I had worked up to heavy poundage while performing the Leg Press. After I finished my last set with twelve 45-pound plates on each side of the machine, I stepped out of it and stood by its side to answer some questions regarding training from a gym member. I wasn't paying attention to what was happening behind me. While on the opposite side of the machine, another gym member started removing all the 45-pound plates from one side. Since the machine was not designed to stay upright with a tremendous amount of weight only on one of its sides, it came crashing down and hit my back like a giant boulder falling off a cliff. The 500 plus pounds that remained on the side I was standing whipped the machine towards me while sending its top metal plate-holder ripping into my back like an axe. Instinctively, I fell downward with the machine's force to avoid breaking my back in two. As I hit the ground, I rolled out of the machine's way and heard it crash loudly to the floor while I watched the 45-pound weight-plates fly in different directions. As the crash echoed throughout the gym, its members suddenly became quiet. I rose from the ground and looked over to see who had stupidly removed all the weight-plates and nearly crippled me. All I could see was a couple of fellows sprinting towards the exit in fear of what might have happened to them. I never did find out who they were, probably a couple of beginners that knew to quit while they were ahead. Because of the incident, I received some serious muscle pulls as well as deep scrapes from the machine as it tore against my flesh like sharp blades. My sweatshirt was soaked in blood and my back burned from the torn flesh. It was time to call it a day and heal my wounds. The one thing that I was reminded of from the experience was always to expect the unexpected. Since gyms are very dangerous places that could cause some serious pain and suffering, I should have known better than to let my guard down. Another lesson well learned!

ALL IN THE FAMILY

Bodybuilding has been a big part of my family's life. About a year after my father introduced me to weight training he got my brother, Johnny, started on a muscle-building regimen. The muscles came naturally for Johnny and as the years passed by, he developed a physique worthy enough to step onto any local muscle dais. Johnny was also a heavy bench presser who could out-lift just about anybody at the gym. Later in life, he raised two sons named John and Nicholas. The brothers also shared the same passion as their father and followed his example by training alongside him in the gym.

Domenic was next in line. Although thin, he too started at a young age to develop his body to the max. In time his physique became muscular and his pressing power explosive. In the 1970s, I introduced Domenic to the fitness industry. I watched his knowledge in the field grow as he managed several health food stores within the metropolitan area as the years went by. Eventually, Domenic's connections in the industry would help bring many sponsors to the shows that I promoted. Domenic also has a daughter named Stephanie who made fitness a big part of her life through the sport of karate (where she is a ranking black belt). Domenic's wife, Cynthia, is also a black belt. One day she demonstrated her striking technique with a broomstick by hitting me several times across my left wrist as I blocked her unprovoked attack (long story).

Since Johnny, Domenic, and I started training at such young ages it came as no surprise when our eight-year-old brother, Philip, took to

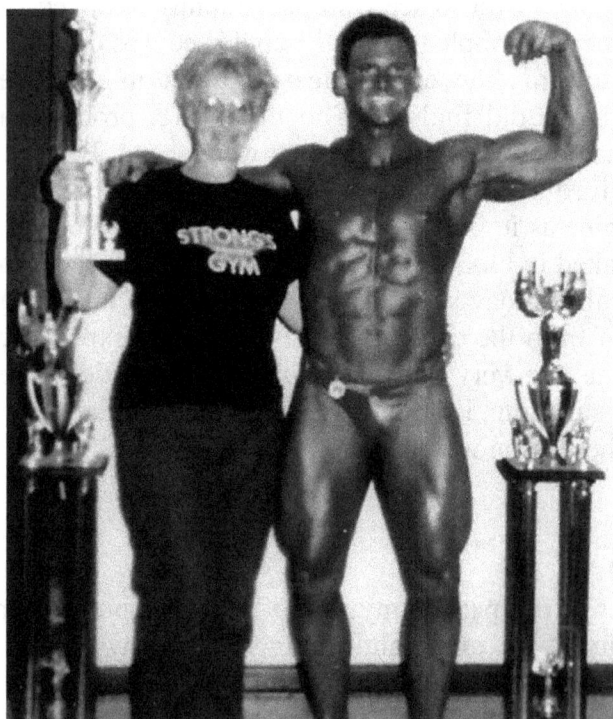

the iron so early in his bodybuilding career. At first, Philip trained in our home's basement gym but eventual made his way to my club when he turned ten. Three times a week, my mother would drive him to the gym straight from school to train under my guidance. For the first couple of years, he trained with light weights and performed high repetitions, using a complete range of motion for all exercises. As his muscles began to take shape, I increased the poundage while lowering the repetitions and had him taking more rest between sets. Eventually he became an advanced bodybuilder and trained instinctively to further continue his gains. Other than myself, Philip (see photo – with mom) is the only other person in my family who has competed in a physique competition.

Philip entered his first bodybuilding show at the age of thirteen. He competed in the 1982 Mr. Staten Island show. While posing at the evening finals the crowd continuously cheered him on. It motivated Philip so much that he continued posing until the show's expediter ran out of patience, walked onstage, grabbed Philip by the neck and yanked him away. This little incident did not detract Philip from future competitions. He went on to take home a number of trophies.

However, this was not the first muscle mishap for Philip. A year earlier, Philip had a post workout accident at my gym. After completing a high intensity training session with his workout partner Keith Miguel, he challenged Keith to some friendly competitive posing to finish their day's efforts. They went at it, pose for pose, flexing their physiques with all their sweat and might for nearly twenty minutes. Neither would give in, until suddenly, Philip collapsed from not breathing correctly and smashed his head onto a 25-pound Dan Lurie weight-plate that was lying on the floor. The impact was so hard that it left an imprint of the weight-plate engraved on Philip's forehead. He was out cold and it took a few minutes before he got some of his senses back. Needless to say, I was shaken up a bit and was relieved when Philip returned to his feet. The next day you could still see the etching of the weight-plate on his forehead. But he still came to the gym for another heavy-duty bombing session.

In his twenties, Philip was still heavily into bodybuilding and went on to open several personal training and diet centers. Being a well-known bodybuilder on the Island, he had a large clientele and was continuously sought after by those seeking to increase muscle mass and become fit.

Another member of the Strong family would find her way to the gym in the early 1990s. During her teenage years, my sister, Carmela, tagged along with me to Gold's Gym on Staten Island. We trained together four times a week for several hours at a time. Gold's was a great gym for her to first experience the sport of bodybuilding. She made fantastic gains within a relatively short period of time. Carmela was consistent with her training and showed no fear when pushed to new limits (see photo). Before we knew it, she was representing the family name proudly. She was Bench Pressing 155 pounds and Leg Pressing 450 pounds with ease for multiple sets and reps. Like her brothers before her, she was a natural for the iron and soon found herself giving advice to others about the benefits of natural bodybuilding. Today, Carmela is more into cardio than weight training and maintains an athletic physique.

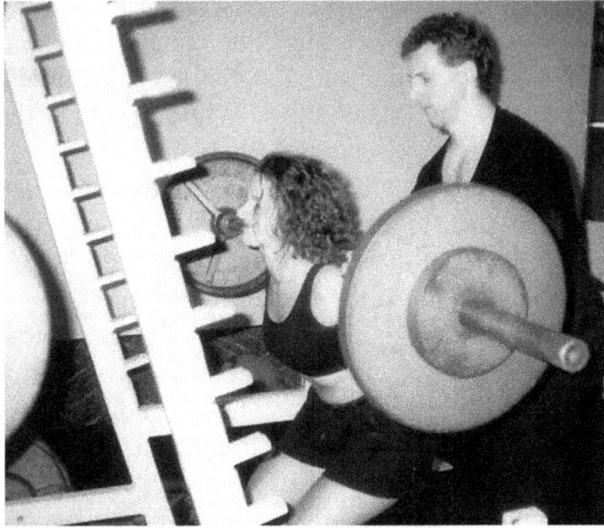

SHAKE, RATTLE, AND ROLL

During the early 1990s, I not only weight trained at the Palms Fitness Center on Staten Island but also participated in their high impact aerobic classes. I wanted a change from my running program and needed some form of cardio to really stimulate my heart and lungs. I chose high impact aerobics. Twice a week, after weight training for two hours, I would jump into an aerobics class. Before I knew it my head was going one way, my torso the other, and my legs opposite of each other. The classes were extremely challenging since I was weighing in at a muscular 225 pounds, while the rest of the class (mostly of women) weighed one hundred pounds less than me. It was easier for me to bang out a thousand pounds on the Leg Press than it was to keep up with these gals. Nevertheless, I stayed with it and eventually found myself soaring at the same rate as the students and instructor. I dressed the part too. After working out with the weights I changed from my sweats into neon blue spandex and a tank top that outlined my proportioned physique. (Richard Simmons had nothing on me!). The high impact aerobics not only conditioned my heart and lungs but also helped me maintain a body fat level of eight percent. The classes were a great compliment to my weight training but after several months of sweat, I had to stop participating in them. I was experiencing continuous injuries in both feet. At 225 pounds of bodyweight, the stress was too great for the tendons of my feet. They were being torn apart by the hard pounding and quickly building up scar tissue. I had to stop while I still had two good feet to stand on. As much as I enjoyed this form of cardio, it was doing me more harm than good. I went back to running outdoors. Foot placement is a more controlled movement as opposed to the violent twisting and turning of high impact aerobics. The one good thing that did come out of all this pain was that I had the pleasure of enjoying some hot dates with the high impact gals. Such is life!

IF I DIDN'T SEE IT, I WOULDN'T BELIEVE IT

While training at Gold's Gym on Staten Island during the early 1990s, I witnessed an unbelievably funny but dangerous incident. A well-known and highly publicized strongman of the era came to the club to give an amazing Bench Press demonstration. His name was Jimmy "The Iron Bull" Pellechia. He was touring the country to perform at gyms and physique competitions. Jimmy was a heavily muscled guy that looked the part and his feat of raw power caught my undivided attention.

What would have won top prize on America's Funniest Videos wasn't so funny for one of the strongman's spotters. After doing several moderately heavy sets of the Bench Press, Jimmy increased the weight to a jaw dropping poundage. With the whole gym watching, he loaded the barbell to nearly 1,000 pounds as he had three spotters (on both sides and the rear) standby to assist if needed. The guy who spotted The Iron Bull from the rear made a big mistake by deciding to secure himself to the barbell with wrist straps. All three spotters helped the strongman get the tremendous weight off the rack. Once the barbell was free, the two side spotters stepped away while the rear spotter remained in place. Jimmy was able to support the weight and with some help looked as if he might just rep the monstrous poundage. However, as Jimmy was completing the lift the enormous weight suddenly crashed down and pinned his body to the bench. Seeing he was in serious trouble, the side spotters tried to lift the weight off

Jimmy but were unable to do so. As this was occurring, the rear spotter remained attached to the barbell because the wrist straps he was wearing were still tightly wrapped around the bar. Immediately, other gym members jumped in to help and dragged the heavy barbell towards Jimmy's thighs. Then in a desperate attempt, they yanked the mighty weight over his legs and sent it crashing to the floor with the rear spotter still tied to the barbell. As the weight was thrown, the rear spotter actually went flying over Jimmy. He then crashed to the floor and smashed his head on a pile of weight-plates. For his assistance, the rear spotter received several bruises from the impact and an 8x10 photo, compliments of The Iron Bull. If only I had a video camera.

THE AWAKENING

On the last day of the Staten Island Bodybuilding Club's existence, one of the members, John "The Viking" Delin, hung a poster high on one of its mirrors. The poster read STRONG WILL RETURN. Like a prophecy, the Viking's words came true several years later.

In 1995, I received a phone call from bodybuilding promoter Mark Delio. Mark told me he was taking over promoting the Staten Island physique competition and wanted to start giving an annual award for bodybuilding excellence. The award was to be titled the "Mario Strong Staten Island Bodybuilding Award." It was for those who made positive contributions to the Staten Island bodybuilding community over the years. He also told me that I would receive the first annual plaque for my contributions to the sport. Since the closing of my gym in 1986, I had remained out of the bodybuilding limelight. My only connection to the sport was training at different gyms on and off the Island. Now a sleeping giant had been awakened within myself and a new era was about to begin.

The 1995 Staten Island Bodybuilding Championships was billed as the day of champions. Many former Staten Island bodybuilding champions were invited and attended. The show's program booklet had a section dedicated to me and the pressure was on to live up to the image. During the second half of the show, Mark Delio gave a great speech about my years in the sport. He talked about the Staten Island Bodybuilding Club, its rich history, and all the champs I had trained along the way. I reflected on the good memories as he spoke and looked forward to the many great years to come, as I once again, felt truly inspired.

After handing me the Staten Island Bodybuilding Award (see photo) Mark Delio summed it up with these words to the audience: "When I first trained at a gym it was STRONG'S GYM. For those who trained there back then, and whenever we train today, we try to attain the same psych as we had there. We felt magic in the ANIMAL ROOM as the theme from *Rocky* echoed in harmony with the sounds of iron pumping. It was the man, who created the magic, and you can never recreate that atmosphere, you cannot buy it, you cannot fake it. It comes from the heart, and none has more than MARIO STRONG!" With that, the audience stood up and cheered in appreciation for what I had done for bodybuilding on Staten Island. I thanked them with a special treat, not seen on the Island in years.

As I walked towards center stage, I waved to the DJ and signaled him to play my favorite tune. Suddenly the theme from *Rocky* exploded loudly throughout the auditorium. As the trumpets flared with the tune of *Gonna Fly Now*, a sense of history repeating itself flooded the auditorium. The captivated crowd stood up from their seats and began to cheer my name repeatedly. I raised the hot water bottle to my lips, sealed it tight, and began blowing air into its thick walls. The more air I forced into it, the larger it became and the louder the fans cheered my name. Once again, it felt great being onstage in front of my hometown Staten Island bodybuilding crowd. I gave it my best and I pushed myself to the limit. After a minute or so of forcing extremely large breathes of air into the hot water bottle it exploded with a thunderous bang and sent pieces of

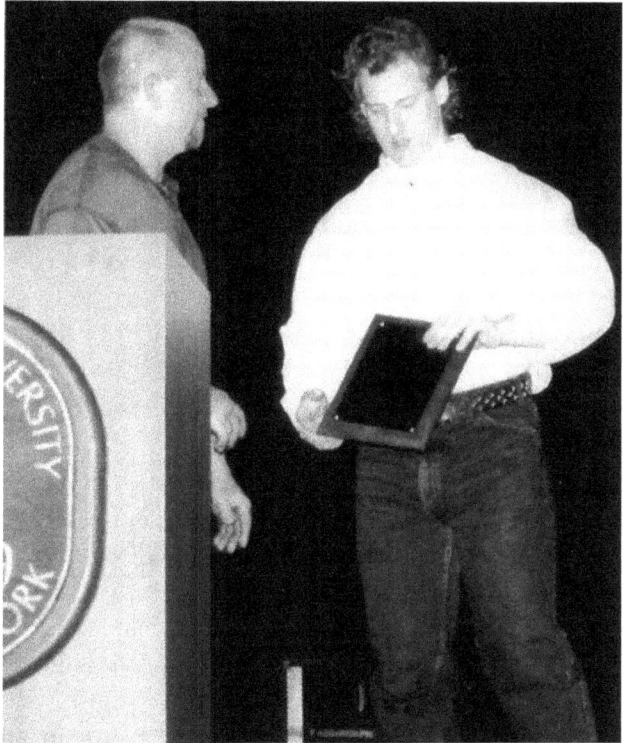

stretched rubber throughout the auditorium. The crowd roared as their cameras flashed to catch the moment, knowing that I was back where I belonged.

A legend from bodybuilding's golden era, Leon Brown, was also present that night and received the Staten Island Bodybuilding Award for his excellence in the sport of bodybuilding. After exploding the hot water bottle, I stepped over to the microphone and gave the following speech:

"Tonight I would like to begin an annual tradition on Staten Island. A tradition that recognizes Staten Islanders for their accomplishments in the sport of bodybuilding. Tonight's award will be presented to a bodybuilder who is not only a champion onstage but also a winner in the eyes of his peers. This bodybuilder's journey has touched many lives. His dedication and perseverance in the sport are legendary, going back to the days when Arnold was the king, Sergio the myth, and gyms looked more like chambers of horror than neon-lit nightclubs. Today this bodybuilder's presence in the gym ignites enthusiasm among the muscle builders. He is a positive force, electrifying all those who follow in his path. Bodybuilding is in this man's heart. It is his reason to smile, his reason to dream, and his reason to live. On behalf of the Fit Physique Health Club, The NPC, and myself, I would like to present the Staten Island Bodybuilding Award for excellence in bodybuilding, to the original Mr. Staten Island, the living legend himself, Staten Island's very own LEON BROWN."

With that, the Brown Bomber walked onto the stage and waved to the standing-room-only audience. Leon Brown was in his element. The stage was his home; on Staten Island, he was as American as apple pie. He was well-respected by his fellow Staten Island muscle builders and a legend throughout the muscle-building world. He had trained with some of the greats of bodybuilding's golden era and was a constant sight at physique shows in the metropolitan area. After receiving the award, Leon mounted the posing platform. He performed a posing routine that displayed his flawless symmetry and proportion. He was a living work of art that captivated the audience with every move he made. The Brown Bomber was back and better than ever!

THE 1995 OLYMPIA FITNESS WEEKEND

On September 8, 1995, I flew to Atlanta, Georgia with my sister, Carmela, to attend Joe Weider's Olympia Fitness Weekend. The trip was a comp, thanks to my brother, Domenic. It was a gift for my 40th birthday, which was the following day. In all my years of training, I had never attended an Olympia competition. I decided this would be a good time to visit bodybuilding's premier event. More than any other reason, I wanted to see all nine (past and present) Olympia champions take the stage with Joe Weider to commemorate the 30th anniversary of the competition. Although I did not share the same philosophy towards bodybuilding as most of the Olympia winners, I was nevertheless inspired by them during my earlier muscle building days and was eager to see and meet with some of them.

The 1995 Olympia Fitness Weekend was more than just a muscle show. It was also the inauguration of women's fitness competitions to the IFBB. It attracted vendors from the bodybuilding and fitness industry to market their products at the Expo. About a mile from the show, a Marriott hotel housed everyone related to the Olympia Fitness Weekend's festivities. The Marriott had a lobby area that was encircled by 30 plus floors of guest rooms and balconies. The majority of the hotel was booked with Olympia guests and it must have felt like being on another planet to those that were there for reasons other than seeing bodybuilders flex their stuff. There was wall-to-wall biceps, pectorals, quads, and abdominals every which way you turned. It was truly muscle-heaven for those who were into the hard-core muscle scene.

For me the highlight of the weekend was on the 9th. Not only because it was my birthday, but because I got to meet with quite a few big names in the industry for the first time and enjoyed conversing with them about our similar passion in bodybuilding.

One fellow in particular I enjoyed meeting was the first Mr. Olympia, Larry Scott. As a teenager, I had always idolized Larry Scott and purchased all of his training booklets to help further my gains. During his prime, Larry had been an inspiration to tens of thousands of young men and at one time was the most famous bodybuilder in the world. While speaking to Larry you could sense his true love for the sport as he went out of his way to spend some time with me to discuss the art of muscle building. Many other past champions echoed that same hunger for the sport that evening, as they too all shared Larry's deep passion for bodybuilding. No matter what philosophy they followed to make it in the sport, they all shared a common denominator. The sport was in their blood and had brought them all together for this historic Olympia weekend.

The day's events went off without a hitch as the many competitions concluded. Then the time for the big moment had finally arrived. All weekend long, the question was asked as to whether or not Arnold Schwarzenegger would show up. The Mr. Olympia's 30th anniversary was filled with thousands of spectators who had come to see him. Arnold had been in another state filming a movie. There were doubts if he would be able to break away from the movie set to be with Joe Weider and the other legends onstage for this historic occasion.

The theater was packed to the rafters that evening. It was a sold-out event and the crowd was drooling in anticipation of seeing all past and current Olympia champions onstage together for the first time in history. About an hour into the show, the MC walked over to the microphone and announced that Arnold had arrived in Atlanta, and was being escorted to the theater by a police motorcade. After several minutes of entertaining the audience, the MC once again addressed the crowd and told them that Arnold Schwarzenegger was in the building. The fans erupted into a huge vociferous roar that was heard for miles away as the houselights dimmed. One by one, the MC announced all nine Mr. Olympia winners as they took their rightful position on this historic stage; Larry Scott, Sergio Oliva, Arnold Schwarzenegger, Franco Columbu, Frank Zane, Chris Dickerson, Samir Bannout, Lee Haney, and Dorian Yates. The standing-room-only, crazed auditorium was in an uproar. This moment was not to be missed and the best was yet to come. As the nine Olympia champions stood there smiling and waving to the crowd, Joe Weider walked onto the stage and thanked each one for their contributions to the sport. After several minutes of sustained applause, the audience returned to their seats and listened to the words of each legend. As expected, Arnold stole the show with his humor and antics but for the most part stood respectfully as Joe Weider worked the lineup from Scott to Yates, reflecting on the many good times he shared with each individual champion. As history unfolded, the audience absorbed its true meaning. Onstage were the men who had helped shape the course of bodybuilding history. The men of the Olympia inspired not only themselves but their images and training concepts motivated millions of others over the years. It was a fitting tribute to those iron-men of muscle who thanked the fans for the years of support while they were on their quest to be the best.

For me, the weekend was one of those times in my life that I will never forget. Being a bodybuilder from the Iron Age, it was a great way to remember this milestone in my life. My 40th birthday also marked the 30th anniversary of the day my father first introduced me to bodybuilding. So many good times in the sport had passed before me and so many more were yet to be realized. Bodybuilding was in my blood!

THE OLD GANG

In May of 1996, Joe Carrero flew from sunny California to Staten Island to be honored at the Staten Island Bodybuilding Championships. Joe was a bodybuilding legend on the Island and had become a dominant force on the national physique stage. His friends respected him and it was great to see his smiling face after so many years away. Through his shirt and tie, you could see Joe came to the show in top form. Even though he had not competed in several years, his muscles were still bulging at the seams. At the show, a long time friend of his named John Versera stepped onto the stage and gave a heart-warming speech about Joe's history in bodybuilding. When John finished speaking, he handed Joe Carrero the Staten Island Bodybuilding Award for excellence in the sport. As the sold-out audience respectfully stood and applauded loudly, Joe walked over to the microphone and thanked them for their kindness. It was a well-deserved moment for the Muscle Wonder of Staten Island, who along with Leon Brown, were the two most famous bodybuilders ever to come from the Island of Mario's Monsters.

After the show, Leon, myself, and several other muscle buddies took Joe out for a dinner celebration. We reminisced and laughed about some of the things we had shared along the way. During the dinner, someone got the bright idea to take Joe to an adult nightclub for a few laughs.

At the club were strippers who occasionally walked by us while passing their hands across our physiques in bewilderment. Leon had a bit too much fruit juice and was like a lion seeking its prey. As he guzzled his drinks down, a hot blond-haired Russian babe asked him if he would like a lap dance. As the Brown Bomber stared at her luscious anatomy, he began to drool in excitement. He immediately dropped his slacks to reveal his statuette physique to the horror of the Russian woman who had the look of a deer caught in a car's headlights. As she performed her dance for Leon, his face grinned like that of a kid on Christmas morning. Every time she said she was finished and would try to get away, he would yank her back for more and more. The funny scene caught the attention of everyone in the club as the bouncers laughingly ran over to save this damsel in distress. For us, it was pure hysteria seeing Leon in a different light.

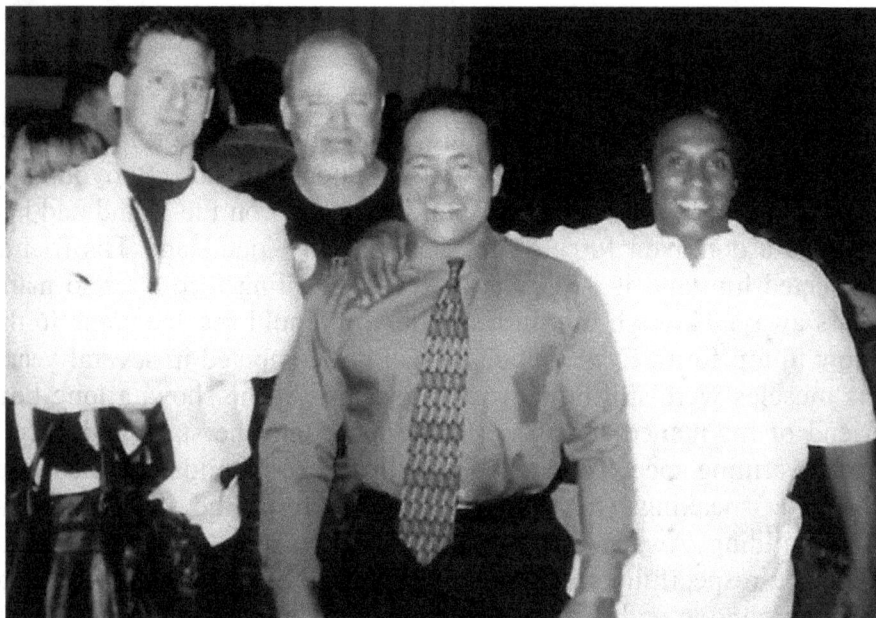

Mario Strong, Charlie Williams, Joe Carrero, and Leon Brown – 1996

At the end of the evening, we all said goodbye to Joe and wished him well. We had shared many good times together and we all looked forward to many more good times to come. For one night, the old gang had reunited for some laughs and good times: it was evident our friendships were still strong.

MORE THAN JUST A LIVING WORK OF ART

As bodybuilders, we wear our earned masterpieces wherever we go. Our physiques are different from that of average mortals and most of the time we stand out in a crowd. In my mind, bodybuilding is more than just being a cosmetic form of art. To me, it also means being ready and able to meet any physical demands that may come my way. I have always been athletic. As a teenager, I played all sports and enjoyed the competitive edge that came with the games. Bodybuilding helped me excel on the field and made me somewhat of a dominant player within the teams I joined. While attending classes at the College of Staten Island, I found myself winning the intramural fitness championships in 1973. In my twenties, I was able to outrun NFL players in the 100-yard sprint while barefoot. In my thirties, I was setting pushup records while at the police academy in Albany, New York. In my forties, was able to leg press 1000 pounds for ten complete repetitions. Now in my fifties, I am still exploding hot water bottles for the fans and able to excel on or off the field as the need arises. While physical excellence is important in the competitive side of things, it is even more important when it comes to protecting yourself or others from possible bodily harm.

My life has had its share of violence. Living and working in New York City, violence is sometimes hard to avoid. One night, during my early twenties, I was standing on a street in front of the home of my then-girlfriend, Denise. As we stood there talking, a car with four or five jerks drove towards us at a high speed. As we moved to get out of the car's way, one of its occupants stretched his arm out of the back passenger window and grabbed onto Denise's handbag, pulling it from her as she crashed to the ground. Shocked and enraged, I made sure she was okay and then yelled for neighbors to call 911 as I jumped into my car to catch up with the creeps. They had about a two-block lead on me, but with a fast car and great driving skills; I took off after them like a rocket. About a half mile down the road, I caught up to them as they swerved in and out of traffic. They drove over sidewalks and lawns while nearly killing several innocent bystanders. About five minutes into the chase, I pulled into the Midland Beach parking lot and blocked their escape with my car. As I jumped out of my car and rushed towards them, one of the idiots grabbed a metal sanitation can and threw it at me. As the can flew over my head, I heard it crash loudly against my car. Instantly I felt an enormous "hulk rage" overcome me. Steaming, I grabbed the punk that threw the can and body-slammed him to the ground like a splattered tomato. He screamed in pain and yelled for help. As his accomplices ran towards their car, they tossed Denise's handbag towards me in hopes that I might leave peacefully. I picked up the same sanitation can that dented my car and flung it through the front window of their car as they hurriedly drove off. I left the parking lot as a curious crowd began to gather. Several minutes later, I returned the handbag to a shaken Denise and drove back to the parking lot with several NYPD officers that had responded to the incident. Upon our arrival, we found the parking lot vacant. Everyone, including the curious, was gone. There was nothing more to do so I said thanks to the officers and called it a night.

Another incident that required my muscles to be more than a showpiece occurred during the late 1970s, when I was talking to a friend in front of my house. A car carrying four unknown faces stopped next to us. These guys were in their twenties and looking for trouble. Without warning, one of them sucker punched my friend and sent him crashing to the ground. With brute instinct, I jumped in to help my friend and found myself in an all-out brawl with the gang of toughs. After a couple of minutes of trading punches and kicks the crew decided to run for their car as I continued to give them a smack down. As they sped off, my friend told me that the incident was mob related and that I was lucky I didn't get whacked. After hearing that, I punched my friend in the head and sarcastically thanked him for getting me involved in his crap. Luckily, nothing else ever came of it.

Being a crime fighter in the state of New York since 1985, I have had my share of violent altercations over the years. I have had baseball bats, chairs, pipes, punches, kicks, bottles, and knives directed at me in an attempt to do me bodily harm. Throughout my years of law enforcement, I rose from the ranks of officer to lieutenant. There have been dozens of very physical interactions with individuals who have had little respect for others, let alone the law. Some of these individuals have been quite big, strong, and intimidating. Although I have had my share of injuries while encountering such perpetrators, I have always managed to enforce a takedown and make an arrest, no matter how violent the battle became. Thanks to the combination of bodybuilding and karate, my physique is more than just a display piece. It is mobile, hostile, and agile! At least, that is what I tell my fellow officers and friends. But seriously, it is very dangerous out there and you never know when the call will come for you to encounter or respond to a violent incident. You can be in your house, on the street, or at the job. Living in these times, being physically fit is a requirement that should not be taken lightly because you just never know when trouble will come knocking on your door.

DOWN FOR THE COUNT

On Father's Day of 1996, I experienced a catastrophic injury that brought my training and life to a crashing halt. While making an arrest of a violent and huge perpetrator, I suffered the rupturing of two spinal disks in my lower back. An intense pain burned down my left leg from hip to heel. I had experienced injuries before. Over the years, I had pulled muscles in virtually every part of my body. I had my share of spasms, strains, sprains, and even herniated disks in my back and neck. Nevertheless, nothing compared to the immense, paralyzing fire that now raged throughout the lower left side of my body.

I was down for the count and unable to stand, sit, or walk for any length of time. As if things couldn't get any worse, I had my first annual NGA Eastern Regional Bodybuilding Classic scheduled for the coming September. Due to my serious injury, doubts began to arise as to whether or not the show would even take place. At first, I visited a chiropractor's office several times a week, where I received adjustments and ultra-sound treatments. Unfortunately, after three weeks, my pain and physical immobility showed no signs of relief and I was forced to try a physical therapist. The therapist treated me with traction, acupuncture, and massage. He also had me wear a back brace and perform some simple exercises to help improve my flexibility. He advised me that there was a chance I might need surgery down the road; I might never train again with the same intensity as before. What the physical therapist said to me really hit home. He was straightforward and to the point. It was then that I realized how bad my injury was and that I had a mountain to climb. I became completely focused on climbing that mountain and standing on its peak. I had a goal to conquer! After a month of dedicated treatments I saw some marked improvement as I was now able to sit for several minutes and walk for a couple of blocks before the pain stopped me in my tracks. When the pain returned, I would lie down on a large cold pack for an hour or so to simmer its fire.

Eventually, my condition improved over the months and I was able to walk, sit, and stand for longer periods, but not able to train with weights. In September I was able to attend my show but not without some pain. At the show, my suit hung like a curtain because of the loss of muscle mass from the weeks of limited mobility and no weight training. It would not be until late November that I would near the mountain as I returned to the gym with the motivation to succeed. When I resumed weight training again, I learned how weak and frail the left side of my body had become. The weights that I once warmed up with felt like tons of steel and the atrophy of the muscles felt as if I was in Pee Wee Herman's body. It did not matter for I knew deep inside my heart that this was just another obstacle in my life to conquer. I gladly accepted the challenge! By late winter of the following year, my body and strength had finally recovered to its former self and I felt better than ever. It had been a long tough battle with an enemy that I persistently fought against and the victory was sweet. I had been knocked down for the count but got up before the final bell. I was bigger and stronger than ever before, and ready to climb more mountains.

THE EASTERN REGIONAL CLASSIC

In 1996, I got the urge to once again promote bodybuilding shows on Staten Island. Years earlier, I had walked away from my role as a bodybuilding promoter because of the anabolic drug scene and the politics within the sport. Now, I eagerly wanted to return to promoting, but without the drugs and politics. I contacted my friend Andy Bostinto. Andy was the president of the National Gym Association (NGA), an organization dedicated to natural athletes throughout America. I met Andy in 1979 when he first formed the NGA, and I knew he was an honorable man who was committed to his cause. After meeting with Andy and his wife Francine, it was decided that I would promote the first natural bodybuilding and women's fitness competition ever held on Staten Island. The show was called the Eastern Regional Classic. I hired Gregory Baker, a well-known artist, who under my direction, created a dramatic drawing of a Herculean muscle builder soaring through the galaxies on a comet with a fitness woman riding its dusty tail. The drawing became the show's logo and was printed on posters, fliers, and magazine ads. The logo was also used on the official Eastern Regional Classic t-shirts, which was complimentary to all the competitors and sold to the audience.

The tone was set and the premiere event would be held at the College of Staten Island's Center for the Arts. The auditorium was a professional theater used for plays and musicals. The sound system was state-of-the-art and the lighting was excellent for physique competitions. Both the audience and competitors were in for a exciting evening.

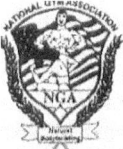

MARIO STRONG

NATIONAL QUALIFIER

PRESENTS THE 3rd ANNUAL

1998 NGA
EASTERN REGIONAL
NATURAL BODYBUILDING CLASSIC

& FITNESS**AMERICA**

P A G E A N T

FEATURING THE HOTTEST WOMEN IN FITNESS!

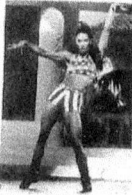

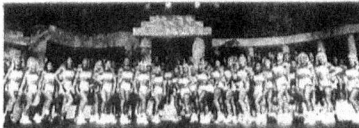

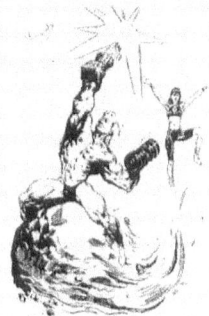

Hosted by

MET-Rx
ENGINEERED NUTRITION

TIGER SCHULMANN'S KARATE
Martial Arts Expo

September 19, 1998

LOCATION:	DIVISIONS:
College of Staten Island 2800 Victory Boulevard Staten Island, N.Y. 10314 **FREE PARKING**	★ MEN'S OPEN ★ WOMEN'S OPEN ★ NOVICE ★ MASTERS ★ TEENAGE ★ FITNESS AMERICA PAGENT

TIME:		AWARDS:
PRE-JUDGING	1 PM	TOP 5 EACH CLASS PLUS OVERALL
FINALS	7 PM	

TICKETS:		ELIGIBILITY:
PRE-JUDGING	$10	PHYSIQUE COMPETITION 5 YEARS DRUG FREE
FINALS	$20/$25	

For those who dare to be...NATURAL!

FOR TICKETS • INFORMATION • APPLICATIONS CALL (718)

TWINLAB
The Leader In Sports Nutrition

ACTIONLABS

METAFORM

TOTALLY FIT

AMERICAN

TRY US ON FOR SIZE SPORTSGEAR
Flexo.

Country Life

TREE OF LIFE NORTHEAST
P. O. BOX 482
NORTH BERGEN, N.J. 07047

CORNUCOPIA
Health Foods
World Trade Center
212-938-0145

"A NEW WEIGH OF LIFE"
DIET CENTERS
(718) 720-3667

SOLGAR
Since 1947

PINNACLE

D & J DISTRIBUTORS
New York's #1 Distributor
of Sports Drinks & Supplements
718-370-0547

Enzymatic Therapy.®
NATURAL MEDICINES

Colombo

AMERIFIT

Natural
BODYBUILDING
AND FITNESS

FREE
SPORTS SUPPLEMENTS &
BODYBUILDING PRODUCT
• Ticket Holders Only •

NATROL

Universal Nutrition

PROLAB

Nelson Bach USA Ltd.

Poster from the 3rd annual NGA Eastern Regional Classic

My brother, Domenic, also joined me in promoting this historic event and was responsible for getting sponsors for the show. Sponsorship was important for the NGA Eastern Regional Classic as the cost of producing such a competition at the time exceeded $12,000 per event. Domenic was the manager of Cornucopia Health Foods, which was located at the former World Trade Center. He was well-liked by the supplement companies he did business with and was able to get more than twenty sponsors to help cover the cost of running such a big show. The premiere of the NGA Eastern Regional Classic was a huge success. During the opening ceremonies, I gave the following speech to the sold-out crowd:

"I would like to thank all of you for coming here tonight in support of natural bodybuilding and women's fitness. Tonight's event is more than just another competition. It is an historic moment in time! Tonight, in this auditorium, a milestone will be crossed and a new era in the art of physical culture on Staten Island will begin. A long time ago, in September of 1976, I opened the door to the Staten Island Bodybuilding Club, which at the time was Richmond County's first bodybuilding gym. Back then, the bodybuilding lifestyle was not only about muscle and power, it also meant striving for excellence in fitness, health, and longevity. Even though we were, no one was ever called a natural bodybuilder; it was just assumed. Physique competitions on this Island use to be standing-room-only events, with loads of competitors and an atmosphere of camaraderie among the lords of Muscledom. That is the way it use to be! Since the early 1990s, sports enhancing substances have become a staple among this Island's muscle builders. These illicit pharmaceuticals are constantly being supplied by some very enterprising individuals throughout the many gym locker rooms on Staten Island. Today, the world of bodybuilding has become nothing more than a sick lie. It is a game of chemical warfare that has put a dark cloud over every physique stage it has ever touched. Modern anabolic bodybuilders have forced the hand of true physical culturists to evolve and create competitions such as this where competitors can compete on a level playing field. If there is one thing you can be sure of, it is that drugs, lies, and deceit will have no place on a stage that carries the name of *Strong*. Nature has given us the gift of life and tonight we as physical culturists celebrate this gift in our own special way. Ladies and gentlemen, I am proud to present to you the 1st annual NGA Eastern Regional Natural Bodybuilding and Women's Fitness Classic. Enjoy the Show."

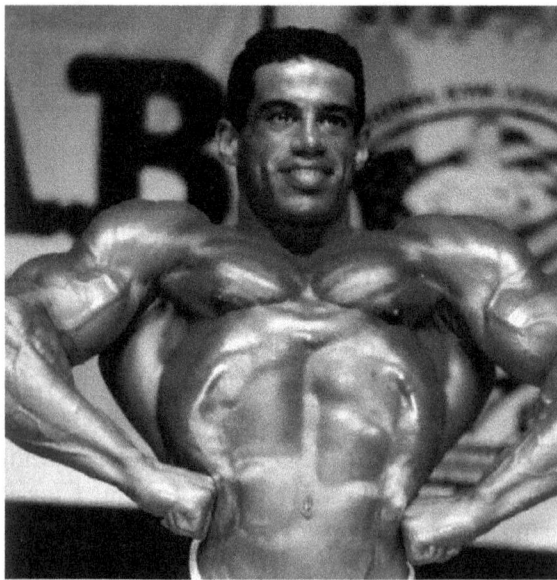

As I finished the speech, the crowd erupted into a loud sustained applause, not only for me, but also for all the competitors who sacrificed to compete that historic night. As the theme from *Rocky* blasted off the walls, the excitement in the room rose – history was in the making. In all, we had seventy-two competitors and several star attractions to help promote natural bodybuilding on my home turf. WNBF World Bodybuilding Champions Eddie "The Rock" Hernandez, and Kathy Unger (see photos) guest posed to standing-room-only applause and the WNBF Fitness Team performed so flawlessly that the crowd demanded an encore. The anti-steroid tide was rising all across America and now its surge was splashing onto the shores of Staten Island. The show was a huge success; the Staten Island audience and media outlets loved it. All the competitors were winners that evening. Each and everyone performed with pride in knowing that they were healthy and natural. It could not get any better than that!

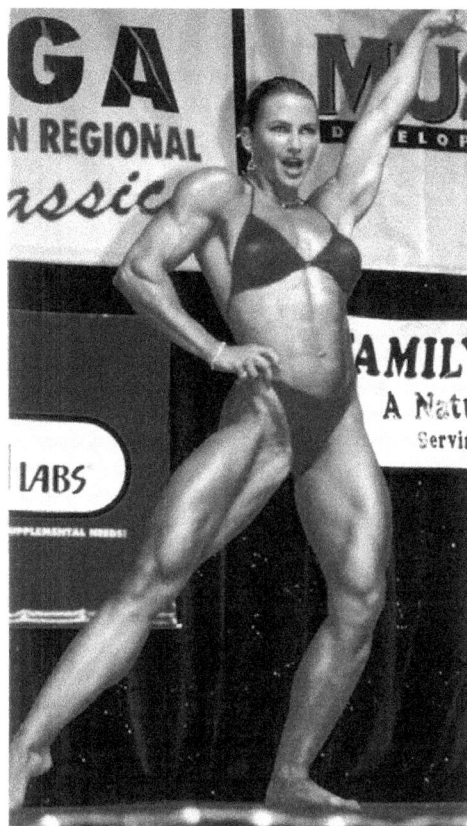

I'M GOING TO SHOOT YOU

Promoting a bodybuilding competition takes a considerable amount of time, expense, and footwork. In August of 1997, I was in the midst of promoting my second upcoming NGA Eastern Regional Classic scheduled for September. I placed full-page ads in natural physique publications and saw to it that fliers and posters were sent to hundreds of gyms and competitors throughout the metropolitan area. Another avenue for promotion was to visit other physique competitions that took place prior to mine in an effort to recruit competitors.

One Saturday afternoon, I had my brother, Domenic, and his team visit a bodybuilding competition in Manhattan to promote my show. I was due to arrive later that day. A well-known, national bodybuilding figure ran the competition.

My brother and his team had done an excellent job handing out fliers to competitors and hanging posters on street poles. It was nothing out of the ordinary, just your standard promotion of an upcoming show. When I arrived, I stood outside the building where it was being held to chat with my brother before I went in to watch the event. As I was talking to Domenic, the promoter of the show flew over to us in a rage, wanting to know who was handing out the fliers and hanging posters. I responded to him that it was my show and I was promoting it. I also welcomed him to promote his shows at my events. My words went in one ear and out the other as every explicative syllable known to man came my way. As this promoter continued in his verbal rage, he tore down several of my posters that hung within shouting distance.

As a crowd began to form, he came within striking distance of me and fumed that he was going to kill me. He repeated this threat several times and after awhile I got tired of his unprofessionalism and shouted, *Go For It!* as I raised my arms in a fighting stance. While everyone watched, he backed down and said, "Not here and now." He said he was going to get a gun and shoot me when I least expected it – blowing my brains out so that even my mother would not recognize me. He made these statements in front of my brother and other witnesses. If I had wanted to, I could have had him placed under arrest for harassment and other charges. However, having witnessed his bad behavior before at other physique competitions, I did not take his bad temper too personally. What I did do afterwards was to make sure I was always armed while off-duty, just in case this maniac decided to make good on his promise. Thankfully, nothing ever came of the threat. On several occasions after the incident, we would come eye-to-eye at different bodybuilding functions but never said a word to each other. About a decade after the incident, we both had the unfortunate experience of attending a mutual friend's wake. Others that came to mourn surrounded us and we broke into a conversation about our lost friend, making small talk about the bodybuilding world. After an hour or so, we shook hands as we both departed the funeral home and went our separate ways. I was glad that after all these years we were able to exchange good wishes, instead of bullets.

SUGARPLUMS

On December 20, 1998, while training at the Dolphin Fitness Center on Staten Island, I looked up to the gym's second level and saw a familiar face peddling away on a Life Cycle. It was an old friend of mine named Aida, whom I had known since attending New Dorp High School and through a mutual friend. As I continued to look up, she caught me glancing towards her and gave me a friendly wave. After I finished training, I went up to the cardio room where she was cycling to say "Hello" and to see how she had been since I last saw her in the early 1980s. On occasion, I would run into Aida's twin sister, Maria, but never her.

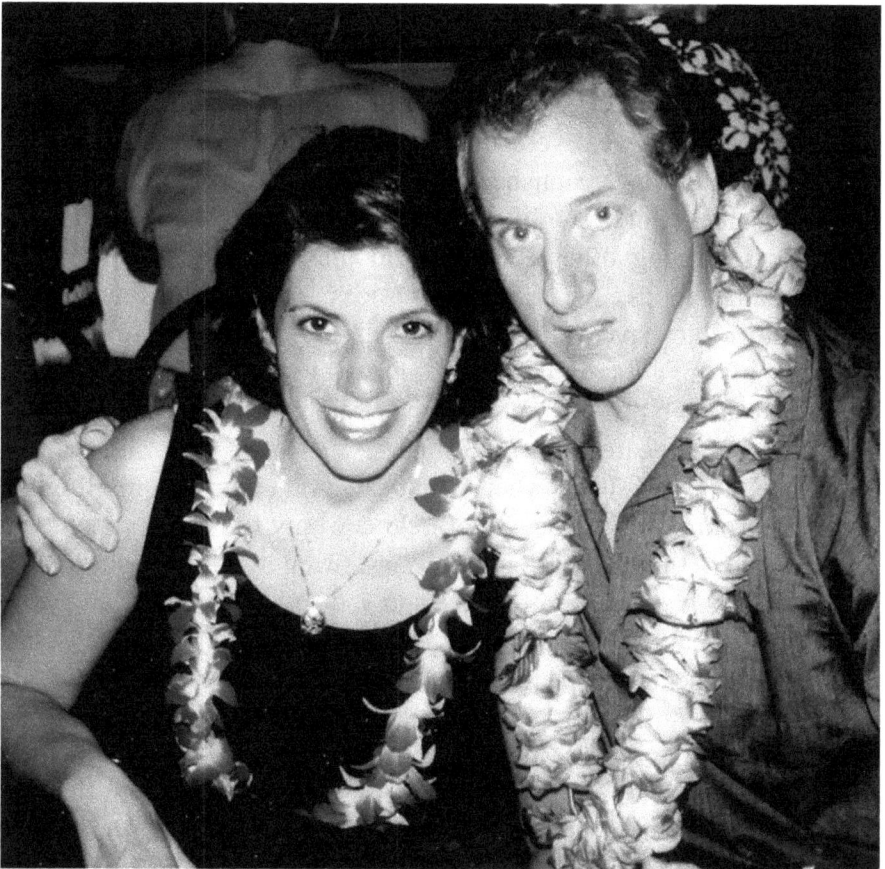

Aida & Mario enjoy the Aloha spirit while in Waikiki – 2001

Everything changed on that day. Before we knew it, we were dating exclusively as we both enjoyed each other's company immensely. I also began to train Aida personally and watched with pride as she made excellent gains while under my guidance. In return, she brought a smile to my face and warmed my heart with her beauty as she slowly wove her love into my life.

It had been a long time since my last serious relationship and I was in no rush to get into another. I was also very particular and needed someone who could understand my dedicated bodybuilding lifestyle. Before Aida came along, I dated women that always had two desires on their minds – marriage and family. At the time, those two words just did not fit into my vocabulary.

With time, Aida and I both learned that we had many things in common. After a year of dating, we decided to give our relationship a serious go by having her move in with me. Now, even though Aida is a sweet person, I didn't realize that she would be stocking my cupboards with all kinds of tasty goodies. Before her arrival into the Strong household, my shelves were mainly stocked with grains, beans, and nuts. Those items were pushed aside to make room for pasta, flour, oils, and spices. Since she liked to cook for others, I soon found these ingredients (among others) stocked on the shelves once filled only with organic foods. Milk, cheese, juices, and lobster invaded the refrigerator. No space in my kitchen was spared. Nevertheless, relationships are a lot about compromise so I let it go. Besides, I never consumed these types of foods so what rational argument could I have with the woman I care about?

Since that fateful day when I first saw Aida pumping her thighs in the cardio room, she has become the love of my life and someone who I cherish very much. Although I don't want to bring a little baby Strong into this world, both Aida and I do plan to marry and enjoy many more healthy decades together. She is a unique person with a warm heart and together we compliment each other's lifestyle very well. Throughout the years, we have enjoyed many trips to Hawaii and have attended dozens of social gatherings, cruises, theme parks, and even a few Broadway plays. Through me, she has been introduced to the world of bodybuilding and has seen the good, bad, and ugly sides of the sport. As our relationship continues to grow, I look forward to many more good years with *Sugarplums*, both in our personal life and in the gym, as we continue to train together like there is no tomorrow.

THE COURAGE OF MR. STATEN ISLAND

Throughout the decades, many men have been crowned Mr. Staten Island. Some became national names, others local Island legends. In 1987, an individual stepped onto the physique stage whose popularity was high amongst his friends, peers, and the local Staten Island muscle scene. This man of iron trained relentlessly for one year in the gym and with one goal in mind – to become Mr. Staten Island! When he stepped onstage that historic night, you knew he was the winner long before the awards were presented. By the end of the show, he had out-muscled all those that dared to challenge him. As he raised his arms in a victory salute, he received cheers of approval and acclamation along with a standing ovation. However, more importantly than winning the title that night would be the example of honor and bravery this modest champion set forth when it counted the most.

I remember first hearing about the events of September 11th from my fiancée, Aida. She worked in lower Manhattan and was getting off an express bus just outside the Brooklyn Battery Tunnel that morning when she saw people running through the streets as tiny silver pieces of metal streamed down from the sky. At the time, she did not realize what was happening and frantically called me from her cell phone at 8:53 AM to tell me what she was witnessing. Immediately, I turned on the TV and to my shock saw a tremendous dark hole filled with flames and smoke in the North Tower of the World Trade Center. I advised Aida that it was a terrorist attack and that she should quickly go to her office, which was several blocks away. As the events unfolded that morning, I shockingly watched on live TV the second attack on the World Trade Center, as well as the destruction to the Pentagon in Washington, DC, and the crash of Flight 93 in Pennsylvania. I remember standing outside my house and seeing this long thick line of black smoke pour into the eastern sky as I heard the thunderous echo of the South Tower come crashing down. It was a horrific morning that served as an awakening for America as it became very apparent that we were no longer safe in our homeland.

That fateful morning in American history saw the best and worst of humanity, as thousands of innocent souls were lost that day. Afterwards, millions of people would live in fear, not knowing what was to come next. For Staten Islanders the pain was all too real. Hundreds of Islanders went to work on that sunny Tuesday morning, just like any other workday. They had plans and dreams about their futures and looked forward to many tomorrows to come. However, for many of my fellow Staten Islanders, tomorrow was not to be as the toll of that day became very apparent by nightfall. The days after September 11, 2001 brought more questions than answers. I remember returning to the gym later that week and feeling guilty for being there. Some of my gym mates were not present and would never be seen again. The Island's close-knit bodybuilding community had suffered a major blow on that day, as the deaths of several well-known iron men gradually became known. One of those brave men was a representative of the many that would make the ultimate sacrifice that morning. He was FDNY Lieutenant Eddie D'Atri (see photo). Eddie was a consistent and well-known Staten Island bodybuilder. He was a dedicated leader at Squad 1 in Park Slope, Brooklyn and was off-duty the morning of September 11th. Immediately upon hearing about the attacks, the former Mr. Staten Island champion made a courageous decision and rushed from his home in Staten Island to help his squad battle the towering inferno at the World Trade Center in Manhattan. Eddie D'Atri was last seen going up a staircase in Tower 1 to be with his fellow firefighters.

In a published interview with FDNY Sergeant Jimmy Canham, the following was recalled about his experiences on that day: "I had passed a Lieutenant Eddie D'Atri from Squad 1. He saw me and said, "Jimmy, where are my guys?" (This is on the 11th floor after the first tower had fallen). He had made his way up. He had said, "Jimmy, did you see our guys?" I said, "No, Eddie. Some bad shit just happened." He said, "Yeah, I know. I don't know where my guys are." He had gone up, and I had made my way back down the hallway. This is after the last civilians had gone by, just prior to me going back to look for the cops. I believe Eddie stayed on the floor with me for a minute. We gave a quick search. Then he made his way up. After that, I didn't see Ed anymore."

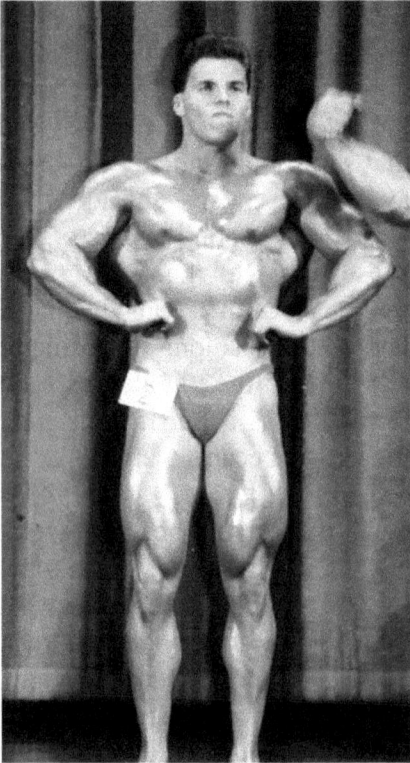

Eddie D'Atri was always looking out for his men and putting his own safety last. I will always be saddened by the loss of Eddie and all those murdered that day and can only hope for a time when cultures and nations can live in harmony. At the 2002 Staten Island Bodybuilding Championships, local bodybuilder and FDNY firefighter, Jimmy White, talked about Eddie's bravery. He also reflected on the more humorous times he shared with Eddie as well as the seriousness Eddie took towards bodybuilding. It was a heartfelt speech about a man that touched many lives in many ways, and none could be more deserving of such a moment. After the speech Jimmy White presented Eddie's two sons, Anthony and Michael, with the Staten Island Bodybuilding Award in honor of their father's heroic sacrifice. As all those in attendance stood in silence, Jimmy spoke about the other Staten Island FDNY firefighters that lost their lives. One by one, he announced their names as the tears flowed from the audience. It was one of those moments in Staten Island Bodybuilding history that brought everyone together in unity – the way it once was here on the Island – a long time ago.

THE CURTAINS CLOSES

I can still remember all the great bodybuilding competitions that took place on Staten Island vividly. I recall the hundreds of competitors that trained with every ounce of energy they had and all the people who helped present such great events. I can still hear the screaming fans and the music that filled the many auditoriums with the magic of bodybuilding. I still see the oil-filled stages that shined with rows of trophies and the smiles of those competitors lucky enough to receive one. And I can still remember all the dieting my students sacrificed for those Staten Island shows: how I helped each one of them on their quest for the elusive title. All I can do now is remember the great competitions and good times shared by the thousands who witnessed history unfold on Staten Island. Memories are all that remains, because that show's curtain has closed forever. In 2002, the long running Staten Island Bodybuilding Championships came to a crashing halt. It was the end of a great era that had witnessed the rise of many local legends and the fall from grace of a few. The standing-room-only crowds that once cheered on their favorite local muscle builders were gone, and so too, was the honor of being titled Staten Island Bodybuilding Champion.

Gone are the days of fame and glory. Gone are the cheers and applause for those that sweat blood to perform before massive crowds. Gone are the dreams that once inspired the Island's bodybuilders to higher levels of achievement. Gone are the promotional posters, media coverage, and stories about the Island champions. Gone is the magic that kept the Staten Island Bodybuilding community a close-knit group. All gone, but not forgotten.

The Staten Island Bodybuilding Championships lasted half a century and saw some of the greatest national level physiques on its stage. After so much history, the local legends were now nothing more than a memory. All ended by a storm that overshadowed the sport in every town and on every corner in America. A storm, whose vast dark cloud was scandalous in nature and deadly to those that sought its illicit power. It is a storm that rages on even today as its horror continues to destroy lives and careers.

The steroid rage that plagued the sport of bodybuilding since the early 1960s had finally taken its toll on the Staten Island bodybuilding community. The crowds that once admired the Island's muscle champs for their hard-earned efforts no longer filled the seats to cheer on the local muscle builders. Many potential competitors refused to follow the same path as the anabolic androids. As a result, the respect for bodybuilding competitions on the Island vanished. The new drug oriented breed brought in a wave of disgust from the local bodybuilding community and the support – gone. The show was dead on arrival. A competition that had boasted dozens of bodybuilders on its stage in past events shamefully dwindled down to a mere handful of competitors. The show was over and I was not about to save it. It needed to die, as does every anabolic competition today. As much as I would like to bring it back, I realize that my attempts to change it would be futile so I will just let it rest in peace.

The sport that I had lived for and dreamed about since I was a young teenager had transformed into a nightmare. I needed a way to warn the masses about the dangers of steroids and to declare that natural bodybuilding was real. Most of all, I wanted to rid drugs from the sport of bodybuilding. But how?

MARIOSTRONG.COM

In June of 2002, I received a phone call from my brother, Philip, who told me that someone was using the name *Maria Strong* on the Internet to promote personal training on Staten Island. I had never heard of Maria before that time and looked at her Web site at MariaStrong.com. After reviewing her Web site, I had no objections to her using the widely recognized *Strong* name since she was helping to promote fitness and well-being on Staten Island. Her Web site awakened me to the growing popularity of the World Wide Web. That same day I bought the domain name MarioStrong.com along with several others to protect my brand. I also contacted Maria's brother, Phil, at Formulaconcepts.com about developing my first Web site. Since he had done such a great job in developing hers, I figured he was the man to see. I was right!

I was no stranger to cyber space. In the early 1970s, my father was a successful investor in the stock market and took the time to teach me the rules of the game. Eventually, I became an avid reader of the Wall Street Journal and tracked stocks for him as I charted several companies over the years to help him realize optimum gains. When the 1990s came around, I relied on my previous market experience to take advantage of the booming economy by day trading on the Internet. I saw the opportunity to make some easy money and jumped in forearms first to cash in on the over exuberance of the times. The Internet had become a resource for entertainment, information, and commerce. Moreover, I welcomed its potential.

By 2004, the Internet had finally caught on with the American bodybuilding public. Although it had been around for some time, it was becoming a major player with consumers and those seeking information. Bodybuilding Web sites grew more sophisticated as their numbers increased. Nevertheless, I did not like what I was seeing on the Web. The freedom of the Internet was bringing the knowledge of how to take steroids and where to purchase them right into the homes of our American youth. At the time, there were a few natural bodybuilding Web sites on the Internet but nothing explosive enough to dampen the ever-increasing drug use among bodybuilders. The time had come for me to help show the horror of steroid abuse in bodybuilding through this new media so I joined the fight to make a difference.

For this reason, I stepped into the battle and created MarioStrong.com. For years, I had written for physique magazines and preached the benefits of natural bodybuilding. I had tons of experience in many aspects of the bodybuilding spectrum and had frequently witnessed both the good and ugly sides of the sport. I was more than qualified to take up the challenge. Not only did I preach the benefits of proper nutrition and exercise: I was a natural bodybuilder for life. And I was as mad as hell for what the sport had become. Bodybuilding had been good to me. It had inspired me towards a better life and given me hope for longevity. It was a way of life with so much potential that I just could not sit back and watch the anabolic freaks destroy its true meaning.

I created MarioStrong.com using my history in the sport to demonstrate the benefits of natural bodybuilding. The Web site is full of muscle building knowledge. Not only does it provide sensible bodybuilding workouts and fat losing advice, it also has an historic gallery of Staten Island's physique champions, plus videos and slideshows of the Island's many well-known muscle builders. Most importantly, it shows the horrors of anabolic steroids. There are dozens of pages filled with articles on the abuse of drugs in the sport of bodybuilding and plenty of real examples of those who have suffered and died from the side effects of these dangerous substances.

MarioStrong.com has hit a raw nerve in America! Every day its mailbox receives e-mails from viewers. Most viewers praise the Web site, calling it a breath of fresh air and thank me for being a guiding light in this dark battle. Others curse it and send me threats of lawsuits and punishment for shining a light on this infectious anabolic plague. MarioStrong.com has become a premier natural bodybuilding Web site, not only with natural muscle builders but also with all athletes looking for a correct path towards health and longevity. Its popularity is a stamp of approval on the growing force of natural bodybuilding and the need for a return to the sports roots of physical culture. Thanks to this modern age of technology, I am able to do my part in reaching such large and vast audiences around the world as the dark cloud of anabolic bodybuilding begins to fade into hell.

AN ARTISTIC CREATION
By the end of 1979 I had sold thousands of gym t-shirts with many different logos, but was looking for something truly symbolic and everlasting to better express my feelings towards the sport of natural bodybuilding. For several weeks, I sat back and tried to envision what

was mighty and just, with Herculean overtones and yet righteous in nature. This creation had to challenge the impossible while expressing an endless journey towards a noble quest. I thought about it long and hard, and then suddenly one morning it hit me like a bolt of lightning. I would have a painting commissioned of the Natural Olympian! An image of a being that best represented what I believed bodybuilding should be. At my gym was a member named Hugh McMunn who was an accomplished painter. He had created several excellent works of art of well-known bodybuilders. He seemed very talented and knowledgeable about physique art. I approached him about creating such an artistic painting for me. As we sat down and discussed my vision of what I was looking for, Hugh smiled with confidence in knowing that he had the skill to create a masterpiece I was looking for.

About a week after our discussion, Hugh brought his camera to my gym to take some photos of me in various poses so he could better understand my muscular physique. The photo shoot took place after gym hours to accommodate both the photographer and myself. As I positioned my body for the photos, I stretched my right arm out to the side and my left arm overhead while I kneeled into a side lunge. Hugh snapped away and took about twenty photos. From these photos and my concepts of how the Natural Olympian should best be represented, he spent the next several months meticulously working on my creation. I was patient and optimistic, since Hugh was not only an accomplished artist, he was also a muscle builder who had a love for the sport.

Finally, one day Hugh came to my gym smiling. With the painting wrapped in brown paper, he placed it in my hands and told me to unwrap it. As I slowly removed the brown paper away from the painting, I saw a shining silver metal frame that proudly held its contents secure. As I continued to pull the paper away, I began to see the brilliant colors of the painting. It was truly magnificent! On the canvas was my concept of the Natural Olympian. I gasped in awe and happiness, for Hugh had captured the symbolic essence of what I believed best represented what natural bodybuilding was meant to be. He had created a Herculean image in oil that shined in confidence, and whose purposeful meaning presented itself in fierce determination. The painting had my likeness and I marveled in disbelief at how accurately Hugh had transformed my vision and concepts onto reality.

The Natural Olympian glowed in honor and shined in strength. There he was, this noble, Herculean figure, soaring through the galaxies on a green comet while on his quest to the Olympian Zone. With one mighty arm raised high, he held a shining beacon to light the way for the masses to follow. With the other arm to his side, he held the cold steel that had transformed his physique from that of a mere mortal to a never seen before entity. You could feel the radiant energy while staring at this work of art.

From that day in 1979, to the last days of my gym, the painting would proudly hang high in the main lobby of my gym for everyone to see. During my gym's era, it was seen by thousands of Island bodybuilders who came to recognize its symbolic importance of what my Staten Island Bodybuilding Club represented. When the gym closed in 1986, I placed the painting back in wraps to help preserve it until it was time to hang it once again.

A decade later, I began to promote the NGA Eastern Regional Classic. This was a natural bodybuilding and fitness competition and I needed a symbolic drawing for its posters and T-shirts. I hired a commercial artist named Gregory Baker to create a black and white artistic drawing of the Natural Olympian soaring through space on an icy comet and with a fitness girl on its dusty tail. Gregory studied Hugh's painting of the Natural Olympian and said he was up to the challenge. His drawing was an excellent representation and captured the essence of my vision in much the same way Hugh McMunn's painting had done. When it was completed, Gregory's creation became a big hit with the hundreds of competitors that received a free T-shirt and with the patrons who believed in the natural bodybuilding movement.

In 2004, I placed the image of the Natural Olympian on the homepage of MarioStrong.com to be seen by Internet viewers throughout the world. The painting once again came to life, but this time, to a much broader audience, many of whom I would never meet or hear from. Today, as the Natural Olympian continues to shine on my Web site's homepage, its image has also been placed on the cover of this book. In my eyes, it best represents excellence in the sport of natural bodybuilding as it continues to grow in popularity with those seeking a healthy lifestyle. The Natural Olympian is an artistic creation that has been with me for several decades and with a little luck will be with me for many more to come.

THE HALL OF FAME

Every year, I visit Hershey Park in Pennsylvania with Aida. Hershey Park was founded by Milton Hershey in 1907, and is billed as the "Sweetest Place on Earth." Even though I have not had a piece of chocolate since 1969, I do enjoy the theme park's rides and attractions. I am big on rollercoaster rides, and to me Hershey has the best thrills in town. After spending a weekend at Hershey Park in 2006, I took a ride to the York Barbell Company, which was located a short distance away. Being a man of iron since the 1960s, I grew up reading about the champions from York Barbell and took this opportunity to visit their Weightlifting Hall of Fame Museum.

The museum contains a diverse history of the strength sports – from their evolution in Greek mythology, early Olympic Games, from the 19th and 20th century amateur and professional strongmen – to the current specialized sports of Olympic weightlifting, powerlifting, and bodybuilding.

As you drive up to the York Barbell Company, you are greeted by an enormous statue of an Olympic-lifter that sits on the rooftop of its office building (see photo). It is an awesome sight to watch as this Olympic-lifter holds tons of steel upwards while turning in a clockwise manner to inspire all who see it. At the entrance of the museum stands a 7-1/2 foot bronze statue of Bob Hoffman, the founder of the York Barbell Company, and considered by some to be the Father of World Weightlifting. Inside the museum are displays of a variety of plaques, trophies, sculpture, and vintage barbells. Some of the highlights of the weightlifting exhibit include a statue of Louis Cyr (a 19th century professional strongman), his actual 220-pound stage dumbbell, and the seven-foot Travis dumbbell (weighing more than 1,600 pounds, named

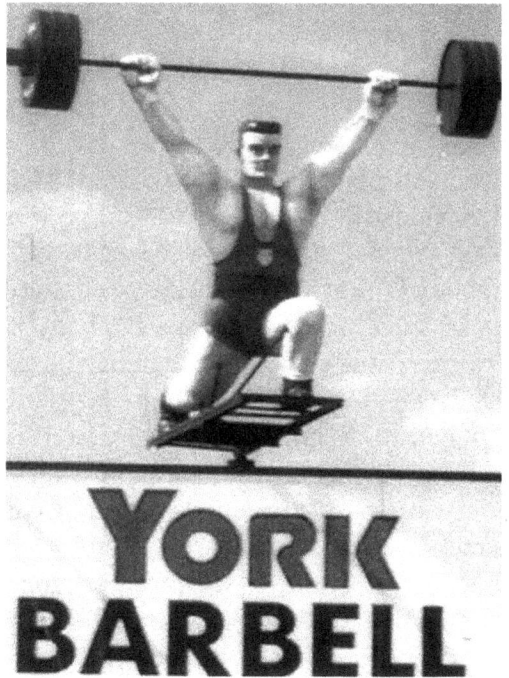

after Warren Lincoln Travis). Travis' exploits as a strongman in the early 1900s included lifting more than 3,000 pounds in the harness and back lifts of people and objects.

As you continue walking through the museum, you enter its bodybuilding section and come upon a full-size body cast of Eugen Sandow, one of the historical pioneers of physical presentation early in the 20th century. Eugen Sandow is generally considered the recognized link between the traditional bulky strongman and today's well-defined muscular bodybuilder. Next to Sandow's statue stands a life-size marble sculpture of John Grimek, a long-time employee of York Barbell, who was an Olympic weightlifter on the 1936 Olympic team. Grimek holds the titles of Mr. America (1940 and 1941), Mr. Universe (1948), and is the only well-known bodybuilder to retire undefeated from competition. John Grimek was dubbed "The Best Built Human" in the first half of the 20th century. Also, in the bodybuilding section of the museum were dozens of posters and photos of all the legendary physique artists of that same century. From Reeves to Schwarzenegger, every historic figure was well represented with his and her image engraved in a metal plaque for all to admire. A fine tribute to the muscle-building branch of the iron game, which made me pause to reflect on those who inspired me throughout my bodybuilding career. I will always be thankful to these men and women of iron whose images and likenesses shine proudly within the walls of the Weightlifting Hall of Fame Museum.

NEVER MADE IT TO THE ARNOLD EXPO

On Thursday, March 1, 2007, I flew to Columbus, Ohio to attend the first annual Iron Age Legends Dinner. Shawn Perine and the moderators of the Iron Age Web site had worked together for over a year to bring the legends of bodybuilding together with a special awards dinner. Being a member of the Iron Age forum, I shared the same passion for an era of bodybuilding that had long been lost. I wanted to thank those who inspired me throughout the decades. The dinner was being held in conjunction with the Arnold Schwarzenegger Classic Expo Weekend. A section was dedicated at the expo for the legends to meet and greet their fans. Since I had always wanted to attend this event, it sounded too good to pass up. Past bodybuilding champions such as Bill Grant, Anibal Lopez, Dave Mastorakis, Joe Meeko, Steve Michalik, Leon Brown, Vince Anello, Sergio Oliva, and many others were scheduled to attend this historic occasion. Besides, I had a personal reason to be there. My good friend, Leon Brown was turning 60 years young that weekend. I did not want to miss his surprise birthday celebration.

The dinner lived up to its billing as past and present champions gathered to share their common bond in bodybuilding. Leon Brown, one of the legends of bodybuilding's Iron Age, was shocked when he heard host, Jeff Preston announce from the stage that it was Leon's 60th birthday. As Jeff and everyone in attendance began to sing "Happy Birthday" to the Brown Bomber, a waitress walked over to his table carrying a large birthday cake. When the cake arrived at its destination, Leon could be heard muttering at how surprised he was while smiling ear to ear. The Brown Bomber was among his peers for this special occasion.

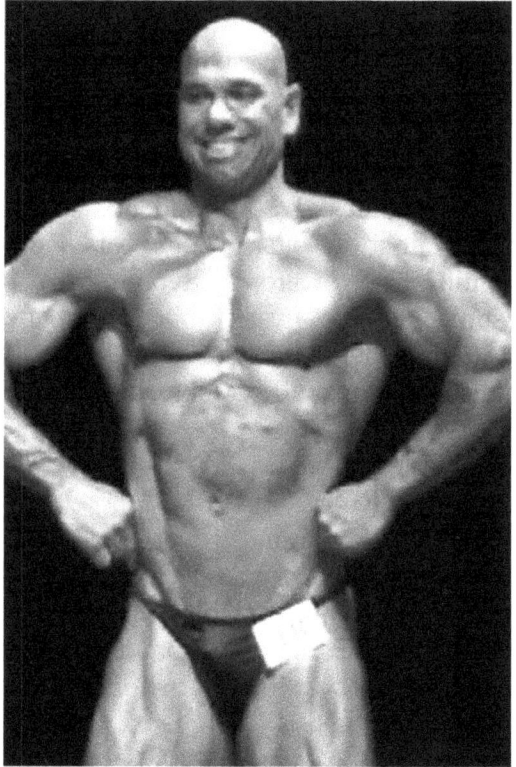

However, Leon's happy birthday celebration was cut short after he received a distressful phone call from fellow Staten Island bodybuilder Joseph Baglio (see photo). Joseph was also in Columbus that evening and called Leon from his hotel room to tell him that he was experiencing tremendous pain throughout his entire upper body. I also spoke to Joe and asked him if he thought his sudden pain might be heart-related. Joe said no but was unsure of what was causing the pain. Joseph Baglio was scheduled to work the Met-Rx booth at the Arnold Expo the next day. He was also planning to stop by the Iron Age Legends Dinner that evening to celebrate Leon's 60th birthday. Sadly, Joseph Baglio never made it.

Two years earlier Joseph Baglio had undergone a heart transplant due to acute cardiomyopathy and now was on the comeback trail. In early 2007, Joseph stepped onto a physique stage for the last time when he competed in the NPC Eastern USA, placing 5th in the Masters Class. Joe was ecstatic at this monumental achievement and his future began to take new hope. Alas, it was not to be. Joe called again telling Leon that he was in extreme pain. Leon Brown immediately left the Legends Dinner to rush Joseph to a local hospital in Columbus where he stayed by Joe's side until he was admitted at 3:30 AM the next day.

The next morning, unaware of the serious extent to Joe's medical condition, both Leon and I attended the legends section of the Arnold Expo as scheduled. As Leon was signing autographs for his fans and I was exploding a hot water bottle for the crowd, Joseph Baglio was fighting for his life during an emergency surgery. It is still unclear to me what procedure he received in the OR, but Joseph remained in intensive care afterwards, never to regain full consciousness. That Saturday, I had an afternoon flight out of Columbus and called the hospital to see if visitation was permitted. I was told Joseph was in intensive care and was unable to receive any calls or visitors. On March 8, one week after Joseph Baglio first called Leon Brown for help, the 40-year-old bodybuilder passed away due to heart complications. I was saddened to hear about Joe's passing. I had known him for over twenty years. Even though I did not agree with his philosophy towards bodybuilding, I'll always remember Joseph as someone who always smiled, no matter how serious an obstacle was. At his funeral, he was remembered as a friend to many, a loving husband to his wife Debbie, and as an athlete who gave it his all.

CALIFORNIA AND BUST

On Thursday, June 28, 2007, I flew with Aida from the Hawaiian island of Oahu to sunny Sacramento, California to attend the 2007 NGA California Bodybuilding and Figure Championships which were scheduled be held in Folsom that Saturday. The show's promoter, John Carrero, was a former member of my Staten Island Bodybuilding Club. John had invited me to participate as a judge and to receive an award at the event. I was also looking forward to seeing John's brother, Joe, who also was a former student of mine and who went on to become a national bodybuilding champion. On the Friday before the show, I happily met with John and Joe at a meeting held for the judges and competitors. It was good to see the brothers again. It had been many years since I saw them last and it felt like no time had passed in our friendship. At the meeting, we reminisced about days past as the competitors looked on with interest. The hungry athletes seemed ready and eager to flex their stuff as the clock ticked closer to the next day's competition. During the reunion, John planted a seed in my brain by asking me if I would explode a hot water bottle at the show. Having been on vacation in Hawaii and not prepared for this dangerous feat of strength, I was unsure if I should try it and said I would need to think about it.

The following day at the pre-judging, I sat next to the head judge of the show, Joe Carrero. About 25 years earlier Joe and I judged a New Jersey bodybuilding competition together and now, here we were on the West coast in similar roles. One by one, the competitors took to the stage. The competition was fierce and made the judging difficult. To date, this was the highest level of competition the NGA California Championships had ever seen. The mandatory and comparison rounds went off like clockwork and the scores were tallied for the evening's finals.

The evening show was filled with an enthusiastic audience. The crowd had come to cheer on their favorites, and as the curtains opened to a stage filled with competitors, the audience rose to its feet to salute the Star Spangled Banner. During the competition, the athletes battled in their respectable divisions, in hopes that they would place well for their efforts. Presented to the winners would be bronze Herculean sculptures and to the overall men's champion a sword created by Neil Andersen. John Carrero acted as MC and helped the show run smoothly with his professionalism. As the evening's events unfolded, the time came for John to present me with an award for being a mentor to him as well as to many natural athletes throughout America.

John told the audience about how he and his brother, Joe, had started their bodybuilding careers at my Staten Island Bodybuilding Club in the late 70s, and how I had mentored both of them during their early days by setting the correct course for their success in the sport. He then went on to talk about my natural bodybuilding lifestyle, calling me a true Superman. A Superman because I not only stayed away from all drugs in the sport of bodybuilding, but more importantly, because I followed a natural diet, exercised daily, and maintained a positive outlook on life. After the kind words, John announced my name and suddenly I heard the theme from the movie *Superman* echo loudly off the auditorium's high walls. Proudly and with some emotion, I took to the stage as John presented me with a plaque in recognition for being a mentor to many natural athletes across America. I thanked him for the recognition and then gave the following speech:

"It's nice to be here in sunny California. I would like to thank John Carrero for inviting me here tonight to accept this award. I have known John since the mid-1970s, and let me say, he is dedicated to his cause in promoting natural bodybuilding in California. In 1998, John competed in my NGA Eastern Regional Classic and he brought the house down with his symmetrical physique while deservingly winning the best poser trophy that evening. It is because of men like John Carrero, who have the vision and will to take a stand against drugs in our sport that the natural bodybuilding movement continues to grow not only in America but also worldwide.

Tonight I am receiving an award for being a mentor. A mentor can only be as good as the student he trains. Sure, I am knowledgeable in training, nutrition, and the sport of bodybuilding. I have been pumping iron since 1965 and have learned quite a bit through trial and error, and let me tell you there have been quite a few errors along the way. Throughout my many years as a bodybuilder, I have participated in many facets of the sport. I have been a gym owner, trainer, competitor, fitness author, promoter, judge, and just about everything else related to physical culture. I have learned that bodybuilding is the scientific application of proper nutrition, exercise, rest, and positive mental attitudes, and that each individual is unique with different requirements to achieve his or her ultimate goals. Each athlete you see here onstage tonight is unique. Each has sacrificed time, sweat, and pain to flex their stuff before you. Each has a burning desire to win and deserves your applause for being here.

Tonight I am here in large part because of one of my students. This student joined my Staten Island Bodybuilding Club in 1978 at the young age of fourteen. From the onset, he showed enormous potential and a burning desire to achieve, while displaying a positive attitude and confidence as he listened to the advice I gave him. While other members of my gym made excellent gains in their training, it was nothing next to this up-and-coming muscle wonder. Day by day, this new student would come to my gym straight from school while carrying his textbooks in one hand and a protein drink in the other. It was a pleasure to watch him progress as I carefully planned his diet and training to set him on a path for success. In just five months of training, he gained twenty pounds of solid natural muscle and was on a course to set history. In May of 1979, at the seasoned age of fifteen, he entered Dan Lurie's Mr. Staten Island competition and shocked the sold-out audience with his flawless symmetry and dense muscularity by placing a close second in what was probably the greatest lineup the Staten Island show ever saw. At the end of the evening, he was also awarded with trophies for Best Back, Chest, and Poser in the overall Mr. New York City competition, which had a field of 78 competitors. Yes, my new student shined that night and caught the eye of Denie, who was the editor of *Muscle Training Illustrated.* Denie requested I write an article for *MTI* about this new, up-and-coming bodybuilding star. Happily, I wrote the story and titled it "15-Year-Old Muscle Wonder." The spark was lit! The day the story hit the newsstands my new superstar's ego grew faster than the universe. There was no stopping him now! He went on a tear, dominating the bodybuilding stage for a span of fourteen years by flexing his Herculean physique against some of the best bodybuilders in the United States. Today, this former national bodybuilding champion continues with his training; and in 2006, he launched a new Web site in his name that is very informative as well as entertaining. He has also been featured on CNBC as an expert on the California real estate market and in 2007 was the host of an international marketing campaign for a major fitness manufacturer. He is here tonight, as he has been for the past several years helping his brother, John, promote natural bodybuilding in California. He is a long time friend of mine and is the head judge for tonight's NGA California Bodybuilding & Physique Championships, Mr. Joe Carrero. (Upon hearing his name the audience gave Joe a great applause as he walked onto the stage and said a few words to the crowd about our friendship. After Joe spoke, I continued with my speech).

During the past few decades, the sport of bodybuilding has suffered from the use of anabolic steroids, growth hormones, diuretics, and drugs used for the purpose of building muscle and strength. Many well-known muscle builders have died long before their time. Many live on dialysis and with heart ailments, not knowing what their future may bring. Some sell their bodies to afford these dangerous drugs, which can cost in the thousands of dollars annually. The anabolic drug scene has been a dark cloud that has lasted too long over a sport with such great potential. Today, those dedicated to physical culture have begun to prevail as the sport of natural bodybuilding begins to shine through that dark cloud. It is a good verses evil scenario that can have only one positive outcome. I will do my part in this fight against drugs in our sport by setting an example for others to follow as I continue to promote natural bodybuilding throughout America. I invite each one of you here tonight to join me in this battle by helping to promote natural bodybuilding in your local gyms and communities.

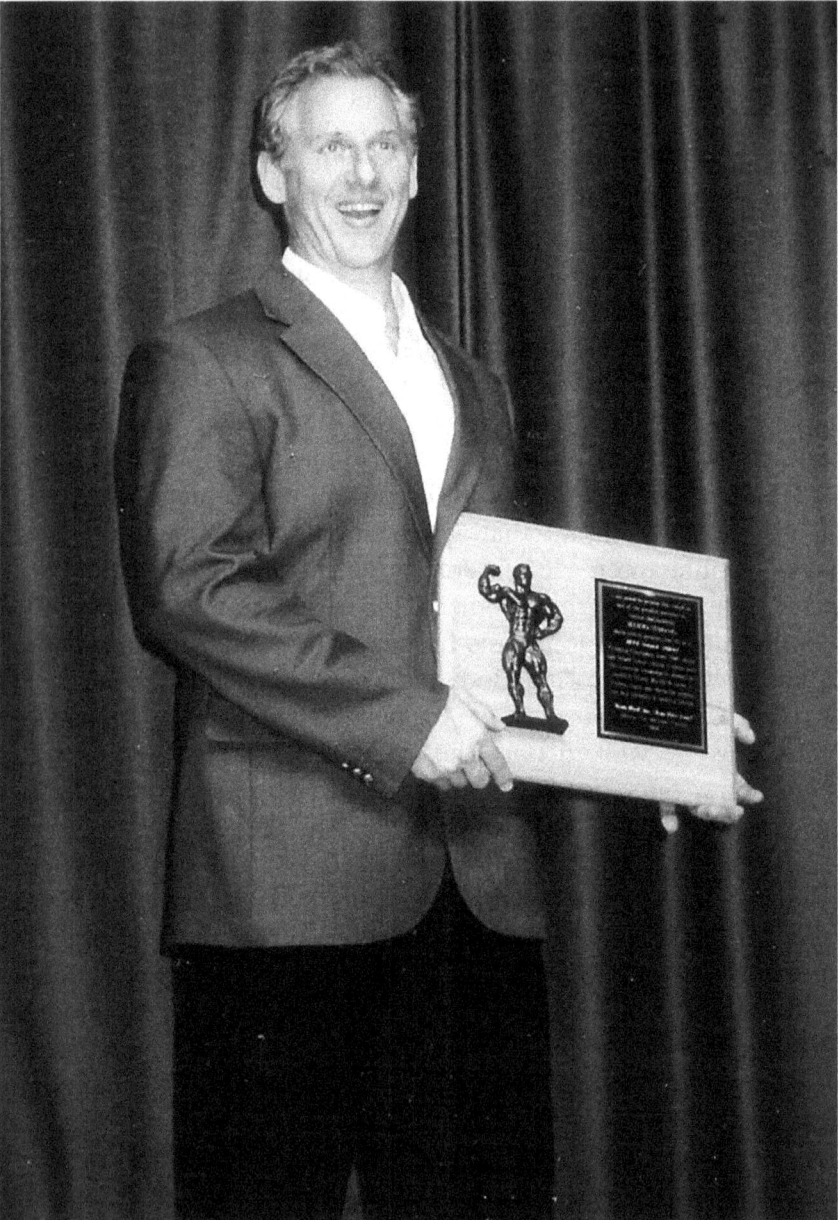

In 2007 Mario Strong was honored at the NGA California show

In closing, let me say that natural bodybuilding is the closest thing you will ever get to the fountain of youth. Not only does it bring quality muscle and lots of strength, but also more importantly, it brings lasting health, vitality, and an inner well being not realized by many. There are no guarantees in life, but all of us should continually strive to improve upon our health and fitness each and every day. Like Rocky Balboa once said, "It's not about how hard you can hit, it's about how hard you can get hit and keep moving forward, how much you can take and keep moving forward." Well that same philosophy applies to all of our lives. In time, we all get knocked down along the path of life. It's those with the inner fortitude to get back up and with the persistence to keep moving forward that will go the distance in this ever changing game of life."

As I finished speaking, John took the microphone and told the audience that I was going to attempt to blow up a hot water bottle. It was an attempt, since I had been on vacation in Hawaii and not had the time to practice for this dangerous feat of strength. The theme song from the movie *Rocky* began to play loudly throughout the auditorium as I cautiously walked towards center-stage while putting on goggles to protect my eyes. I felt good inside. This is where I belonged. The music was loud, the crowd was cheering, and the pressure was on. As I began to force air into the hot water bottle, I immediately began to feel the resistance of the thick latex rubber. "This wasn't going to be easy," I thought to myself. I had performed this feat of strength so many times before, since the 1970s, and here I was again going at it. I continued forcing air into the hot water bottle and with each mighty breath the resistance grew stronger. At twenty breaths, most hot water bottles would explode, but not this one, this baby was going to make me give it everything I had. As the music continued to play, the audience's applause grew louder and louder, inspiring me on as my heart beat in tune to their thunderous cheers of *Go For It*! There was no way I was going to let them, the Carrero brothers, or myself down. With determination and purpose, I forced more and more air in as I battled with this nostalgic moment. At thirty breaths, the impossible began to take shape. Air began to escape from the tremendous pressure and my face felt the pain of its muscles straining. I was in no man's land and was not about to turn back. It was a test of will as I struggled to keep the air from going down my lungs and ripping them apart. As the audience continued to cheer, I dug deep inside my heart and forced huge breaths into the hot water bottle. It continued to expand as I forced in more and more air. At 35 breaths, I zoned out and completely focused on the task. I could no longer hear the crowd or music, as it was do or die…literally. In a violent rage I forced more air into this seemingly endless void... 36, 37, 38, 39, I raised the beast upwards and from deep within myself forced a large blast of air into the hot water bottle, causing it to explode with a loud thunderous burst that sent pieces of the monster flying all over the stage. Suddenly, I focused to where I was and heard the crowd screaming in awe as the song *Gonna Fly Now* framed this historic moment for a lifetime. Yes, this was where I belonged I thought to myself, as I smiled and bowed to the audience and thanked them for their cheers and support during my difficult performance.

At the end of the show, every competitor left with a trophy and smile, knowing that they gave it their best. John Carrero had produced another great NGA California competition and after the show invited everyone to a local restaurant to feast. Of course, I brought my own meal: boiled chicken breast, carrots, celery, and tomato salad. At the restaurant, he presented Best Poser awards to the crowd's favorite competitors. It was a nice time that capped off a great day. Sadly, the night had come to an end, as I said goodbye to my friends, John and Joe Carrero. It had been great seeing them and meeting their sister Margaret, as well as their parents and Joe's fiancée, Jamie. The Carrero family was wonderful, warm, and loving.

GONNA FLY NOW

On Thanksgiving Day 1976, I went to the premier of the movie *Rocky*. While the film itself was unique, it would be Bill Conte's theme song, *Gonna Fly Now*, that would inspire and energize me for many years. The song has magic! Its tune grasps deep within my heart and lights a fire that cannot be extinguished. *Gonna Fly Now* is an original theme that has not only exhilarated me but millions of others to take up the challenge and *Go For It*.

During the mid 1970s, I had an 8-track player at my Staten Island Bodybuilding Club that was there to play only one tape. That tape was the soundtrack from the movie *Rocky*, and it continuously played throughout the day to inspire the muscle builders to train hard and heavy. (I still have that original tape and have stored it in the Strong Archives). The gym contained a multi-level sound system and as you may have guessed, *Gonna Fly Now*, as well as other great hits from the *Rocky* movies would continuously blast off its walls to motivate everyone. Never has there been a more inspiring song than *Gonna Fly Now*! So many years after I first heard its electrifying tune, I can still sense the song's energy deep within my blood and feel the strength it brings me as my mind and body energize for any challenge that may cross my path. Here are the words:

"*Trying hard now, It's so hard now, Trying hard now, Getting strong now, Won't be long now, Getting strong now, Gonna fly now, Flying high now, Gonna fly, fly, fly.*"

Although not a bodybuilder in the truest sense, Sylvester Stallone's character, Rocky, has captured the essence of what every athlete experiences through time. Deep within Rocky's heart is the will to overcome the harshest of obstacles and the burning desire to rise to the challenge on every occasion. I can relate to Rocky as many other athletes can. In the sport of bodybuilding, you get knocked down with time. You experience injuries and setbacks that sometimes last for months or even years. It's those with the same type of drive, fortitude, desire, and heart of Rocky Balboa that not only find the strength within themselves to get back on their feet but to also go further than ever before.

In the thirty-plus years of the *Rocky* franchise, I never had a reason to visit Philadelphia and run up the nostalgic *Rocky Steps*. The *Rocky Steps* is the nickname given to the front steps of the Philadelphia Museum of Art. They are well-known for the role they played in the film *Rocky* and several of its sequels in which the bigger-than-life character runs up the steps to the accompaniment of the inspirational song *Gonna Fly Now*.

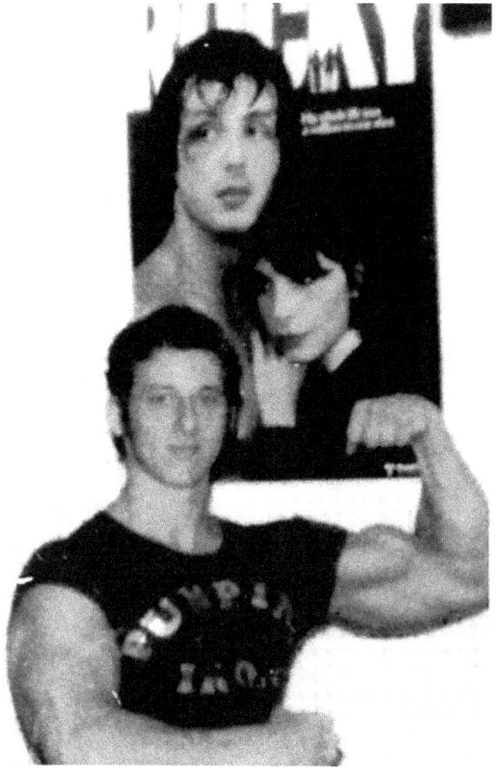

That all changed on Sunday, September 9, 2007, when I got the itch to create another online video and wanted to include the *Rocky Steps* in it. It was my 52ⁿᵈ birthday and I took the ride to Philadelphia with Aida, to first visit Liberty Square and then the Philadelphia Museum of Art. Liberty Square was full of American history and pride. We first took the tour of Independence Hall, where the *Declaration of Independence* was signed in 1776, and then visited the Liberty Bell itself as well as the Betsy Ross house, which were a few blocks from the square. After spending several hours at Liberty Square, both Aida and I felt a renewed sense of patriotism and respect for our country, which offers so much to those that are willing to work hard for the American Dream.

After visiting Liberty Square we drove to the Philadelphia Museum of Art and were in awe at all the commissioned statues and works of art in front of and surrounding its main building. Across the street from the museum's steps was a monumental bronze statue of George Washington riding a horse with other huge bronze statues of moose, bears, and other wildlife encircling the first Commander in Chief. It must have been at least thirty feet high and seemed wide enough to hold a private jet. The view from the top of the *Rocky Steps* offers a commanding view of Eakins Oval, the Washington Monument, the Benjamin Franklin Parkway, and City Hall. One look from its top steps and you instantly realize why Sylvester Stallone chose it as a symbolic place of achievement for his character Rocky.

One special work of art, commissioned by Sylvester Stallone and created by Thomas Schomberg in 1983, stood at the bottom right grassy area of the Museum. It was the two-ton *Rocky Statue* that welcomes visitors to the Philadelphia Museum of Art. After seeing the statue in several *Rocky* films, I was glad to have finally paid tribute to the character that inspired me so greatly since 1976. The ten-foot tall bronze statue of Rocky Balboa is an awe inspiring sight as it stands there with its arms raised victoriously while greeting the many visitors that come to admire and pose with it.

I also had the good fortune to meet the winner of a national Rocky Balboa look-alike competition, who was dressed in full Balboa fashion, wearing grey sweats, white hand wraps, and the Rock's trademark black converse sneakers. At first glance I thought he was some crazy dude who believed he was actually Rocky Balboa, but I soon learned that he was a guy named Mike Kunda (see photo) who was hired to portray Rocky to visitors at the steps of the museum. After mixing a few words with Balboa's younger looking and sounding twin, I became energized to accomplish what I had mainly traveled to Philadelphia for and walked over to the *Rocky Steps.*

As I looked up to the top of the climb, I saw several huge Roman columns that stood proudly at the entrance of the art museum. The *Rocky Steps* themselves are no great task to run as dozens of people did so in my two hours there. Visitors to the museum can often be seen mimicking Rocky's famous run up the steps. The run, which is 72 steps high and has several large, standing levels, symbolically represents the ability of an underdog to rise to the occasion. What I did do that was different from the others that day was to explode up the climb while skipping two, three, and sometimes four steps with every long stride that I took. Every time I ran up those steps I felt a rewarding and gratifying experience as my heart drummed in beat with the tune *Gonna Fly Now*. I could have ran all day if time would have allowed as I felt at home on the steps while seeing others give their best to make the climb.

Filming me running up the *Rocky Steps* actually proved more difficult for Aida to record than for me to run up them. Aida was in charge of capturing the action on video and found it extremely challenging to keep the camera's lens focused on me because of my explosive running speed. It took about forty takes to get enough video for editing and by the time we were finished my legs felt a little wobbly from the tremendous amount of energy they had expelled. Running up the famous steps and hanging out on the grounds of the museum was a heart-warming experience that I will always remember. It was

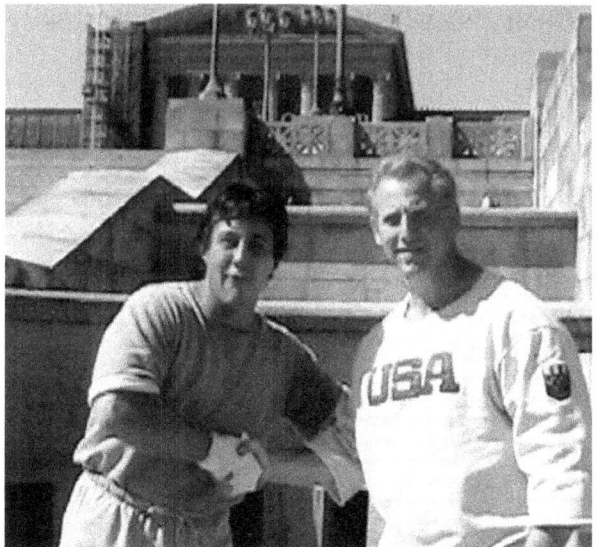

truly a labor of love that I surely will return to enjoy many more times in the many decades to come. Yo, Adrian…I did it!

In November 2006, the sixth installment of the *Rocky* franchise hit theaters nationwide. It had been thirty years to the month since the first movie of the *Rocky* saga played on the silver screen. The latest film, *Rocky Balboa*, had the same dynamics as the original and was widely accepted by fans everywhere. I attended the premiere on Staten Island and was amazed by not only seeing a sold-out theater consisting of an all-new younger generation but also the look of anticipation the now twenty-something crowd had in waiting to see the film. For me, that night felt the same as three decades earlier, when the audience became exhilarated while watching their fighting champ on the big screen, as he fought the odds in much the same manner he had always done. I gave the film two biceps up, my highest rating.

GONE BUT NOT FORGOTTEN

It is weird how life sometimes works. In 1985, while competing in the AAU Eastern Classic I met a competitor named Rick Trimarco, who was in the same division as myself and who also happened to manage his own bodybuilding club. Rick was a natural-for-life bodybuilder who trained hard and championed the physique stage. He was also a promoter of natural bodybuilding competitions in New Jersey and was well-respected among the vast bodybuilding community. I had run into Rick on several occasions over the following years and always found him to be honest and sincere in his approach towards promoting natural bodybuilding and living life to the fullest. Fast forward to the spring of 2007, when I received a phone call from an old bodybuilding friend named Michele Bean. Michele was once a competitive bodybuilder in New Jersey who was helping to promote the upcoming 2007 INBF New Jersey Bodybuilding and Figure Championships, which were scheduled for October. She called asking for my assistance in promoting the competition, which I was more than happy to help with. As we talked about old times, Michele delivered some very sad news that shocked me to the core. She told me that Rick Trimarco (see photo) had passed away a few years earlier after a long bout with cancer. I had always known Rick to be vibrant, healthy, and full of life. He was a fierce competitor who gave it his all and enjoyed celebrating victory on many an occasion. This news just did not seem right or fair. How could someone who was in his forties and took such good care of themselves perish at such a young age? Unfortunately, the longer you live the more you realize that sometimes life's cards are not dealt evenly. It does not matter how much you sacrifice or how hard you try, sometimes you just can't win. At least for Rick, he died knowing that he had never abused his health with anabolic steroids and it was just his fate to have such an illness take him away during his prime.

Michele was intent on bringing back the New Jersey Championships in a similar fashion that Rick once promoted. She was an old school muscle builder who loved bodybuilding and teamed up with Roger Rudzinski, a former winner of my NGA Eastern Regional Classic to promote the show. Roger was also a natural bodybuilder that shared the same philosophy towards the sport as Rick and Michele. I met with the both of them in June of that year to discuss their upcoming event. At the meeting, we developed several strategies to help promote the show. It was also decided that I would participate as a judge that day.

After Rick passed away, the show ceased to exist, which left a giant void in natural bodybuilding competitions in New Jersey. Several years later, his close friends came together and brought the show back to life with the same style and flare that Rick once gave it. On the day of the competition, I was happy to see that all the promotion had paid off. Over fifty athletes had registered to compete within the different categories and the crowd was as enthusiastic as I had ever seen. I was also joined in the judges section by fellow Staten Island bodybuilders Sigrid Taylor, Leon Brown, and Danielle Kalish to assist in scoring the athletes. During the evening portion of the

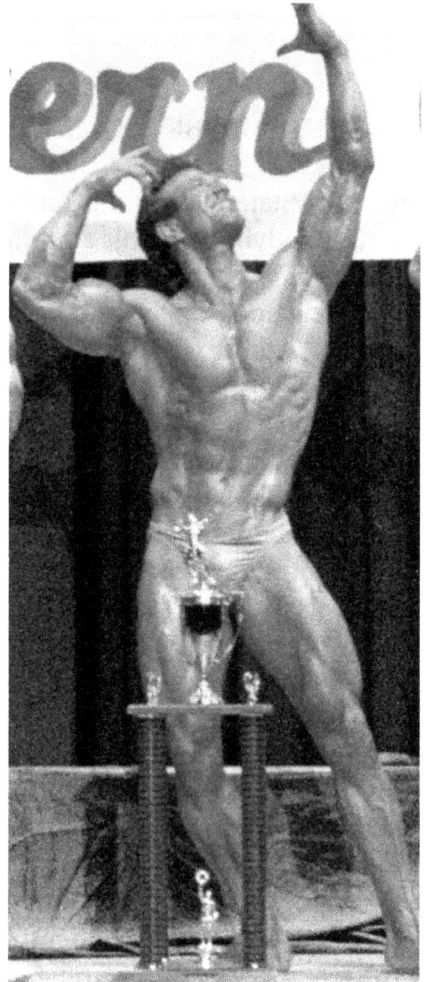

competition, there were plenty of surprise performances from pro-natural athletes. The audience just ate it up by giving the performers thunderous cheers and applause to show their approval. Personally, I had a great time judging the event and met one judge in particular who had been a good friend of Rick Trimarco, and who was nice enough to share some of his remembrances with me about Rick's natural New Jersey competitions. It was clear that all I spoke to that day missed Rick. He was back through the rebirth of the INBF Natural New Jersey Bodybuilding and Figure Championships. It was a fine tribute to a bodybuilder who once shared his passion with others, as they now remembered him in return by bringing back the show he once poured his heart and soul to produce.

Rest in peace, Rick!

STEROID PROBE REACHES STATEN ISLAND

It seems that every few years a wave of steroid abuse crashes onto the shores of Staten Island. In October of 2007, the abuse of steroids in the sport of bodybuilding hit close to home once again when the headlines of the *Staten Island Advance* read; "Steroids Probe Expands to Here." According to the story, a massive, multiyear investigation netted a complex web of pharmacies, Web sites, and doctors that had begun in Orlando, Florida, and ran through several states. The investigation led to the raids of a well-known Brooklyn pharmacy and a prominent doctor on Staten Island. It was reported that the raid in Brooklyn netted millions of dollars worth of human growth hormone and anabolic steroids, and a list of prescriptions for the illicit muscle-bulking drugs. What I found even more disturbing was the mention of a Staten Island doctor who was reported to be a source for the drugs via the prescriptions. I had known the doctor personally through a gym I trained at and had found him to be a pleasant, well-educated person. To make matters even worse was that the gym I knew the doctor from was also linked in the story as a source of referrals for bodybuilders, police officers, and high school athletes looking to get their muscle-bulking drugs. Once again, the ugliness within the evil anabolic cloud cast its dark shadow over bodybuilding. For decades, I have known the practice of taking steroids and growth hormones was common among many bodybuilders throughout Staten Island. Occasionally, I would try to discourage them and others from taking the harmful and illegal drugs, but for the most part all I got was strange glares that meant, "Thanks for the advice, but no way am I listening to you."

Several months after the story was reported in the media, I received a disturbing phone call from a gym buddy named Steve. Sounding upset, Steve requested that I remove an article posted on my Web site regarding the previous story. While I can appreciate the request (the doctor was a friend of Steve's), what really disturbed me was the way Steve tried to defend the use of drugs in the sport of bodybuilding. I had known him for many years and always thought he was stable and sensible, but I thought wrong. In his mind, anabolic steroids and growth hormones were okay as long as they were taken under medical guidance. The first thing I tried to explain to Steve was that all drugs take the body further than nature ever intended it to go. That included drugs for muscle building, drugs to get high, and drugs for medical reasons. Now, if medication is needed to fight an illness, prevent a problem, or help solve one, then of course I understand the potential benefits of drugs in these types of circumstances. However, for bodybuilding purposes, there's no sane reason.

I tried to explain to Steve that most of us are born healthy and to take a chance in losing our health for some added muscle was just not worth the risk, no matter how small a gamble it may appear. He went on to name some famous bodybuilding individuals that were known to use sports enhancing substances but had not yet shown any form of ill health. I countered with several recognizable names within the bodybuilding community whose illnesses and deaths were directly related to the use of muscle-building drugs. His response was; "I'm 38 years old and I don't want to live forever. I'm going to do what I want and I don't care about any possible side effects. Besides, if I take drugs under a doctor's care, then I'm guaranteed not to suffer any medical issues." I tried to explain to Steve that with drugs there are no guarantees on anything, no matter what purposes they are used. Towards the end of the conversation, I told him that if he was lucky enough to live to the half-century mark his thinking would change. Having a dozen years to go, he just laughed and said, "When I get there I'll worry about it." Unfortunately, that same mentality has caused suffering and tears to many bodybuilders and their families.

On Staten Island, the anabolic drug scene has been a brisk business for those enterprising individuals who have little regard for the law or the possible ill effects these powerful drugs can bring. Multiple arrests have been made during the past twenty-plus years over these chemical agents, but that has not slowed down their use by the bodybuilders. Over the years, I have found myself on the receiving end of threats from several steroid dealers on Staten Island whenever I tried to discourage a local bodybuilder from the use of these drugs. I have even had to crack a couple of muscle-heads with my fist to make it known that I would not back down from what was right. The issue of steroids has not only brought me enemies on Staten Island but also the loss of friends who went the way of the dark side and who continue to rely on pharmaceuticals for their gains. However, on occasion I get lucky and am able to get my message across to someone willing to learn and listen. To me this makes the fight all worth it and is a large part of why this book has been written.

In February 2009, when Alex Rodriguez of the Yankees was making the headlines for allegedly using sports enhancing substances, the previously mentioned doctor found himself being indicted on multiple charges. One of those charges was related to a former member of my gym named Joseph Baglio. Apparently, the District Attorney had established an illicit link between the doctor and him. Through the various media outlets, it was reported that between June 2005 and January 2007 the doctor prescribed Baglio anabolic steroids and human growth hormones on more than two dozen occasions, even though he knew how dangerous these drugs could be for the heart transplant recipient (see page 137). I, too, became tangled in the news, when I was contacted by a reporter from the *New York Times* requesting a few quotes on the Joseph Baglio tragedy. During the interview, I vehemently expressed my feelings on the latest anabolic debacle to hit the Island, but was happy to talk about Joe, whom I knew since the mid-1980s. I watched as he transformed his thin physique into Herculean form. Sadly, Joe did it by chemical means and was never able to escape the shadow of the anabolic cloud.

GIVING BACK
In Part Three of the *Godfather* trilogy, Al Pacino's character, Michael Corleone, expresses a deep desire to break free from the Cosa Nostra, which had consumed much of his adult life. Unfortunately, for Michael, he is pulled back into the vicious life of crime, never able to escape. In much the same way as the godfather's plight, I too, find my presence demanded, as my expertise and knowledge in the iron game is constantly sought after. Although I am always happy to contribute to

this world of muscle and steel that I love, I do at times find it consuming much of my free time.

In March of 2008, while shopping at a local supermarket, I had the pleasure to run into a former member of my gym named Phil "The Beast" Thompson. Phil was one of my gym's original members and was hard-core to the bone. During his younger years at my club, he trained intensely and I could see that he was still very much into bodybuilding. Phil told me he was a high school football coach on the Island at St. Joseph By The Sea and asked me if I would one day like to participate in helping the football team. I said, "Sure," and several weeks later received a phone call from Phil requesting my assistance during a powerlifting meet between his school's football team and three other high schools.

On the day of the competition, I arrived at St. Joseph By The Sea early and reminisced about times past, when I was once a senior at New Dorp High School and occasionally took the five-mile bus ride from my school to hangout with friends at the former all-girl school. That was thirty-five years ago. Today, St. Joseph By The Sea has become a co-ed school with a winning football team destined for greatness.

I met with Phil and took a tour of the team's weight training facility. I was impressed to say the least. So much had changed since my high school days when the only pieces of equipment to train on were an old Universal Machine and a sit-up board. The weight room at St. Joseph By The Sea was well-designed with rows of benches, machinery, and racks of heavy steel. It was equipped for results and I thought to myself how lucky the team was to have such a state-of-the-art training facility as well as coaches that believed in the benefits of weight training. As I walked through the weight room, I also recalled how my high school's football coaches were mistakenly against heavy weight training while I was a student. This in itself was the main reason I never participated in team sports. Being a new generation however, I was happy to give back to the community that had been so supportive of me during my reign.

At the competition, I participated as the sole judge for the eager lifters. They came to match their strengths and wills with the dozens of other high school athletes that strained for top honors. It was great to see the hunger and hope in the young eyes of the players and it reminded me of my own burning desire so long, long ago. This was the next generation of iron warriors and to them the world seemed for the taking. The lifting on this day was fierce and intense, and judging the athletes was a pleasure as the crowd cheered loudly from the bleachers for their favorite lifters.

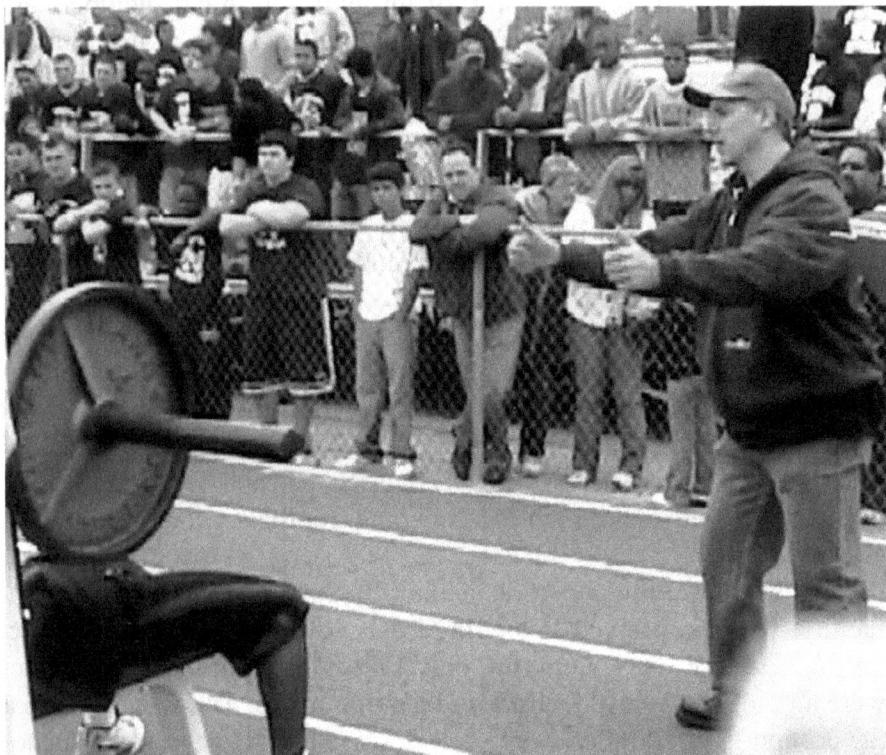
Mario Strong judging athletes at St. Joseph By The Sea High School - 2008

Later that same year, I had the privilege to participate as a judge in Dan Lurie's first annual muscle beach show at Jones Beach. The show was a benefit to help raise money and awareness for the crippling disease of cerebral palsy. I was more than happy to contribute my time to such a worthy cause. It was great to be once again participating in a Dan Lurie sponsored event. It had been many years since I was last involved with Dan's World Body Building Guild and on this day it was like old times, as the "85 years young" bodybuilding legend displayed his relentless humor and quick wit to charm the crowd of hundreds. It was a perfect day that made everyone, including the competitors, relax and have fun as they all united for an important cause. Nature provided some glorious weather. Rays of sunshine provided hope to all those present for this important event.

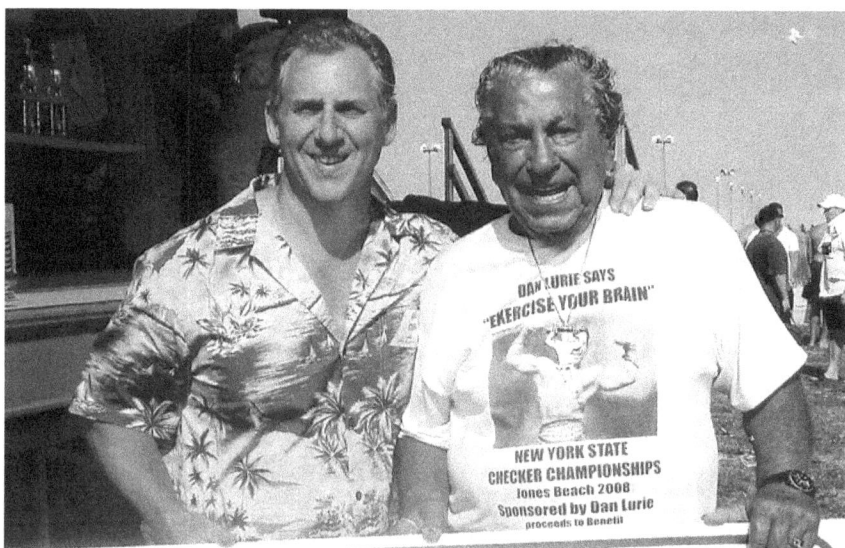

DAN LURIE SAYS
"EXERCISE YOUR BRAIN"

NEW YORK STATE
CHECKER CHAMPIONSHIPS
Jones Beach 2008
Sponsored by Dan Lurie
proceeds to Benefit

Dan Lurie presents

Mr. & Ms.
Jones Beach USA
Bodybuilding Competition

Mario Strong and bodybuilding legend Dan Lurie join forces - 2008

These two events, like so many before, found me in one of the many roles within the bodybuilding spectrum. For years, I had trained and accumulated a wealth of knowledge to share. Now, decades after I first began to train, my time has come to pass on the torch to future generations, in hopes that perhaps some unique individuals might go the distance in the iron game. No matter what event it may be; whether it is a physique competition, a lifting meet, a seminar, or a charity function, I will always be there as a guiding light, planting the seeds of health, strength, and fitness whenever I can. In the end, this is what's important. To give back so that some lives might be better, and just maybe in return, our country's future as well. Who knows, with a little time and care, nature might produce a fine harvest.

STRONG OBSERVATIONS

LOOKING BACK

In the early 70s there was still some innocents left in bodybuilding. We were a subculture within a society of couch potatoes that only a handful of men would dare participate. We went about our daily muscle-building lifestyles as if we alone knew the secrets to radiant health and Herculean physiques because that's how we felt when we trained in the gym. We owned the world and were aiming for the stars. There was no stopping our momentum as we were driven to succeed. We trained as if there was no tomorrow and dreamed of impossible goals that would one day be realized. We may have lost some of that naïveté since then. However, whenever we reminisce about those old days of Guts and Glory, our hearts instantly warm.

Looking back at it all, bodybuilding has been good to me. Not only has it provided me with superior health and vitality, it has also given me the confidence and fortitude to take on every challenge that has crossed my path. Bodybuilding has enabled me to go where most dare not venture. It has given me the drive to test my limits without fear and has shown me how to reach levels of performance I never dreamed possible. The sport has also taught me the power of positive thinking and has given me the ability to zone in on the task at hand. Most of all, bodybuilding has provided me with the keys to success, and for this I am grateful.

I am a natural-for-life bodybuilder. Always was, always will be! Throughout the years, there have been many individuals who have motivated and inspired me to excel in my chosen sport. Many were natural bodybuilders while others were not. Some were world champions, others local muscle builders. Whatever their philosophy or title, I am better because of them and will always be grateful for the inspiration they gave me along my life's journey.

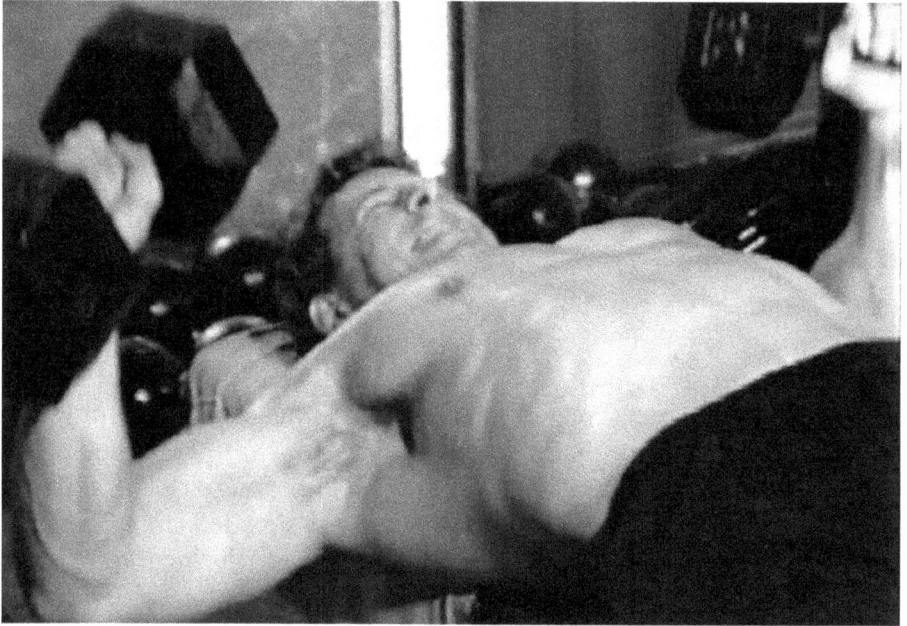

Mario Strong pumping the iron at his home gym – 1992

Throughout my many years in the sport, I have collected and read just about every muscle magazine ever published. From my early training days as a teenager, when I first visited Dan Lurie's Barbell Company in Brooklyn and bought every current and past issue of *Muscle Training Illustrated*, to the late 1990s, when I could no longer tolerate the enormity of anabolic androids and images of T&A that graced the covers and filled the pages of just about every modern physique publication.

Bodybuilding magazines were very inspiring back in the 1960s to the 1980s. Men who had bodybuilding in their hearts published those magazines. When the muscle-builders of the day read the stories about the eras top bodybuilding champions, they absorbed every written word into their own training and lifestyles. We all followed the workouts of the champs, ate as they did, and took the same supplements that they endorsed. The magazines of yesteryear were also very informative and provided sensible training and nutritional concepts, while the publications of today seem to rely chiefly on anabolic androids and big-breasted gals on the covers to make sales.

You name the magazine and I had it. I had every *Muscle Builder & Power, Iron Man, Strength & Health, Muscle Mag, Muscular Development, Health & Strength, Mr. America, Muscle Training Illustrated, Muscle Digest, Flex,* and so on. I had several decades' worth piled ceiling-high in my basement as their numbers reached into the thousands. Not only did I possess so many issues, but I made it a point to read and memorize every fact and theory printed in them.

If it was not for the physique publications of the 1960-80s, I doubt I would have gotten very far in bodybuilding. The inspirational images of the champs during the sports golden era helped to fuel my drive each and every day. Whenever a new magazine would hit the newsstands, I was first on line to get a copy. I was hungry to succeed and got my fill through reading the bodybuilding magazines of the day. So many Herculean covers have motivated me to succeed. So many dreams were created and realized thanks to the physique publications. Early in the 21st century, I gave away thousands of the muscle magazines to friends who shared the same passion as I did. Today, I have a few hundred of my favorite issues left in my archives to remember what muscle building was really like during the Iron Age of bodybuilding. Sorry e-Bay, they are not for sale!

During my era, I purchased many training booklets published by the champs of the day. I had and still own all of Pearl's, Schwarzenegger's, Columbu's, Zane's, Park's, Sipe's, and Scott's complete training sets of booklets, along with many more from the other champs of yesterday. When it came to bodybuilding, I was well-read. If you asked me about a particular champion, competition, or what training principles were best, I knew the answers. I absorbed the physique publications word for word and came to my own conclusions of what worked best for my students and me.

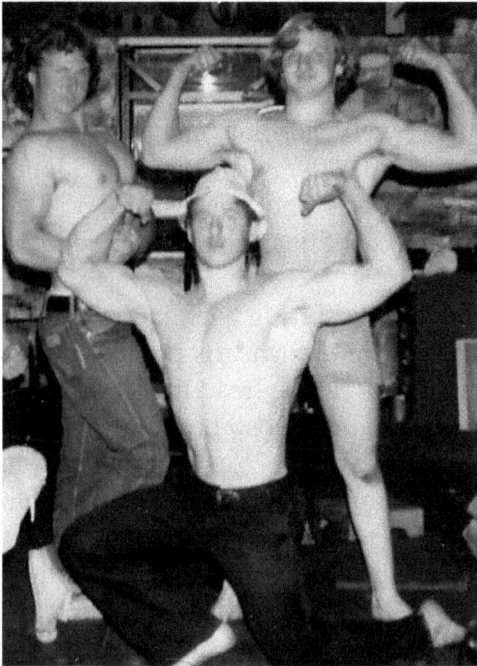

I remember my home's basement gym. My brothers, Johnny, Domenic, and I (see photo – 1976) first started to body build with my father's original barbell set. Gradually, as we became stronger and more developed we purchased additional weights and equipment to fill our needs. Eventually, the basement in which we made great gains during our youth became obsolete and was replaced by our home's spacious garage. Soon, neighbors and friends joined us in our quest for muscle and then the inevitable followed with the opening of my Staten Island Bodybuilding Club. I have made many great friends because of bodybuilding. I remember all the good times as well as the bad. I remember all the loves that came my way and the few that were lost because of it.

Yes, bodybuilding has been a big part of my life. It is a lifestyle that I will continue until my last dying breath. Today, my main focus in bodybuilding is to inform others of the potential dangers of drugs within the sport and to set an example for others to follow. Bodybuilding is a never-ending battle. For me, it is a war worth waging and whose victory is worth savoring. It's a lifelong journey towards fitness and longevity. It is like a painting that is never finished, as there is always something more to be added to the masterpiece. In some ways bodybuilding is a living form of art that changes with every repetition, every set, and every workout that is performed. As the days, months, years, and decades tick by, I will continue to improve upon my creation.

WHAT'S CHANGED
Today, everything in bodybuilding has been amplified to the max. There are many more muscle builders, spectators, self-proclaimed experts, training philosophies, methodologies, and exploitation of the bodybuilders. Manufacturers of exercise equipment and nutritional supplements promise muscles fast in exchange for a few hard-earned bucks. The sport where once common sense principles governed the iron lifters has seen a radical shift by today's muscle pumpers who demand instant results by any means.

Long gone are the small storefront gyms of the 1960-70s. Bodybuilding today has evolved into a billion dollar industry. In days past, a few hundred steady members was enough to keep a gym afloat. Today's multipurpose fitness centers enjoy memberships into the thousands, which brings large sums of cash into this ever-growing industry. During the golden days of bodybuilding, gyms primarily consisted of a few basic exercise machines, benches, and several tons of steel. Today, smooth nylon belts that glide with ease have replaced the thick steel cables that once tugged on some exercise machine's pulleys. The raw angle-iron benches of days past now come in an assortment of powder-coated colors with strong square tubing. Although the steel is still present in today's modern clubs, it has been accompanied by rows of treadmills, elliptical trainers, recumbent bikes, aerobic classes, personal trainers, and corporate owners. The big named companies have replaced the personal touch, with most clubs looking similar in design. In the old days, individuals who lived for bodybuilding owned hard-core gyms. Their gyms had the magic! As soon as you would step into clubs such as Vince's, Gold's, or Pearl's, you would feel the atmosphere. It was so thick that you could bounce a barbell off it. These gyms had members that were highly motivated because someone they believed in led them. Someone that not only knew how to build muscle, but also looked the part and lived the life. Those were the days! The gyms of yesteryear were not built to see how big a bankroll they could create but mainly for the purpose of building proportioned muscle and strength.

In many ways, the sport has changed. In some aspects for the better and in some ways for the worse. The cold steel weight-plates and dumbbells are now rubber coated. The plates themselves have holes for better gripping. The huge posters of the bodybuilding champions that once hung in every gym have been replaced by artful drawings for those more fitness-oriented. The hard-core atmosphere that once energized the training floors of the Iron Age have been replaced with TVs and iPods. Sometimes change is good. For me, today's multi-purpose fitness centers are a welcome change to the muscle-head gyms. After bombing and blitzing for over four decades it is nice to be able to bang out some heavy sets in an environment whose clientele is more than just muscle. Now don't get me wrong, I am still hard-core within my heart and continue to train vigorously. It is just that I am self-motivated. Once I am finished training I exit the gym, leaving my hard-earned sweat behind. At this point in my life, it is all about my own self-satisfaction and health that keeps me coming back for more. Leave the rest for the gym-rats.

Another thing that has changed to meet the demands and dollars of today's fitness buffs is the evolution of the supplement industry. Volumes could be written on this, but to be brief, health foods and supplements have become a billion dollar industry in America. What began as a few bottles of supplements on the store shelves has grown into aisles of designer products. The marketing of these products in the bodybuilding and fitness publications help support some of today's pro-bodybuilders and athletes through endorsements. Today, you can find designer supplements being marketed as having the same size and strength-building capabilities as anabolic steroids. It's all fair and legal, I guess, and I wouldn't have any problem with it except for one question. Why is there such a demand for these products? Supplements are just that – supplements. For our purposes, they were designed to enhance a properly balanced diet and not become the main source for one's muscle building needs. Proper nutrition is not that complicated. You don't have to be a rocket scientist to figure out how much protein, carbohydrates, fat, and calories you need. As Americans, our understanding of nutrition has never been better, yet supplements have become a mainstay in our land of plenty. Go figure!

THINGS I WILL NEVER UNDERSTAND

Being a person that has spent quite a bit of time in bodybuilding gyms, I have come across some behaviors that range from absurd to idiotic. The list of bad behavior includes not putting the weights back after use, using foul language in front of the ladies, and spitting on the gym floor. These are sure signs of an inconsiderate person but I can understand the limited mentality. I will never understand, however, is when a trainee is "lifting heavy" on the Bench Press, Squat, or some other exercise and needs a strong spotter to perform every repetition with him. I don't know about you but I rarely ever use a spotter. Not having someone assist me during my workouts ensures that I'm going to push the steel very hard and with everything I've got in order to complete my reps. It also tells me exactly how my training is progressing, unlike someone that is using ten spotters and a crane to set a new personal record and has no clue of how much they could actually lift on their own. I remember back in the mid-70s when I would assist guys at my gym with their training. Every day there was always a member or two that would load a barbell with more weight than they could possibly handle and have a spotter assist them in performing their exercises. Most of the time these members couldn't even complete one repetition on their own, but with the assistance of a spotter they would bang out several reps and receive high-fives for their "big accomplishments." On more than one occasion, I fell into the trap of assisting these over-zealous trainees with their lifting and was rewarded with severe strains in both forearms for my efforts. After getting tired of being injured while spotting some of these guys during the Bench Press, I came up with a solution to make them stop asking me for assistance. That solution was simply to drop the barbell on them! I'm always willing to help a trainee complete his final rep but if he can't get at least one good rep on his own, after he told me he wanted a clean set of six, than he had better not ask me for assistance.

The same bad habits and behaviors that existed over thirty years ago in bodybuilding gyms still exist today. In 2009, while training at a gym, I watched a member perform squats while receiving a spot from a workout partner that stood behind him. This workout partner assisted the trainee by wrapping his arms around his upper torso. It looked as if the workout partner was doing more lifting than the trainee was. He pulled the trainee up on every rep performed. What kind of help is that? Unfortunately, this is something I see all too often in our gyms.

Another thing that boggles my mind is watching bodybuilders on completion of their workouts exit the gym and smoke cigarettes with their friends. With all the educational materials available about the dangers of smoking and with the media continually advertising the benefits of quitting, you would think that today's generation would get the hint. Bodybuilding is supposed to be a healthy way of life, but I guess for some, it is just a way to get big biceps and pectorals. Years ago, there was a member of my gym named Warren that was a regular at the club. Warren was always joking around and did not take his training too seriously. One day, while in my gym, he decided to light up and smoke a cigarette, thinking it would be funny. He was wrong! As a couple of members voiced their disapproval, I walked over to where the smell of smoke was coming from and told Warren to exit the gym immediately. While laughing he blew smoke in my face, which caused me to respond in a very angry manner. Without hesitation, I smacked him across his jaw and sent him flying over an exercise bench. After several gym members helped him to his feet, I terminated his membership and threw him and his cigarettes out of the club. About a year later, Warren came back to my gym and apologized for his stupid behavior. He also stated that he had kicked the habit and was looking to get back into shape. I was glad to see he had the strength to beat the nicotine addiction and signed him up for another year of quality pain.

There is an old Strong saying that every now and then needs repeating. It goes like this: "Of all the senses, common sense is the least common," I think those words say it all when referring to some of the odd behaviors within our gyms and society in general. As bodybuilders, if we cannot act properly in a place where fitness and health shine, then what hope is there of us ever becoming well-rounded individuals that not only seek respect but show it as well?

STILL THE SAME OLD PROBLEM
Something that has not changed is the continual use of drugs for the purpose of building muscle and gaining strength. After decades in the sport, I am tired of hearing stories of friends who have died or are suffering with medical ailments. I will never understand the human mind. It can posses such great knowledge to survive and yet can be so self-absorbed and destructive. Some of the current crop of gym-rats would have made great chemists if they only had applied their intellect in a more positive manner. Moreover, what is it all for anyway? In the end, when the barbells are laid to rest and the trophies collect dust in the closet, who really cares how big your arms were or how much you once were able to Bench Press? The answer is hardly anyone. Recently, a fellow Staten Island bodybuilder died from following the wrong path in bodybuilding. He was a good guy and was admired by his gym buddies and friends. Unfortunately, the meaning of his passing was lost on those too narrow minded to change their ways. In as little as six months after his burial, those who paid their respects at his funeral were flexing their stuff on a physique stage loaded with steroids, growth hormones, and diuretics.

Time has afforded me the ability to look back over the decades and see what has transpired in the sport of bodybuilding. What I see is two very different philosophies on how the sport is practiced: one camp promoting natural bodybuilding and the other actively using sports enhancing pharmaceuticals. This drug craze is really out of hand and its effects are now being felt by mainstream America. Most professional sports have put a bright spotlight on the abuse of sport enhancing drugs.

Another disturbing trend is the increased use of anabolic agents among our nation's teenage population. Both boys and girls now partake in the use of steroids for the purpose of sports enhancement and physical appearance. Several years ago, I attended a pro-bodybuilding show and was shocked at not only how freaky the anabolic androids looked onstage, but more importantly, on how the young crowd cheered them on and idolized its hormone-filled heroes. In the old days, we were somewhat naive to steroids in bodybuilding as it was rarely discussed. But today it is all out in the open for the world to see. It makes me wonder about the common sense and morals within our sport. I guess it is just a sign of the times and I am afraid very little is going to change to rid this dangerous practice from our sport any time soon.

On a positive note, I have met plenty of former steroid users who openly admit to using these drugs during their early muscle building years and now curse the day they ever heard of the stuff. Sadly, most have suffered side effects, including permanent damage to their hearts, kidneys, and other vital organs. It is these fellows who are able to reach the younger minds by telling of their horrors derived from steroid abuse.

Personally, I no longer buy the hard-core muscle magazines or attend the pro-shows. The steroid scene has completely turned me off to that aspect of the sport and today my only connection with bodybuilding is in the gym and through my Web site MarioStrong.com. Occasionally, I am asked to make an appearance at a natural competition to give a speech or act as a judge, but that is as far as it gets. I have seen and witnessed enough to make me sometimes wish that I never heard of bodybuilding. Moreover, I am not alone in my thinking. Thousands of long-term bodybuilders throughout our nation have also voiced their disgust to the sport to which they were once proud to be affiliated. They also no longer purchase the magazines or attend the shows and their only connection with bodybuilding is through their own personal training. Although I will continue to promote natural bodybuilding, I realize that it is a battle that will last past my lifetime. These days, I am more into enjoying the other fruits of my life, such as studying the universe through my telescope and hiking tall mountains in my spare time.

Is it any wonder when we live in a society that supports self-deviant behavior to such an extent that harmful abuse can occur in our sport? Look at people who smoke cigarettes, for example. They know by smoking they are subjecting themselves to all sorts of serious illnesses and deadly effects and yet many continue this sick practice to their deathbed. Before we can ever hope to get drugs out of the veins of bodybuilders, our society must first take a good look at its own ill practices and make a drastic change for the better. Sad to say, I am afraid nothing will change in our lifetime and it will be the same story 100 years from now.

THE SACRIFICES

Bodybuilding is the scientific application of exercise, nutrition, rest, and positive thinking. Having stated that, I look back in amazement at the tens of thousands of hours and workouts that I have spent toiling away towards an endless goal. Bodybuilding requires time! It demands our presence in the gym and our sweat on the barbell. It does not care if you have a party to go to or a meeting to attend. It is with us twenty-four hours a day. Looking back over my life, I realize that bodybuilding has cost me dearly, not only in monetary numbers, but also within my social circle.

In my younger days, while on vacation in the Catskill Mountains or on the Jersey Shore, I use to pack my car's trunk with 300 pounds of weights so I could train. God forbid if I missed a workout and instead, joined my friends and family at the pool or on the beach. On Friday nights, when a girlfriend wanted to go out dancing, I was bombing my thighs until I could not stand any longer, let alone do the hustle. At dinners and special occasions, while everyone else was feasting on some delicacy, I always brought my own food and munched on skinless chicken breast as the guest glared oddly at me.

Because of my bodybuilding lifestyle, I have found myself on the receiving end of some loud verbal rages from those I cared about. My "way of life" has ruined many good love relationships and put much stress on several friendships. Earlier in my bodybuilding career, I made sure to get my scheduled twelve hours of sleep every night. Even though it was great for muscle repair and looking young, you can imagine how that went with others wishing to share their time with me for a night out on the town. I had to skip trips with friends that I couldn't attend and spoil romantic dinners by peeling a banana under the soft candlelight. At the local theme parks, when friends were allowed entry, I was treated like a terrorist and denied access because I brought my own prepared food. The security guards didn't care what my story was and in a way, it was discrimination against someone trying to take care of his health. But hey, I had a lot of training to do so I didn't have the time to tell it to the judge!

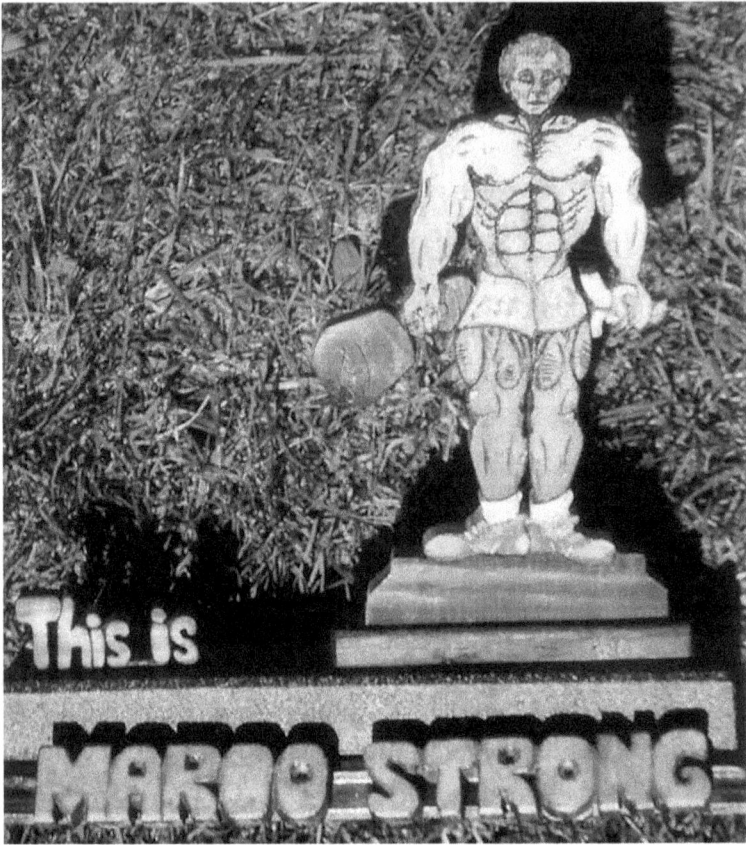
This is MAROO STRONG

Nobody understands or cares what your thing is unless they have lifted the same dumbbells and worn the same posing trunks as you. This sport is a science that gets in the way of our social lives. It forces us to juggle our lifestyles, trying to get it all in without sacrificing something else. But, it is virtually impossible to do. In reality, we all have to work, attend school, and fill our daily commitments. It is a choice we each have to make and live with it. It has been a real revelation to live life differently from most people I know. Although they respect my efforts, it is not something they would ever want to try or can even understand. Bodybuilding is my choice. It is something I believe in and as the years go by, I see how right I was to choose this path. As I look around, I see those that I have known since childhood, both family and friends alike, aging poorly with the seasons that pass before them. Although I am not immune to the clock, my secondhand moves much slower than those whose lives tick faster because they follow the same path as the masses. Yes, I am different and have sacrificed many good times to be who and what I am today. It is what I know. It is my destiny. It is my means to an end.

TRAINING LIKE THERE IS NO TOMORROW

I am a quiet, unassuming, somewhat composed type of guy. I constantly monitor the world around me. Like most people, I perform my daily chores and bear the stresses that life can sometimes bring. However, when I enter the gym I leave the world's problems outside its doors and ignite with enthusiasm. Bodybuilding, for me, is a glorious and painful experience all wrapped into one. The feeling of self-satisfaction the weights bring me energizes my body and mind to train extremely hard and with great intensity. I am a guy that likes to train heavy. Sometimes the poundage is so monstrous that my muscles feel like their ripping off my body. By training in this manner, I am constantly putting myself in the danger zone, which forces me to give it everything I have. It is the way I've trained since my teenage days and it is the same principle I follow today. In the iron game, you have to constantly push the limits of the mortal man and enter the superhuman level of bodybuilding. That's how true lasting results are realized and it's the way I have trained for decades.

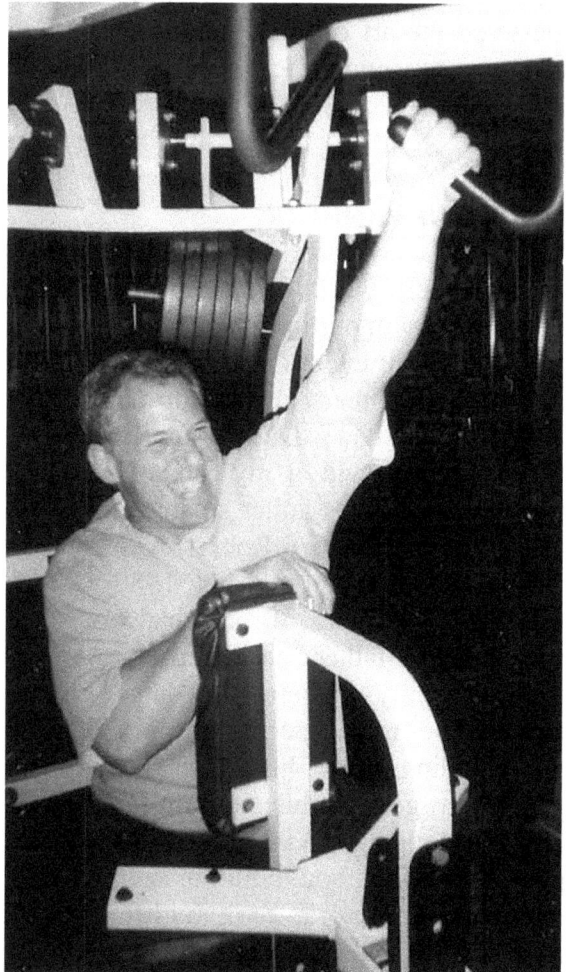

Training in the manner I do can be quite intimidating to the average fellow, but at the same time, inspiring to those willing to go the extra mile. Through my bodybuilding career. I've had dozens of training partners and have often found myself in competition with them during our intense workouts. The workouts became a game of *can you top this,* as my training partners would load the barbells or machines with tremendous amounts of steel in an effort to outdo me. I have never been one to throw in the towel and have always pushed myself beyond the limits. There is nothing greater than the feeling of conquering a new exercise or setting another milestone in the gym as the gains realized from such efforts can last a lifetime. These days, while I continue to *train without pause,* I find myself training alone as I am able to enjoy the solitude within my pain more deeply. After so much time in the gym, I find little need for training partners. I have mastered the art of muscle building and have learned to use my raw instincts to guide me on my endless journey to the realms of Muscledom.

GONE FULL CIRCLE

We often take life for granted as the years pass by. With today's fast-paced modern world, it is easy to lose focus on the important people and moments in our lives.

While training at LA Fitness on Staten Island in the summer 2007, one of the members of the club named Robert approached me to ask for training advice. During our conversation, he mentioned that his father once trained at my Staten Island Bodybuilding Club. I asked him his age and his father's name. He replied that he was nineteen and his father (also named Robert) had trained at my gym for many years during the 1970s through the 1980s. After he described his father to me, I felt like a sack of rocks had just hit me in the head. Thirty years ago, Robert's father had joined my gym when he was also nineteen to train under my guidance. His father followed my advice and became one of the main faces on the Island during its golden days of bodybuilding. Now, here I was standing with Robert Jr., thirty-plus years later, giving advice to him in much the same way I had given his father so long ago. As I spoke to him, I reflected on the years that had passed by, when bodybuilding seemed so much simpler and yet had a much greater importance in my life. I couldn't help but yearn for those days of Guts and Glory and wondered to myself where all the time had gone. As the years go by it gets a little weird for me, having trained for so long and realizing that once I was the same age as the majority of the today's gym members.

After talking to Robert, I looked around the gym and glanced at the many faces of those training. There they were, the guys and gals, sweating away in much the same way my members had done during my reign in my gym. The thing that stood out in my mind was that I was no longer part of that generation.

Even though I look young for someone in his fifties and could easily out-train most of today's gym members, I am still from a different era and at times feel a little prehistoric. Even in my youth, I knew this time would come.

I made a pact with myself back in the 1970s to train intensely and to live as healthy a life as possible. As a teenager, it was my long-term goal to remain young forever, and I believe I have been successful.

Today, as I continue with my passion, I have become more distanced from those of my generation. Even though I am chronologically older than most members at the gym, I belong there. The gym is like a base camp to me where I stage my quest for lasting health and vitality. Those of my generation are couch potatoes and wither away as the days pass. Today, when I'm at a gym, I tend to reminisce about my own club, and the guys I used to train with. My quest for health and fitness is my lifetime commitment. I welcome the challenge that this commitment brings me every time I place my callused hands on a cold barbell.

DAYS OF GUTS AND GLORY

There is something inherently dangerous about the male youth. Maybe it is the high voltage testosterone that rages within their veins, or the thrill of the conquest to push the envelope to the edge. In many ways, I was no different from most red-blooded American males during my earlier days. Not being satisfied with the status quo, I constantly challenged myself to strive a little further in any endeavor I attempted. During the brutal winters of the Catskill Mountains, I would run barefoot for several miles over its hilly terrain. When behind the wheel of a car, I would always push the speedometer to go a little faster to test my skills. Even at school, if something caught my interest, I would study it until there was nothing left to learn. That is just the way I was and to some degree remain.

It was no different in the gym. For me, bodybuilding brought a realm where limits were tested and broken. Barriers of pain and suffering were met with joy as new muscle and strength waited behind their doors. It was an endless battle that I gladly pursued, since bodybuilding to me represented the Fountain of Youth. I correctly believed that if I put myself through hell while in my youth that my health and longevity would shine later in life. The fruits of my endless labor have paid off in big dividends, in much the same way as saving for a rainy day.

During my prime, I invested wisely in my health. Today I reap the benefits, whereas others much younger than I am have fallen with the hands of time. While I have mellowed a bit, one constant remains. A fire for the iron burns deep inside of me since day one when I first lifted a barbell and it continues to shine its bright beacon now.

Like so many other bodybuilders and powerlifters, I have spent a lifetime in the gym. I tested every weight training system ever documented and developed a few of my own theories about them. The lack of desire and inability to adapt with age breaks most men down. For me, it is the ultimate challenge. As the years go by, I constantly strive to train heavier and with greater intensity. There is no moderation! What greater quest, what greater victory, but to beat Father Time at his own game and live a long, full, healthy life well past the century mark. This worthy purpose is the reason that I have suffered through all the pain, all the sweat, all the sacrifice, and all the seemingly endless years that continue on at the gym.

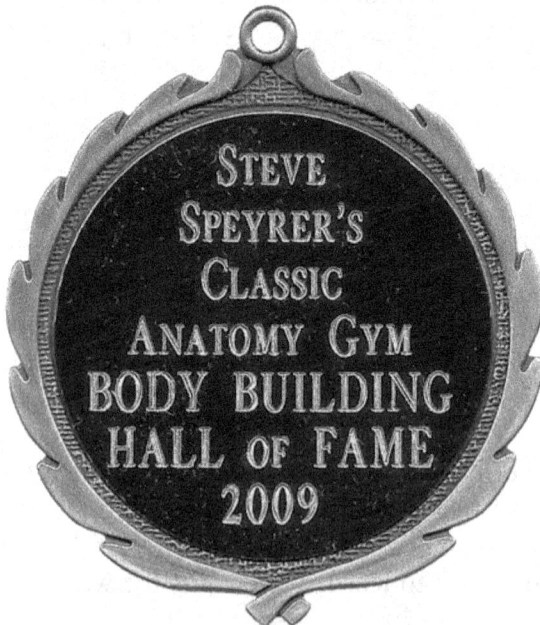

In 2009, Mario Strong was inducted into the Classic Anatomy Gym Body Building Hall of Fame for his hard work, dedication, and selflessness in promoting natural bodybuilding.

THE ROAD AHEAD

A CELEBRATION OF LIFE

For pure muscle builders, there is something magical in bodybuilding that is hard to explain. The sport contains a force within its lifestyle that constantly summons us to return to the gym. It demands that we watch our diets, get plenty of rest, and *train feverishly*. Natural bodybuilding is a celebration of life. It is because of the radiant health realized through our demanding lifestyles that life itself becomes one big fiesta. As I look at humanity today, with its poor lifestyle choices, I can only feel sorrow because so many people are missing a great opportunity to experience something special.

When I wake up in the morning, I look forward to the day ahead. I know that life is not always "peaches and cream" but hey, I am alive and healthy, so what more can I ask? When you do not have your health, the world does not seem like such a nice place. It doesn't make a difference how wealthy you are or what kind of material items you possess; without your health, your capital is not worth much. Unfortunately, we have seen examples of this played out throughout the media for many years. Many famous people with great wealth and talent have lost their lives to drug abuse and poor health habits.

When I enter the gym, I am electrified. I feel blood pump through my veins in anticipation of the workout to come. I am on automatic pilot and flying high as my cerebrum's memory bank yanks out a fresh tune of *Gonna Fly Now*, long before I ever place my callused hands on a cold barbell. For me, working out is the most rewarding part of my day. It is my way of renewing my vow to continue my endless quest towards radiant health, fitness, strength, and longevity. And it has really paid off.

Recently, I went to the gym earlier than usual and was horrified at what I saw. It seems that the "older crowd" likes to get their workouts completed before the mad rush, and this is fine. However, I was disturbed by what I saw in the locker room. A group of about a dozen older guys in their 60s and 70s had allowed life to beat their bodies to a pulp. They were flabby with potbellies and wrinkled skin that hung like old drapes. Their limbs looked frail and they did not seem to have much pep left in the tank. Although it was good they were attempting at some kind of improvement towards their health, it was a little late in the game for any lasting result. Why had these men let themselves go like that? They all seemed well educated and probably enjoyed a great business career as well as a wonderful family life. Why had they not taken care of their most important asset – their health? It just boggles my mind when I think about the way people just stick their heads in holes like ostriches and wait for life to give them a big kick in the old butt. My friend, John Newman, once said it best: "The masses are asses." If you think that statement is incorrect, just look at the billions of dollars that are spent in this country on tobacco, alcohol, and fast foods. Although they are not the greatest things for your health, they sure keep the medical industry in business. Most of us have a choice in life and are accountable for the path we choose to follow. I have made my choice to celebrate the gift of life, both today and in the decades to come. Thanks to following a natural bodybuilding lifestyle, I am able to reap the benefits of my dedication and look forward to the challenges that lie ahead.

WHAT'S IN A NAME

During my senior year in high school, I was somewhat popular with the girls and had one friend in particular who use to flirt with me by feeling my biceps and calling me her "Strong Man." Sometimes between classes, she would see me walking in the hallways and shout, "Hello, Strong Man!" causing me to turn her way and smile back at her. She continued using her special nickname for me and eventually the title began to catch on with the rest of the student body. Since my physique looked the part and I was well-known for lifting heavy steel by my friends and classmates, I began to find myself being referred to as "Strong" more and more often. This suited my ego just fine and I let it go at that. Later in my senior year, I purchased some training booklets from Arnold Schwarzenegger. When the booklets arrived, I noticed that Arnold had changed his last name from Schwarzenegger to Strong. Suddenly, a surge of energy went through me like a bolt of lightning. Arnold was keenly using the surname *Strong* to better market himself to mainstream America. All those in my inner circle already knew me by that name, but like Arnold, I had bigger aspirations of fame and grandeur, so I created the name "Mario Strong." It seemed to make perfect sense to me, since I was already known by that name at school and in the local muscle scene.

It would not be until the late 1970s, during the days of my Staten Island Bodybuilding Club that my name would begin to reach those I had never met. At first, it was through reporters from *the Staten Island Advance,* who would occasionally come to my gym to write a story about one of my members or me. The newspaper would always quote me as "Mario Strong" and eventually I wrote articles for them under the pen name *Mario Strong.* I felt like Clark Kent, with two different identities, living two different lives. When I was in the gym, I was Mario Strong and when I was at home, I was just a mere mortal. In 1978, the name *Mario Strong* would become nationally recognized when I began writing for a syndicated bodybuilding magazine. Now I was directly reaching those who shared my same passion and before I knew it, I had stacks of fan mail piling up at my gym addressed to "Mario Strong." I sold t-shirts by the dozens and promoted physique shows under the *Strong* name. Every billboard, poster, or advertisement I created had the name "Mario Strong" boldly printed on it. The name became so popular that my gym was constantly being referred to as Mario Strong's, both by its members and the media.

Eventually, I changed the name of my gym from the Staten Island Bodybuilding Club to Mario Strong's, and began to live larger than life, as my name was everywhere. Every day, thousands of Staten Islanders would see the name *Mario Strong* as they drove by my gym. As thousands of cars drove by on the main road, a huge sign stared back at them. High on my gym's front exterior wall, the words MARIO STRONG'S were painted in Superman-type lettering. I was being marketed twenty-four hours a day, and everywhere I went on the Island, everyone knew me. Whether I was at the bank, at a store, or giving a guest performance, I was Mario Strong. The one down side to all this marketing was that I had very little privacy. I had marketed myself to such great popularity that even the old women feeding the pigeons at the local park knew me. Such is the price of stardom!

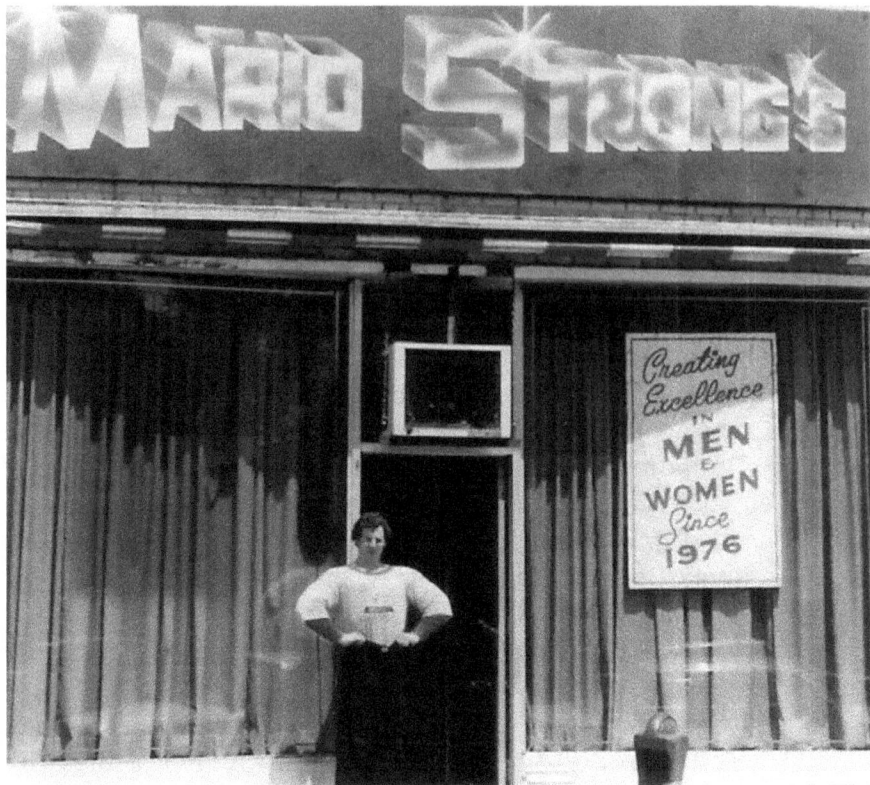
Mario Strong proudly stands in front of his bodybuilding club – 1985

In 1986, when I closed my gym's doors forever, I tried to resume a more normal life. It was not so easy. People still called me "Mario Strong" in and out of the physique world. I was branded for life with a title that evolved from high school to the present day, and to be honest, I am much more comfortable living the life of a superhuman. Mario Strong is the person who I really am. Deep inside me is a pure burning passion for health and longevity. My professional name has long been respected among my peers and has a record of accomplishment attached to it in the sport of natural bodybuilding. Bodybuilding is deep inside my blood and it energizes me every day. It is the power of Mario Strong that has prepared me for life's challenges and it is his heart that will lift me when I am knocked down. Thanks to a cute girl who once called me her "Strong Man," I have become someone who has been able to help many people in the fitness industry. I have a deep desire to correct some of what has been wrong in a sport with such great potential. As long as I can breathe, the name Mario Strong will stand for health, fitness, strength, and longevity.

LOOKING FORWARD

Although I continue to enjoy training at gyms, I have no desire to open another one any time in the near future. I also have no desire to be a personal trainer. I have been there and done that. If someone needs my advice, I will always be glad to offer it but as far as doing it for a living, well, I have better things to do with my time.

Today, after decades of bodybuilding, the fire in my heart for the iron still burns. Although my passion for the sport aspect of bodybuilding has simmered, my personal drive to excel at the gym still rages on. As the years go by, I see those I have known since childhood whither and age with each sun that sets. It is my goal to slow this process down within myself as much as possible. I remember as a child, looking out of my grammar school's class window and staring at the graves in the cemetery across the street. So many headstones, so many past lives, so much history gone forever. I remember vowing never to die and have my name carved into stone. Dying did not make sense to me back then and it still does not. It is a process that I am determined to deny for as long as I can. To me, the thought of dying always left me asking why. I know it is an inevitable end for every living thing, but hell, I am sure not going to make it easy for the Grim Reaper!

On my property in the Catskill Mountains, there is a cemetery with gravestones that date back to World War I. Some of the marble stones can barely be read because of the many seasons that have worn away the names of those buried there. It is a somber place, surrounded by nature. Above the graves live the animals and plants; the sky is blue, and the stars shine at night. Below the ground is the hand of death and eventually it comes knocking on everyone's door.

I come from a big family, and unfortunately, I have mourned at too many funerals. It is heartbreaking to see those you care about suffer from an illness and perish before their time. Especially, when you know deep in your heart, if they would have followed a different path in their lives, they might still be alive today. I know there are no guarantees, but when it comes to living a full and healthy life, I am not going to chance it away with poor habits. I am not a gambler and will do everything humanly possible to live as long and as well as I can. When I see the abuse others inflict upon themselves through their poor lifestyle habits, I just keep it to myself, because I know my words of advice will only be ignored. Human nature is what it is and to get someone to change his or her ways is next to impossible. If "beings" from another galaxy were ever to visit our little place in the solar system, they would take a look at the way most humans abuse their health and hightail it out of here faster than you could say "Scottie, beam me up."

For me, natural bodybuilding is a celebration of life; I meet every day with a smile. I truly enjoy the life I live. Life exhilarates me. I look forward to each and every day with happiness and take in the marvels of my world. To be a living entity in the vastness of our universe is such an honor that it calls for the highest efforts to be strong and live long.

I find natural bodybuilding more fulfilling and rewarding than anything I have ever accomplished. It is something that I live with twenty-four hours a day and look forward to continuing throughout the rest of my life. What is better than being so full of life that each day feels like a paradise? What greater feeling is there than to possess vibrant amounts of endless energy? What is better than knowing that you are on the correct path towards longevity? Nothing! Natural bodybuilding, through the scientific application of proper nutrition, exercise, rest, and positive thinking is the optimum way to living long and being strong...always.

It has been more than half a century since I first laid eyes on a barbell. The weight-plates that I once rolled around my home as a child have gradually evolved into tons of steel. For years, I have pushed and pulled these irons to transform my frail body into Herculean proportions. I cannot calculate how many reps, sets, and workouts I have pained through to bring me where I am today. I have spent so many hours, weeks, months, years, and decades doing seemingly torturous rituals at the gym that it amazes me how I lived through it all. I have trained with hundreds of bodybuilders in my lifetime and have learned something from each one of them. In return, I have also had the pleasure to teach thousands about what I learned as I continue to help those willing to listen. Bodybuilding has taken me throughout the United States, sometimes to support a student or friend and other times to be a participant in a physique event. Competing fiercely on the stage, I have enjoyed the big thrill of winning. I have also had the good fortune to meet some of the big names in bodybuilding. Some were well-known champions that inspired me throughout my muscle building career and others were the main players that helped shape the evolution of modern bodybuilding. There is so much good in this sport and I am thankful to have had the opportunity to be a part of it. Bodybuilding has been a way of life for me for as long as I can remember and wherever I go in the future, it will always be there as a reminder of what has transpired in my life.

I have experienced many sides within the sport. Unfortunately, some of it has been a dark cloud of lies and deception, serving the ugly greed of those who prey on the weak. But I know what is right and true in a sport with such great potential. I witnessed the impossible become reality, as those with burning dreams and desires pushed themselves beyond their normal limits to reach unimaginable heights of achievement. Because of bodybuilding, I tasted the love of many tender lips and shared many fun times. Bodybuilding has been a true journey, and it feels like just the beginning. I will continue to pursue my goals of health, strength, muscle, radiance, and longevity.

I train to live. I want to live for a long, long time to come. Natural bodybuilding is the means to this end. I want to be the strongest centurion that ever lived. I aim to climb mountains when I am well past a hundred. I want to surf the tropical waters of Waikiki Beach in 2055. I want to keep bodybuilding for the next 50 years... and I will! You are all invited to my 100th birthday celebration at the top of Diamond Head Crater on the Hawaiian Island of Oahu. See you there...Aloha!

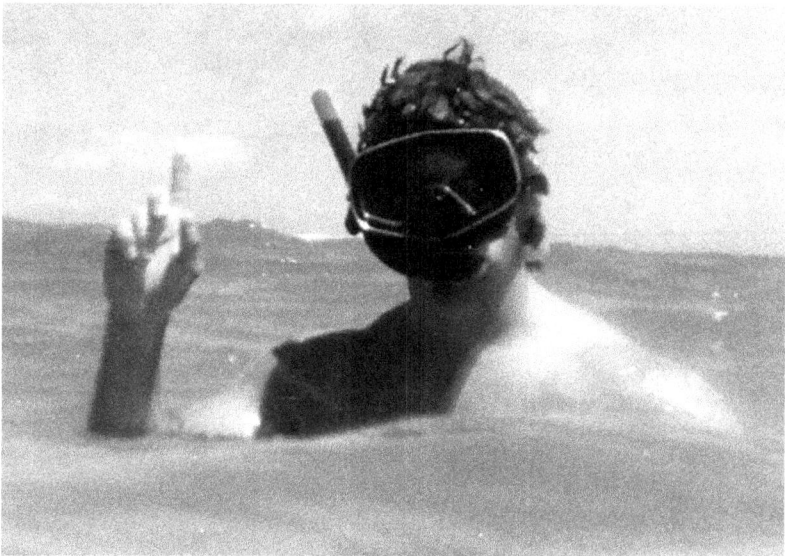

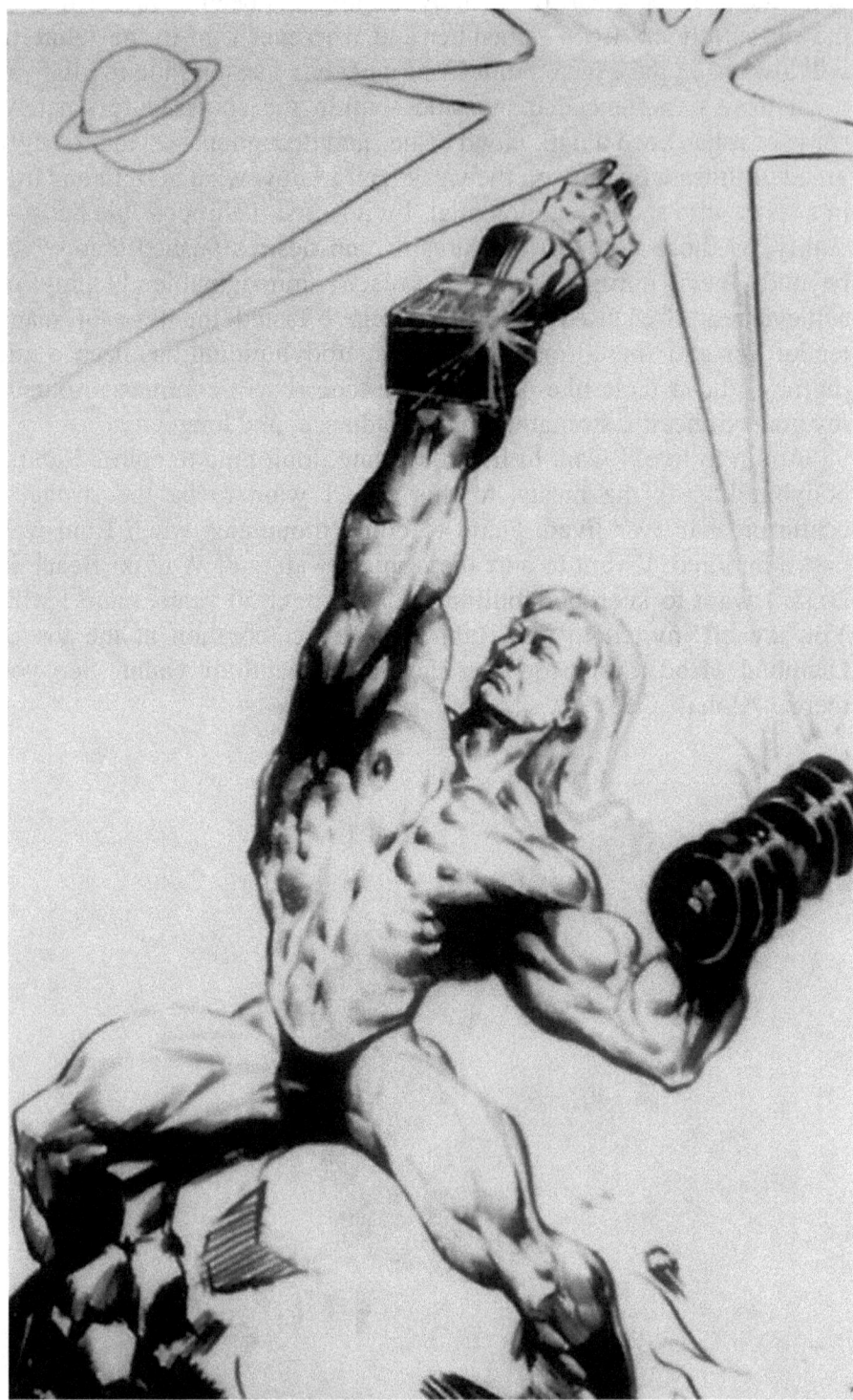

PART 2

JOURNEY TO THE OLYMPIAN ZONE

In a world where many men exist
Few stand alone
Chosen to go beyond
To stand up and challenge
What is right and what is wrong
To live life to its fullest
Destined to be
What they were meant to be
Natural Bodybuilders

INTRODUCTION

What is Man but the dust of the earth?
He is nothing more than a mere mortal that has evolved over the eons into a state of self-awareness while giving way to the disappearance of much of his natural instincts. Man, whose presence over the millenniums has changed the face of our world forever. Through his capabilities and ever-increasing knowledge, he has taken the human race out of its natural state and brought it to the point of no return. Man's genius and progression was supposed to make a better world for all. His talent and hunger to survive gave rise to civilizations whose peoples and cultures would coexist amongst each other, sometimes in harmony and sometimes at war. The evolution of humanity has been nothing less than extraordinary, both in the grandeur of its accomplishments and the disappointment of failures. Today, dreams of distant light years to come help propel humanity forward, while memories of the past vanish with the dead, leaving the search for its final destiny unknown.

Natural bodybuilders have the opportunity of a lifetime. In this 21st century, the latest state-of-the-art gyms and fitness centers are at their disposal. Decades of research and application in theories of exercise, physiology, nutrition, and healthy living have been documented into thousands of volumes for us to study and learn. Natural bodybuilders are the masters of their lives. Every day there are new opportunities to be bigger, stronger, and more vibrant than ever before. There are no limits. Welcome the challenges that stand before you now. By applying the advice you are about to read in this book to your life and by continually searching for your ultimate destiny, you, the natural bodybuilder, are on your *JOURNEY TO THE OLYMPIAN ZONE*!

NUTRITION AND THE BODYBUILDER

Planet Earth contains an abundance of food, thousands of farms, and millions of acres of natural wildlife. Earth's skies were once clear, and its waters were once pure. The knowledge, skills, and capabilities developed by humanity have gradually evolved and created an artificial environment not fit for any living being. From the air we breathe, to the foods we eat, and the water we drink, humanity has been slowly poisoning its future generations. The air we breathe is filled with biochemical combinations of pollutants such as sulfur oxides, hydrocarbons, toxic metals, and carbon dioxide. These and other pollutants find their way into our respiratory system, causing all kinds of havoc upon our health. They also add to the ever-increasing threat of global warming and may one day be partly responsible for the death of countless lives throughout our planet.

Our oceans, rivers, and lakes are becoming unsafe from the millions of tons of garbage we have dumped into them. From human waste to radioactive materials and hazardous toxic substances, these vast bodies of water have become ticking time bombs that potentially could one day kill most life below its surface. Because of pollutants from agricultural waste such as fertilizers and pesticides, our drinking water must be treated with chemicals such as chlorine, fluorine, phosphates, alum, sodium aluminates, soda ash, carbon, and lime to help purify it. However, questions have been raised as to the possible dangerous side effects of these substances. Will we ever learn?

America the plentiful! From the beaches of Waikiki to the shores of Staten Island, our nation is flourishing with an over abundant supply of food, resulting in over indulgence by the American consumer. Our country has tens of thousands of supermarkets, grocery stores, delis, restaurants, and fast food outlets to satisfy our taste buds, twenty-four hours a day, every day of the year.

Our nation's diet is loaded with tons of sugar, salt, artificial coloring, additives, preservatives, flavorings, emulsifying agents, stabilizers, and other artificial ingredients. Whatever happened to good old-fashioned wholesome meals? This country's health statistics show an ever-increasing danger. Illnesses such as cancer, heart disease, stroke, and high blood pressure are on the rise at an alarming rate. Is there a relationship between this civilization's diet and its poor health? You better believe it!

Many of our people live sedentary lives. Our high tech society has become a nation of couch potatoes whose major exertion is moving from the TV to the PC. Before our eyes, we are witnessing a culture emerging into bodily proportions never seen before. It is up to you, the individual, to get on the highway to health. As you travel along its path, you will learn about nutrition, exercise, rest, proper mental attitudes, and all the facets necessary for a healthy lifestyle. By applying these basic concepts of health into your lifestyle, you will become more in tune with nature and thus become more vibrant and positive about yourself and the world in which you live.

NUTRITION IS BODYBUILDING

Nutrition is bodybuilding! The foods you eat will not only help to determine how fast and strong your muscle tissues will replenish after a big workout, but more importantly, they will help to determine how healthy and long a life you may live. Since nutrition is of the utmost importance to the bodybuilder, it should be clearly understood, that to develop and maintain a muscular body, he or she, must be sure that all the essential nutrients, such as carbohydrates, fats, proteins, vitamins, minerals, and water are supplied and utilized in an adequate balance to help maintain optimal health and well being. If inadequate amounts of the essential nutrients are not provided for a period time, deficiencies may occur, resulting in poor – organ development, reproduction, growth, maintenance, health, working efficiency, and resistance to infection. This may lead to disease and the inability to repair injury and build muscle.

No single substance can maintain vibrant health. Although specific nutrients are known to be extremely important in the functions of certain body parts, they too are dependent upon the presence of other nutrients to function properly. Since our health is similar to a

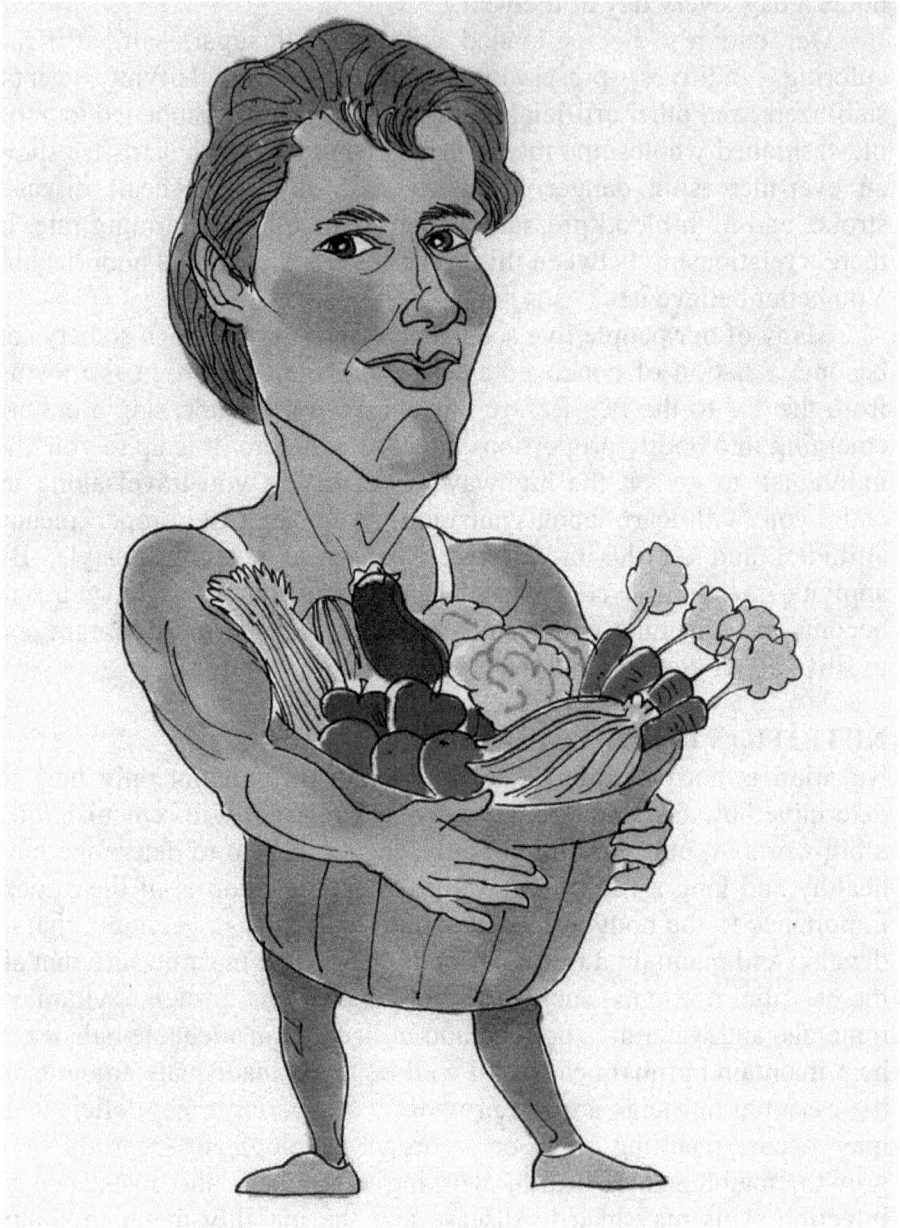

Whatever happened to getting one's nutritional needs from natural foods? Nature provides us with all the ingredients necessary for building and maintaining a muscular, strong, and healthy body. Whenever possible consume foods in their natural form; free of preservatives, additives, coloring agents, etc. Keeping your nutritional intake basic is the best way for lasting health.

puzzle, we should make every effort to acquire all the pieces needed to help maintain an adequate and balanced daily intake of all the necessary nutrients throughout life.

I can still remember the diets I use to read about in the old muscle magazines. Foodstuffs such as pasta, ice cream, cakes, cheeseburgers, and hero sandwiches were at the top of the list. Let us not forget the old protein malteds. A mixture of corn syrup, strawberry preserves, ice cream, honey, peanut butter, protein powders, and gallons of whole milk were among the ingredients. It's amazing how some bodybuilders didn't explode with all the gas created within their intestinal system.

I'm sure we have all seen bodybuilders with fantastic physiques that live on diets loaded with all kinds of junk foods. It is true they look good now, but how are they going to look in twenty years? After a while, their poor lifestyles are going to catch up with them. Chances are their health will become impaired as their vital systems experience various illnesses, causing their once mighty muscles to weaken and become nothing more than a shadow of their former selves. Bodybuilding's ultimate goal is to build a super strong body, glowing with radiance and sparked with health, and to create a positive attitude towards life. When planning your meals, remember you are not living to eat, but eating to live.

With this thought in mind, I myself follow a well-planned nutritional program, consisting of just the right amounts of all the essential nutrients. Through decades of endless research and natural living, I have brought my health to a state of near perfection. It did not come easy. I tried and experimented with many different food variations. As time went on, I eliminated more and more artificial foodstuffs from my diet. I bought and read dozens of books on nutrition and eventually my knowledge on the subject became paramount as I evolved into a living chemistry set, calculating my nutritional intake day by day.

UNDERSTANDING NUTRITION

It is important for bodybuilders to know and understand the many sources from which calories are obtained. Our primary sources of energy come from carbohydrates, fats, and proteins. These essential nutrients supply the fuel necessary for our bodies to produce energy and body heat. Their fuel potential is expressed in calories, a term that signifies the amount of chemical energy that may be released as heat when food is metabolized. Therefore, foods that are high in energy value are high in calories, while foods that are low in energy value are low in calories. Fats yield approximately nine calories per gram, and carbohydrates and proteins yield approximately four calories per gram. The natural bodybuilding lifestyle requires more calories in the diet than that of an average person. Natural bodybuilders also need sufficient calories, proteins, carbohydrates, fats, vitamins, and minerals each and every day to help regenerate muscle tissue after tearing it down through intense training. Let's look at these essential nutrients.

FATS

Having lived in America all my life I have come to some disturbing conclusions regarding its poor nutritional culture. It seems to me that the vast majority of people in our country are overweight. If you have not been following a well-balanced nutritional program and getting your quota of the required exercise for the past several years, chances are you are carrying an excess amount of body fat. Even a person who appears to be thin may still have unwanted bodyweight. You do not judge the amount of excess fat you have just by pinching the side of your belly. There is more to it than meets the eye. Internal fat accumulates in all kinds of places. Modern research has shown and proven that substantial amounts of excess fat can cause obesity, arteriolosclerosis, indigestion, and many other conditions. Now, before you decide to go on a nonfat diet, let me warn you, although it is unlikely to occur, a fat deficiency could also result in nutritional deficiencies.

The most concentrated source of energy available for a bodybuilder comes from fats. When oxidized, fats create more than twice the number of calories than carbohydrates or proteins do per gram. Fats act as carriers for the fat-soluble vitamins A, D, E, and K. They also play a major role by insulating and protecting our vital organs. Fat deposits surround, protect, and hold in place certain organs, such as the kidneys, heart, and liver. They act as insulators, preserving our body's heat from environmental temperature changes. Fat molecules are made up of simpler units called fatty acids. Fatty acids can be either saturated or unsaturated. Unsaturated fats can be either mono or polyunsaturated. In general, the more liquid the fat or oil, the more unsaturated it is. Unsaturated fat may decrease blood cholesterol just as saturated fat may increase it. It should be clear that fats are important to our lives as well as our workouts. Therefore, the last thing we want is a deficiency. Fats are an essential part of any nutritional program and to eliminate them from the diet would interfere with many normal bodily processes. A bodybuilder who trains intensely has to be particularly careful not to follow an extremely low-fat diet for an extended amount of time because this could prevent his or her body from burning subcutaneous fat stores. This is because the human body has developed a survival mechanism (base level) and it will stubbornly hold onto body fat if it senses inadequate amounts of fat in the diet.

The important thing is to receive our fats from natural sources. The reason a great majority of our country's population is overweight is its poor nutritional habits. As newborns, infants are weaned on milk so they may receive all their nutritional needs. It is true that healthy babies need mother's milk to help start them off right in life, but in my opinion, that is the only form of milk a healthy child needs. In this country, we have the habit of consuming cow milk. We drink hundreds of gallons of it every year. Milk from a cow can be extremely hard to digest; many people are lactose intolerant, which means they find it difficult to breakdown milk's simple sugars. Some are even allergic to casein, a byproduct of milk. Therefore, the intake of this substance can possibly do more harm than good. The way I see it, if cow milk were meant for human consumption, we would all be sucking on their udders. Personally, I have not had any milk since my teenage years. Today, I am well into my fifties, and look and feel as strong as I ever have. I have also never broken a bone in my body from lack of calcium. In fact, on rare occasion when I need to take an x-ray of an injured body part, the attending doctor would always notice the thickness of my bones. To me it is just common sense. Nevertheless, here we are in the 21st century and our society, both young and old alike, are still relying largely on cow milk as a source of protein.

Besides milk from cows, Americans consume all kinds of dangerous fats from various food items throughout their lives. Chicken skin, hot dogs, butters, burgers, and sweets, are some sources of unhealthy fats. Through time, we store up huge amounts of fats externally, but more importantly, internally. We build up excess amounts of fat not only because we eat tremendous amounts of them but also because we eat the wrong types. The body was made to handle natural foods, not artificial foodstuffs. By eating foods that were not made for human consumption we run the risk of serious medical issues. To avoid this, one has to follow a diet consisting mostly of natural foods in their raw state. The natural bodybuilder needs energy for workouts. Both strength and endurance are required to train at maximum levels. By eating natural foods in the form of nuts, seeds, beans, grains, and yellow vegetables, there's a better chance of sustaining energy force throughout the entire workout. When the proper balance of natural food is consumed and oxidized, its nutritional values are stored throughout the entire body in correct amounts. Mother Nature would not have it any other way. By applying the laws of nature to your diet, you'll come out a winner.

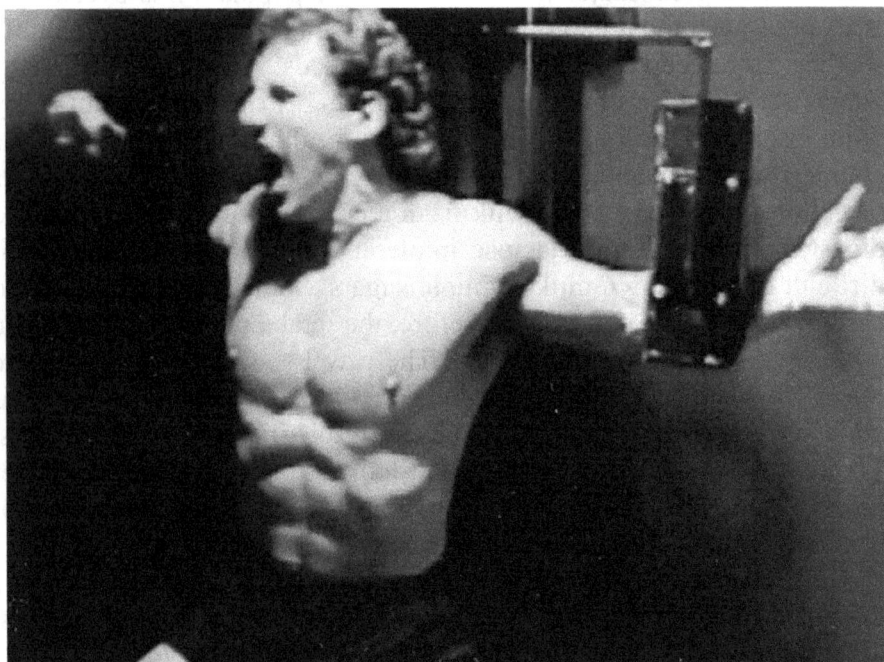

ACHIEVEMENT COMES TO THOSE THAT DARE THE PAIN DARE TO STRAIN AND DARE TO GAIN... NATURALLY

The following are some selected items for comparison:

AMOUNT	FOOD	CALORIES	FAT (g)
1 cup	whole milk	150	8
1	extra large egg	86	6
1 cup	egg whites	122	0
3 oz	salmon	121	5.50
3 oz	flounder	77	1
6 oz	tuna (in water)	200	1.40
3 oz	lobster meat	77	.80
4 oz	chicken breast	187	4
4 oz	turkey breast	214	8.50
4 oz	chicken thigh	237	12.25
3 oz	shrimp	90	1.50
1 oz	almonds	164	14.40
1 oz	brazil nuts	186	18.80
1 oz	peanuts	160	14.00
½ cup	filberts	396	36.80
½ cup	cashews	374	31.35
1 cup	oats	311	5.10
1 large	potato	159	.20
1 large	bagel	310	2.23
1 large	bran muffin	209	6.25

THE SKINNY ON TRANS FATTY ACIDS

Trans fatty acids are considered dangerous by many in the medical field because of their double-barrel impact on cholesterol levels, yet they are still widely consumed. Trans fatty acids are created when hydrogen is added to vegetable oil through a process called hydrogenation. Since they are more solid than oil and are less likely to spoil, trans fatty acids are used in foods to help give them a longer shelf life and have a less greasy feel. When trans fatty acids first reached the dinner table it was believed that they were a healthy alternative to animal fats because they are unsaturated and come primarily from plant oils. In 1990, scientists sent shock waves through the food industry when they concluded that trans fatty acids appeared to both increase LDL cholesterol and decrease HDL cholesterol levels. More studies over the years confirmed this. Commercial baked goods such as crackers, cookies, cakes, and many fried foods such as doughnuts and French fries may contain trans fatty acids. Shortenings and some margarine may also be high in trans fats. Trans fatty acids use was more common in the past, as food manufacturers have begun to use it less. Since early in the 21st century, manufacturers in the United States have been required to list the trans fat content on nutrition labels. Manufacturers in other countries have taken similar steps. As a result, more and more companies are now using little or no trans fat in the manufacturing process. In the United States, the labeling requirement has a caveat. Trans fatty acids that amount to less than 0.5 grams per serving are listed as 0 grams of trans fat on food labels. Even though that is a small amount of trans fat, if you eat multiple servings of foods with less than 0.5 grams of trans fatty acids, you could exceed recommended limits.

OMEGA-3 FATTY ACIDS

Omega-3 fatty acids are an essential nutrient for human health and must be obtained from food since the body cannot manufacture it. It is important for every bodybuilder to maintain an appropriate balance of omega-3 and omega-6 fatty acids in their nutritional plan as these two substances work together to promote health and vitality. Also known as polyunsaturated fatty acids, omega-3 and omega-6 fatty acids play important roles in brain function as well as normal growth and development.

There are three major types of omega-3 fatty acids that are nutritionally supplied and used by the body. They are alpha-linolenic acid (ALA), eicosapentaenoic acid (EPA), and docosahexaenoic acid (DHA). Once these nutrients are consumed, the body converts ALA to EPA and DHA, which are the two types of omega-3 fatty acids more readily used by the body. Studies have shown that omega-3 fatty acids help reduce inflammation and prevent certain chronic illnesses such as heart disease and arthritis. These two essential fatty acids are highly concentrated in the brain and appear to be particularly important for cognitive and behavioral function.

It is very important to maintain a balance between omega-3 and omega-6 fatty acids in the diet. Omega-3 fatty acids help reduce inflammation and most omega-6 fatty acids tend to promote inflammation. An incorrect balance of these essential fatty acids may contribute to the development of disease, while a proper balance helps maintain and even improve health. Researchers believe that a healthy diet should consist of roughly one omega-3 fatty acid to four omega-6 fatty acids. The average American diet tends to contain eleven to thirty times more omega-6 fatty acids than omega-3 fatty acids, and many in the medical field believe this imbalance is a significant factor in the rising rate of inflammatory disorders in the United States.

In contrast, a Mediterranean type diet consists of a healthier balance between omega-3 and omega-6 fatty acids. Many studies have shown that people who follow this type of nutritional program are less likely to develop heart disease. A Mediterranean type diet does not include much meat, which is high in omega-6 fatty acids and emphasizes foods rich in omega-3 fatty acids such as whole grains, avocados, soybeans, pumpkin seeds, walnuts, pistachios, fresh fruits, vegetables, fish, olive oil, dark leafy greens, and garlic.

CHOLESTEROL

Cholesterol is a soft, waxy substance found among the lipids (fats) in the bloodstream and in all the cells of your body. It is an important part of a healthy body because it is used to form cell membranes and some hormones. It is also vital for many bodily functions. Unfortunately, when cholesterol levels in the blood become too high they can present a major risk factor for coronary heart disease, which can eventually lead to a heart attack.

Cholesterol comes from two sources. Your body's liver naturally produces about 1,000 milligrams a day. The second source is animal products such as meats, poultry, fish, seafood, and various dairy products. Foods from plants, such as fruits, vegetables, grains, nuts, and seeds do not contain cholesterol. The main factor in causing cholesterol levels in blood to rise is fatty acids, which increases the risk of heart disease. Another factor is dietary cholesterol. The average man in this country consumes about 360 milligrams of cholesterol a day, the average woman consumes between 220 and 260 milligrams. Some of the excess dietary cholesterol is removed from the body through the liver. The remainder builds up in the walls of the arteries that feed the heart and brain, possibly resulting in a heart attack or stroke. Since cholesterol is present in all foods from animal sources, people with severe hypercholesterolemia may need to limit their consumption of meat, fish, poultry, etc. to no more than six ounces per day. In these cases, proteins from grains, beans, and nuts may be good substitutes for proteins derived from animal sources.

Since cholesterol and other fats cannot dissolve in blood, special carriers of lipids and proteins called lipoproteins must transport them to and from the cells. There are several kinds of lipoproteins, but the ones to be most concerned about are low-density lipoprotein (LDL) and high-density lipoprotein (HDL). Low-density lipoprotein is the major cholesterol carrier in the blood. A high amount of LDL cholesterol circulating in the blood can slowly build up within the walls of the arteries that feed the heart and brain. LDL cholesterol is often called the 'bad' cholesterol because a high level reflects an increased risk of heart disease. About one-third to one-fourth of blood cholesterol is carried by high-density lipoprotein. Some in the medical field believe that HDL carries cholesterol away from the arteries and back to the liver, where it is passed from the body. Experts also believe HDL removes excess cholesterol from atherosclerotic plaques and helps retard their growth. Since a high level of HDL seems to protect against heart attack, it is known as the 'good' cholesterol. The opposite is also true: a low HDL level indicates a greater risk.

Regular physical activity has been shown to affect blood cholesterol levels in people by increasing their HDL level. High HDL levels have been linked with decreased risk of heart disease. Physical activity helps to control bodyweight, diabetes, and high blood pressure. Exercise that uses oxygen to provide energy to our muscular system raises the heart and breathing rates. Such vigorous, regular physical activity as cycling, jogging, and swimming also condition your heart and lungs. Physical inactivity is as a major risk factor for heart disease. Even mild activities, if done daily, help reduce your risk.

DIETARY FIBER

Dietary fiber is the term used to describe several, soluble or insoluble, materials that make up the parts of plants your body cannot digest. Soluble fiber increases the diet quality and decreases the risk of cardiovascular disease when eaten regularly as part of a nutritional program low in saturated fat, trans fat, and cholesterol. It also reduces LDL cholesterol beyond levels achieved by a diet low in saturated fat, trans fatty acids, and cholesterol alone. Oats have the highest proportion of soluble fiber of any grain. Foods high in soluble fiber include oat bran, oatmeal, beans, peas, rice bran, barley, citrus fruits, strawberries, and apple pulp. Insoluble fiber may decrease cardiovascular disease in high-risk individuals. Foods high in insoluble fiber include whole-wheat breads, wheat cereals, wheat bran, rye, rice, barley, most other grains, cabbage, beets, carrots, Brussels sprouts, turnips, cauliflower, and apple skin. Dietary fiber may promote fullness by slowing gastric emptying, leading to an overall decrease in calorie intake.

TRIGLYCERIDES

Triglycerides are the chemical form in which most fat exists in food as well as in the body. They are also present in blood plasma and, in association with cholesterol, form the plasma lipids. When you eat, your body immediately uses some of the calories consumed for quick energy. Remaining calories are turned into triglycerides and stored in fat cells, regardless of what type (protein, fat, or carbohydrate) of food is consumed. If you regularly eat more calories than you burn, you may have high triglycerides and be at risk for heath disease. High triglyceride levels are associated with a condition called metabolic syndrome. Metabolic syndrome is the combination of high blood pressure, high blood sugar, too much fat around the waist, low HDL cholesterol, and high triglycerides. This syndrome does increase your risk for heart disease as well as for diabetes and stroke. Triglycerides are measured as part of a blood test that measures your cholesterol. Normal triglyceride levels are below 150, while high levels top 200.

BODY COMPOSITION

In today's ever-increasing world of obesity, a person's body composition in regards to their health and fitness is often questioned. One way of measuring a person's overall physical fitness is through his or her body composition. The others are cardiovascular endurance (fitness of the heart and lungs), muscular strength, and flexibility. The first two parts are linked with the risk of heart and blood vessel disease. Obesity is a major, independent risk factor for heart disease.

One test to determine a person's body composition is the Body Mass Index test (BMI). The Body Mass Index test is a mathematical calculation used to determine whether a person is overweight. BMI is calculated by dividing a person's bodyweight in pounds by their height in inches squared. The number can be misleading, however, for very muscular people, or for pregnant or lactating women. Being obese and being overweight are not the same condition. A BMI of 30 or more is considered obese and a BMI in the range of 25 to 29.9 is considered overweight.

BODY MASS INDEX FORMULA

Table 1 - Men
Prevalence of Medical Conditions

Medical Condition	Body Mass Index Range			
	18.5 to 24.9	25 to 29.9	30 to 34.9	≥ 40
	Prevalence Ratio Percentage			
Type 2 Diabetes	2.03	4.93	10.10	10.65
Coronary Heart Disease	8.84	9.60	16.01	13.97
High Blood Pressure	23.47	34.16	48.95	64.53
Osteoarthritis	2.59	4.55	4.66	10.04

Table 2 - Women
Prevalence of Medical Conditions

Medical Condition	Body Mass Index Range			
	18.5 to 24.9	25 to 29.9	30 to 34.9	≥ 40
	Prevalence Ratio Percentage			
Type 2 Diabetes	2.38	7.12	7.24	19.89
Coronary Heart Disease	6.87	11.13	12.56	19.22
High Blood Pressure	23.26	38.77	47.95	63.16
Osteoarthritis	5.22	8.51	9.94	17.19

CARBOHYDRATES

Carbohydrates are the body's main source of energy and are responsible for all bodily functions and muscular exertion. When a bodybuilder consumes carbohydrates, he is provided with immediate energy from the calories that are broken down when the carbon in his system combines with the oxygen in his blood. Carbohydrates provide bodybuilders with explosive strength. They also help power muscular contraction and fuel the central nervous system. Intense weight training is an anaerobic form of exercise that requires carbohydrates for explosive energy. Anaerobic exercise is relatively short in duration when compared to aerobic training, which is less intensive and requires more oxygen to fuel the workout. Anaerobic exercise works the muscular system to a greater degree and requires the glycogen derived from carbohydrates to fuel the body for dynamic workouts.

Carbohydrates are not only important for muscle size, but are also needed by the bodybuilder for the recovery and recuperation that takes place after a workout, when the muscles go through the processes of rebuilding and adding new mass. Aside from being a metabolic primer for fat metabolism, carbohydrates also spare protein from being synthesized into glucose. Monosaccharides, disaccharides, and polysaccharides are the three kinds of carbohydrates. Monosaccharides and disaccharides are also called simple sugars or simple carbohydrates, and polysaccharides are called complex carbohydrates. The simple sugars are fructose (fruit sugar), sucrose (table sugar), lactose (milk sugar) and maltose (grain sugar). Complex carbohydrates are starch, glycogen, and cellulose. Complex carbohydrate foods are also made up of sugar, but the sugar molecules are strung together to form longer, more complex chains. Complex carbohydrate sources also include fiber, which makes them more difficult for the body to breakdown and digest. As a result, the insulin response is not as dramatic, and the food is broken down more slowly. The slower digestion rate of the complex carbohydrate translates into less body fat. Regardless of the original form of a carbohydrate, the liver converts them into glucose, which is blood sugar. Some glucose is stored in the liver and muscles as glycogen, some is used as energy, and some is converted into fat.

As you can see, carbohydrates come in many forms. The bodybuilder who requires immediate energy before his workout might consider selecting foods that are loaded with simple sugars. Fruits such as oranges, pineapples, and bananas provide the explosive energy needed for intense workouts. Before every barbaric bombing session, I energize my body with natural carbohydrates, usually in the form of some fresh fruit eaten about 30 minutes before my workouts. This gives my bodily processes just enough time to produce the energy required for my Herculean bombing sessions.

At the gym, I begin my workouts slowly and increase the intensity as I go along. The more my blood pumps through my veins the more energy my body creates. I begin to feel as if I am a powerhouse stored with millions of electrical kilowatts. As the workout progresses my intensity increases more and more. After a short time, I am using poundage so monstrous that each repetition I perform feels like an atom bomb exploding inside of me. The carbohydrates I ate just a short while ago are now fueling my system with an optimum amount of energy. This energy is necessary for my intense weight training sessions. After my workouts, I usually refuel my body with complex carbohydrates in the form of rolled oats. The oats are a slow burning fuel that satisfies my sugar requirements while helping to keep my energy level burning steadily as my metabolism continues to burn at a high rate. Moreover, since I train at night I also benefit from their calming effect on my body, thus ensuring me a good night's sleep.

Eating several small meals throughout the day helps benefit the absorption of carbohydrates. Consuming too many carbohydrates at one time spikes the insulin levels in your bloodstream and causes the body to store the excess calories from carbohydrates as fat. In addition, eating complex carbohydrates that contains fiber throughout the day gradually replaces glycogen stores in the muscle cells, which in turn helps refuel the body's energy for the next training session. However, consuming too much complex carbohydrates will result in added fat to your body. As a health conscious bodybuilder, it is important to find the balance that works best for you.

Carbohydrates from fruits are very easily digested and readily available to the body, whereas carbohydrates from starches and cellulose need more time to be broken down. Starches such as those found in whole grains require prolonged enzymatic action in order to be broken down into simple sugars (glucose) for digestion. Cellulose, which can be found in the skins of fruits and vegetables, is largely indigestible and adds little energy value to the diet, although it is a good source of roughage material.

Carbohydrates from fabricated sources such as white sugar disrupt the natural functions of the body. As an example, when you consume white flour, white rice, and artificial sugar products, you run the risk of becoming deficient in the B-vitamins and other nutrients. To show how important that is, carbohydrate combustion may not take place if the B-vitamins are absent. This can result in all kinds of unwanted symptoms such as indigestion, heartburn, and nausea. A prolonged deficiency may lead to a loss of muscle tone, loss of energy, depression, and a breakdown of essential body proteins. It should be clear that bodybuilders must include generous amounts of natural carbohydrates in their diets, with the elimination of synthetic foodstuffs. This must be done if they are ever to realize optimum health in their lives. Nature provides us with all the essentials we need, it is up to each individual to take advantage of this offering.

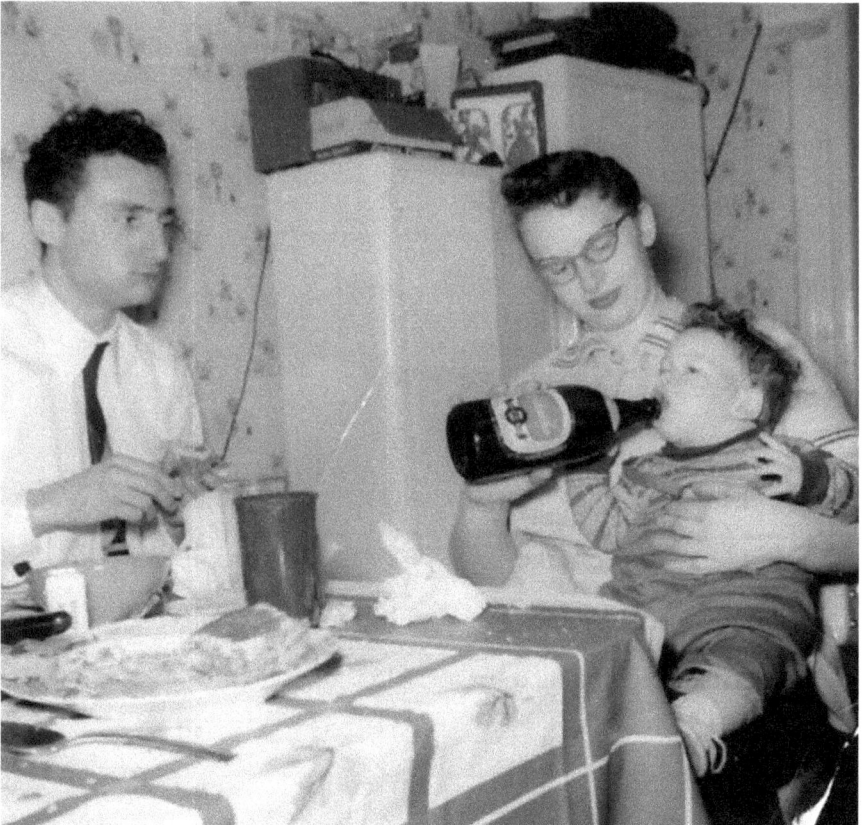

Mario Strong's parents help him carb-up for the workouts to come! - 1956

The following are some selected items for comparison:

AMOUNT	FOOD	CALORIES	CARBS (g)
1 cup	oats	311	54.27
1 large	potato	159	36.32
1 large	bagel	310	52.73
1 slice	wheat bread	70	12.93
1 large	bran muffin	209	37.06
4 oz	pasta - wheat	400	78
1 large	corn on cob	146	28.67
1 cup	beets	58	13
1 cup	brown rice	704	152
1 cup	spaghetti	155	32.2
2 oz	egg noodles	195	36.54
1 cup	broccoli	24	4.61
1 cup	tomato	31	6.91
8 oz	carrot juice	94	21.93
1 med	apple	81	21.05
1 med	pear	80	20.03
1	orange	62	15.40
1 cup	grapes	114	28.40
1 med	banana	125	38
½ cup	raisins	218	57.37

PROTEIN

Certainly, one of the most discussed and misunderstood topics in the field of nutrition is protein consumption as it relates to building muscle. Next to water, protein is the most plentiful nutrient in the body. It is an important element in the maintenance of good health and vitality and is our primary source for growth and development.

Protein is extremely important to the bodybuilder. When taken in the right form and amounts it serves as the building blocks for his muscles, blood, skin, hair, nails, and internal organs, including the heart and brain. Protein is needed for the formation of hormones, which control a variety of bodily functions such as growth, sexual development, and rate of metabolism. Bodily protein also helps prevent the blood and tissues from becoming too acid or too alkaline and helps regulate the body's water balance. Enzymes, substances necessary for basic life functions and antibodies that help fight foreign substances in the body, are also formed from protein.

Protein comes in many forms and is found in every cell in our bodies. Hormones, enzymes, structural and immune components, as well as muscle contractile molecules are all proteins. Amino acids are the building blocks from which protein molecules are constructed. Of the twenty amino acids, eight are called essential. Essential amino acids are called such, not because they are more important to life than the others, but because the body does not synthesize them, making it essential to include them in one's diet in order to obtain them. Eggs have all the essential amino acids. They are also high in the vitamins, A, B, D, E and choline. Lecithin, which is a natural emulsifier of cholesterol, is also found in eggs. Two other excellent sources of protein are fish and chicken. These, along with eggs, contain all the amino acids necessary for human survival.

As you can see, protein is a top priority for the bodybuilder, which leads us to understand why it is consumed in excess amounts. Since bodybuilding is a serious business, many athletes are sure to include plenty of protein in their diets to help guarantee continued gains. This is fine and should be the case, but somewhere along the way, things have gotten out of hand. Many muscle builders advocate eating extremely high amounts of protein to build muscle mass. I have seen two hundred pound bodybuilders consume anywhere from 2.0 to 3.0 grams of protein per pound of bodyweight on a daily basis. This equates to eating roughly between 400 to 600 grams of protein a day. Eating high amounts of protein does not guarantee muscle mass. It is not how much you eat that counts, but what you eat, digest, and assimilate. A natural bodybuilder cannot assimilate the large amounts of protein that a bodybuilder using steroids can. Excess protein will thus be removed as waste or stored as fat. A basic guideline for a natural bodybuilder in training is to consume between 1.0 to 1.25 grams of protein per pound of bodyweight daily, and to spread it out over several small meals throughout the day to help maximize muscle repair and growth. This is the same principle I have personally followed for decades and I find that it helps me maintain my muscle mass as well as my phenomenal strength. At times, when vacationing or just taking a break from training, I will lower my consumption of protein to less than one gram per pound of bodyweight. Calories, carbohydrates, and fats are also lowered, since my body needs less in the way of these nutrients to function normally.

Due to over exposure by the media, advertisements, and numerous articles written by the so-called champs, consuming large amounts of protein has become a daily habit for many athletes. It has come to be believed that daily intakes of large amounts of protein make the body's muscle mass grow at a faster rate. Actually, the opposite is true. Excess protein consumption may cause fluid imbalances and disrupt the body's functional systems, depriving us of our health and vitality. Excessive proteins are also stored as fat, since they are an inferior source of energy as compared to the carbohydrates and fats from foods.

The human body can only digest so much protein at any one sitting. Consuming 30 to 50 grams of protein at one meal is much more efficient than stuffing your body with 70 to 90 or more grams at a time. Learn what your protein requirements are and then design a diet for yourself that helps you realize the benefits of maximum protein absorption from several small meals throughout the day. Multiple small meals not only make it easier to consume the number of calories required to sustain and build muscle, but they also give your body the chance to absorb more nutrients with less chance of waste.

It would seem to me that the best source of protein comes from the egg. It is nature's most natural, complete, and balanced protein; packed with loads of vitamins, minerals, and fat emulsifiers. It even comes wrapped in its own shell, which holds and protects its vital nutrients safely. Next to the egg, chicken and fish are two other sources of high quality protein. If you feel that your body requires animal flesh to keep your health and muscle gains at an optimum, then chicken and fish are the protein sources to fill your needs. Beef products are questionable. As a protein source, beef is inferior when compared with the nutrition derived from eggs, chicken, and fish. Per pound, beef contains more uric acid than either of the aforementioned food sources. Uric acid is a leading cause of gout, a painfully serious illness that plagues many Americans.

Protein supplements are a big business in this country. Consumed by the ton every year, American athletes rely greatly on their nutritional value. While these supplements do work to some degree, questions have to be raised as to their need. Why is it that Americans use supplements at all? Why is it that our people are not educated on nutrition? Through my research, I have found that not only bodybuilders, but also athletes in all sports, feel that protein supplements are needed as insurance towards success. It has been nearly four decades since I last used any form of protein supplement. I solely rely on single ingredient natural foods for my protein requirements, and have enjoyed optimum strength and health, while maintaining my muscular mass well into my fifties. It is through the consumption of natural foods that our bodies experience lasting health and vitality. Why not give it a try?

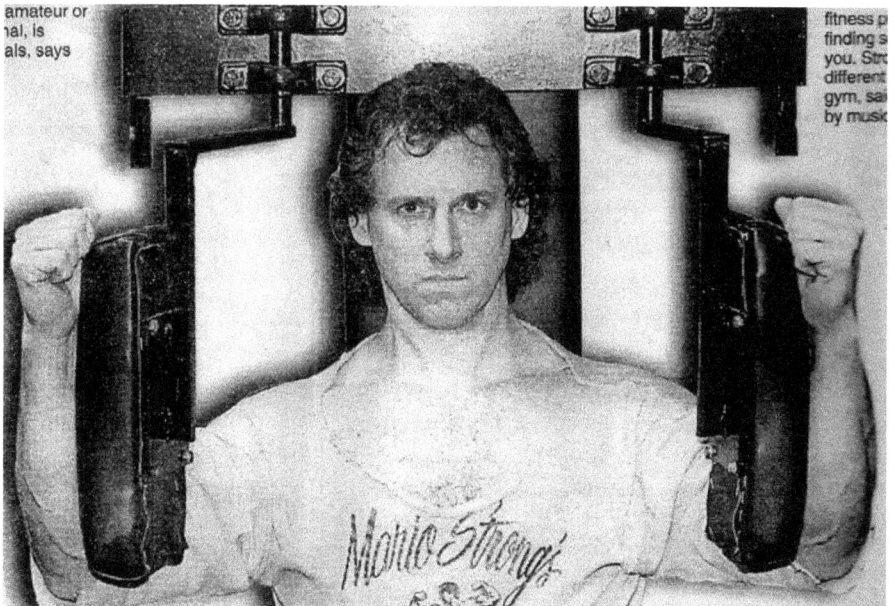
Mario Strong demonstrates an exercise for the Staten Island Advance - 1999

The following are some selected items for comparison:

AMOUNT	FOOD	CALORIES	PROTEIN (g)
1	extra large egg	86	7
1 cup	egg whites	122	25
3 oz	sea bass	82	16
3 oz	cod	75	15
3 oz	salmon	121	17
3 oz	flounder	77	16
6 oz	tuna in water	200	44
3 oz	lobster meat	77	16
3 oz	crab meat	87	17
4 oz	chicken breast	187	35.25
4 oz	turkey breast	214	32.50
4 oz	chicken thigh	237	29.50
1 oz	almonds	164	6
1 oz	peanuts	160	8
½ cup	filberts	396	11
¼ cup	walnuts	180	7
1 cup	wheat germ	414	27
1 cup	oats	311	12.96
1 cup	kidney beans	218	14.4
1/2 cup	lentils	140	16

VITAMINS AND MINERALS

Vitamins and minerals, or macronutrients, are consumed a great deal in supplement form. Like protein supplements, these do work to some degree. However, a healthy person need only rely on natural foods as the chief source of these important macronutrients. Still, there is a problem. Because of modern farming methods that destroy and devitalize many of our fruits and vegetables through soil exhaustion and over use of nitrogen and phosphorous fertilizers, our foods have become somewhat deficient in the vitamin and mineral substances we need. Therefore, vitamin and mineral supplements are useful when taken in correct amounts. They are also helpful because Americans cook so much of their food. Cooking alters the chemical properties of raw foods and reduces the efficiency of certain vitamins and minerals. I consume most of my vegetables raw, but when I desire to cook them, I will either boil or steam them for a short period of time so they do not lose much of their nutritious value. My goal is to eat foods as close to their natural state as possible and for the most part I am able to accomplish this.

When it comes to people's taste buds however, it's hard to understand how we became a society of fast-food junkies. Instead of enjoying fruits, which are a key source of vitamins and minerals, we as a society have chosen to voluntarily consume vast quantities of artificial sweets such as cakes, candies, ice-cream products, and similar foodstuffs known to cause health concerns, but yet, are found in great abundance in our country. These artificial sweets are one of the major causes of heart and bone disease; illnesses that could be prevented if people just consumed fruits such as bananas, oranges, and apples, instead of the poisons found on the grocer's shelves. Fruits also help to keep the body's colonic tract functioning properly. Their simple sugars are easily assimilated into the body's bloodstream, which in turns helps to keep a persons energy at an optimum level. Fruits are truly one of nature's pleasures.

VITAMINS

Natural vitamins are organic macronutrients, which are found in living things such as plants and animals. Less than twenty substances acting as vitamins in human nutrition have so far been discovered. Each of these vitamins is present in varying quantities in specific foods, and each is necessary for proper growth and maintenance of health. With a few exceptions, the body cannot synthesize vitamins; they must be supplied in the diet or in dietary supplements.

Vitamins and minerals are the guardians of our health. They are responsible for hundreds of functions in our bodies. Here is a brief list of some of the body parts they affect: Bones, eyes, hair, skin, tissues, teeth, liver, mouth, nerves, gastrointestinal tract, brain, nails, muscles, blood, kidneys, heart, tongue, glands, membranes, arteries, lymph, and circulatory systems.

BASIC VITAMIN GUIDE

Vitamin A / Beta Carotene
Biological Functions: Maintenance of healthy skin, eyes, bones, hair, and teeth. Beta Carotene is an antioxidant.
Sources: Eggs, Carrots, Squash, Broccoli, Green Leafy Vegetables, Pumpkin, Sweet Potatoes, Winter Squashes, Cantaloupe, Pink Grapefruit, Apricots, Broccoli, Spinach, and most dark green Leafy Vegetables.

Vitamin D
Biological Functions: Assists in the absorption and metabolism of calcium and phosphorus for strong bones and teeth.
Sources: Egg Yolks, Fish Oils, Exposure to sun enables the body to make its own Vitamin D.

Vitamin E
Biological Functions: Helps in the formation of red blood cells as an antioxidant, protects against abnormal breakdown of fats and vitamin A, and inhibits formation of nitrosamines (a suspected carcinogen).
Sources: Oils from Corn, Soybean, Vegetable and Cottonseed, Brown Rice, Nuts, Wheat Germ.

Vitamin K
Biological Functions: Needed for proper blood clotting.
Sources: Green Vegetables, Liver, also produced by intestinal bacteria.

Vitamin C

Biological Functions: As an antioxidant, inhibits nitrosamine formation, which is important for the maintenance of bones, teeth, collagen, blood vessels (capillaries), enhances iron absorption and red blood cell formation.

Sources: Citrus Fruits, Strawberries, Broccoli, Green Peppers, Red Berries, Kiwi, Tomatoes, Broccoli, Spinach.

Vitamin B-1 (Thiamine)

Biological Functions: Releases energy from carbohydrates needed for normal appetite and for functioning of nervous system.

Sources: Sunflower Seeds, whole and enriched Grains, dried Beans.

Vitamin B-2

Biological Functions: Releases energy from foods necessary for healthy skin and eyes.

Sources: Liver, Spinach, Mushrooms, Eggs, Legumes (peas, lentils), Nuts.

Vitamin B-3

Biological Functions: Releases energy from foods, aids in maintenance of skin, nervous system and proper mental functioning.

Sources: Mushrooms, Bran, Tuna, Chicken, Beef, Peanuts, enriched Grains.

Vitamin B-6

Biological Functions: Releases energy from food, plays a role in protein and fat metabolism, essential for function of red blood cells and hemoglobin synthesis.

Sources: Animal protein foods, Spinach, Broccoli, Bananas, Beans, Seeds, Nuts.

Vitamin B-12

Biological Functions: Prevents pernicious anemia, necessary for healthy nervous system, involved in synthesis of genetic material (DNA).

Sources: Found almost exclusively in animal products such as Fish, Poultry, Eggs, Chicken, and Red Meat.

Biotin
Biological Functions: Releases energy from food, plays a role in metabolism of amino acids.
Sources: Egg Yolks, Cauliflower, Peanut Butter.

Pantothenic Acid
Biological Functions: Releases energy from foods, involved in synthesis of acetylcholine, excitatory neurotransmitter needed for normal functioning of adrenal glands.
Sources: Liver, Kidney, Yeast, Egg Yolks, Broccoli. Fish, Shellfish, Chicken, Legumes, Mushrooms, Avocado, Sweet Potatoes.

Folic Acid
Biological Functions: Necessary for proper red blood cell formation, plays a part in the metabolism of fats, amino acids, DNA and RNA.
Sources: Green, leafy vegetables, Orange Juice, Organ Meats, Sprouts.

MINERALS
Minerals are organic and inorganic macronutrients that exist in the body and in food. Seventeen minerals are known to be essential in human nutrition. Minerals account for a very small percent of the human bodyweight, yet are extremely vital to overall mental and physical well-being of the individual. Every tissue and internal fluid in your body contains varying quantities of minerals. Minerals are constituents of the bones, feet, soft tissue, muscle, blood, and nerve cells. They are vital factors in maintaining physiological processes, strengthening skeletal structures, and preserving the vigor of the heart and brain, as well as all muscle and nerve systems. Our main source of vitamins and minerals comes from vegetables. Vegetables contain the very substances that guard our health against sickness, disease, and other illnesses.

BASIC MINERAL GUIDE
Calcium
Biological Functions: Builds strong bones and teeth, involved in nerve transmission, muscle contraction.
Sources: Broccoli, Turnip Greens, Collards, Kale, Mustard Greens, Almonds, Brazil Nuts.

Magnesium
Biological Functions: Needed in many enzyme systems, especially those involved with energy production, essential for proper heartbeat, nerve transmission, constituent of bones and teeth.
Sources: Spinach, Beef Greens, Broccoli, Popcorn, Cashews, Wheat Bran, Nuts, Seeds, Green Leafy Vegetables, Potatoes, Beans, Avocados, Bananas, Kiwi, Broccoli, Shrimp.

Phosphorus
Biological Functions: Maintains strong bones and teeth necessary for muscle and nerve function.
Sources: Chicken Breast, Lentils, Egg Yolks, Nuts.

Iron
Biological Functions: Prevents anemia, as constituent of hemoglobin, transports oxygen throughout body.
Sources: Liver, Lean Meats, Kidney Beans, enriched Bread, Raisins.

Iodine
Biological Functions: Needed for proper function of thyroid gland and production of thyroid hormones.
Sources: Cod, Sea Bass, Haddock, Perch. Other good sources are plants grown in iodine-rich soil.

Copper
Biological Functions: Essential for red blood cell formation, hemoglobin synthesis, involved in many enzyme systems.
Sources: The richest sources of copper in the diet are Liver and other Organ Meats, Seafood, Nuts, Seeds.

Zinc
Biological Functions: Component of insulin, required for blood sugar control, needed for proper taste and hearing, important in wound healing and enzyme activation.
Sources: Oysters, Shrimp, Crab, Beef, Turkey, Whole Grains, Peanuts, Beans.

Potassium
Biological Functions: Electrolyte needed to maintain fluid balance, proper heartbeat, and nerve transmission.
Sources: Peanuts, Bananas, Orange Juice, Green Beans, Mushrooms, Oranges, Broccoli, Sunflower Seeds.

Selenium
Biological Functions: Antioxidant, constituent of glutathione peroxidase, protects vitamin E.
Sources: Adequate amounts are found in Seafood, Kidney, Liver, and other meats. Grains and other Seeds contain varying amounts depending on the soil content.

Chromium
Biological Functions: As GTF, works with insulin to regulate blood sugar levels.
Sources: Beef, Liver, Eggs, Oysters, Wheat Germ, Green Peppers, Apples, Bananas, Spinach.

Manganese
Biological Functions: Cofactor in many enzyme systems including those involved in bone formation, energy production, and protein metabolism.
Sources: Whole Grains and Cereal products are the richest dietary sources. Adequate amounts are found in Fruits and Vegetables.

Molybdenum
Biological Functions: Required for proper growth and development, plays a role in fat and nucleic acid metabolism.
Sources: Beans, Cereals. The concentration in food varies depending on the environment in which the food was grown.

Boron
Biological Functions: Possibly plays a role in maintaining strong bones.
Sources: Boron occurs in all foods produced by plants.

ENZYMES

There are thousands of enzymes in the human body and each one is essential for life to be sustained. Our best source of enzymes comes from raw food and raw food extracts. Enzymes are found in every cell of every living creature and are the primary chemicals that activate every bodily function. During every second of your muscle building life, enzymes are at work. Throughout your day, enzymes are functioning to allow you to perform such simple tasks as breathing, seeing, tasting, smelling, and hearing. They are also responsible for renewing, maintaining, and protecting your health. Enzyme's proteins are produced by living organisms that consist of amino acids, and differ from other proteins because of the way they behave within the body. Enzymes are catalysts that make many essential biochemical reactions happen quickly and efficiently. Some chemical reactions would happen very slowly or not at all without enzymes. Only a small amount of enzymes is needed to make a big change in a bodybuilder. Every enzyme has a special function and works in a particular way. For example, metabolic enzymes are essential in facilitating reactions that build compounds from the body's raw materials. They are responsible for transporting elements, breaking down substances, and eliminating waste from the body.

When we eat, digestive enzymes are secreted by the salivary glands, stomach, pancreas, and small intestine so our bodies can absorb the nutrients. Every cell in our body is dependent on the raw materials provided by these enzymes. Digestive enzymes influence many health conditions. One important function is to transport nutrients throughout the body so our systems can make use of them. Every food source and nutritional supplement a bodybuilder consumes is worthless if it is not sufficiently broken down and absorbed by the body's systems. Metabolic enzymes are the laborers and assist in many biological and chemical reactions. They are also responsible for releasing the benefits of vitamins, minerals, proteins, and hormones. Some particular enzymes need certain vitamins and minerals in order to function. For example, magnesium participates in hundreds of enzyme reactions. This mineral, as well as other vitamins and minerals are known as co-enzymes. A co-enzyme gives an enzyme the three-dimensional structure it needs to create the active site required to perform its catalytic function. If a needed co-enzyme is not available, the enzyme will not function. Enzymes are found in food, your digestive system, and throughout your entire body. If you do not get or produce what your body requires, you will suffer poor health and put your life in danger.

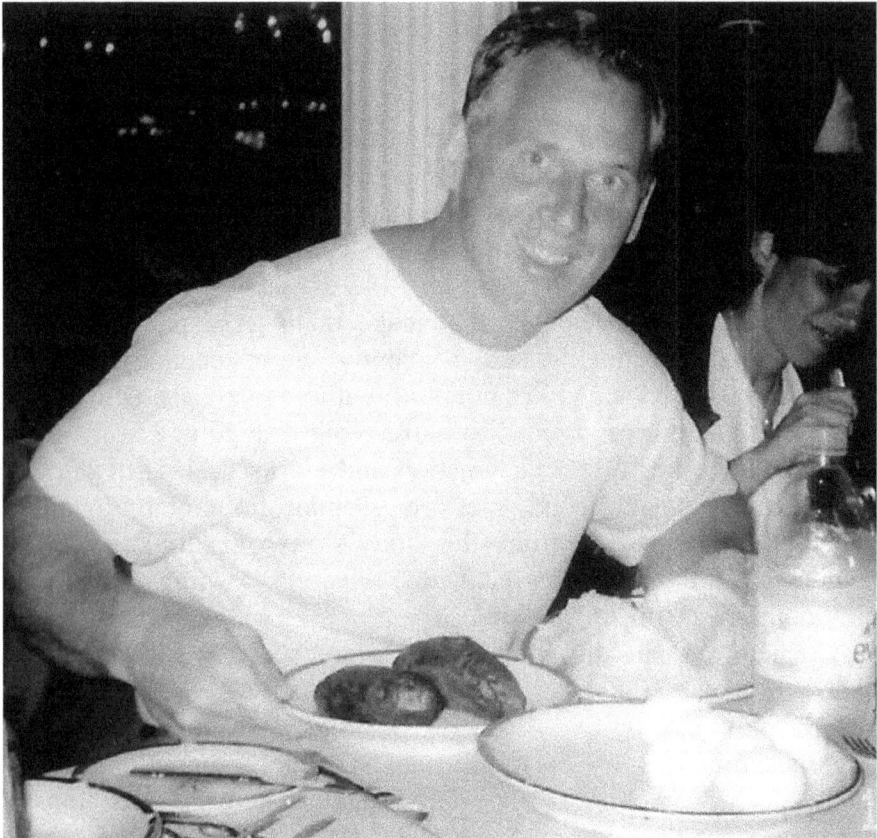
Mario Strong prepares for dinner while on a Caribbean cruise – 1999

WATER
When eating, I limit my consumption of water to just one glass so I do not wash away the acids, enzymes, and other digestive secretions needed for proper absorption of nutrients. If I want to drink a large quantity of water, I do so about an hour before or after my meals. Water enables chemical reactions to occur within the body. It is roughly two thirds of the body composition and is essential for life, as we cannot store it for long periods. Without water, crucial bodily functions such as respiration, digestion, assimilation, metabolism, elimination, waste removal, and temperature regulation could not occur. The digestive system releases important nutrients that are derived from raw materials through the breakdown of food by

enzymes. Water is essential in dissolving and transporting oxygen and mineral salts via the blood, lymph, and other bodily fluids. Water also helps keep the pressure, acidity, and composition of all chemical reactions in equilibrium. Only oxygen is more essential than water in sustaining the life of most organisms. In a moderate environment, humans can live around five weeks without protein, carbohydrate, and fat consumption, but just a few days without water. Water helps bodybuilders eliminate waste products, including the lactic acid produced by their intense weight training sessions. It is of paramount importance that you get your water from natural sources such as a mountain spring or underground well. Drinking sufficient quantities of water after heavy-duty workouts helps bodybuilders recuperate more quickly and reduces the time of post workout soreness.

You can become dehydrated without the proper amount of fluid in your body. Such a condition can result from not drinking enough water, or losing too much of it through perspiration. During exercise, your body temperature goes up and causes you to perspire, thus resulting in the loss of water and electrolytes from your body. Electrolytes are minerals such as sodium and potassium. It is important to replace water and electrolytes lost in perspiration during long exercise sessions. Even a moderate level of dehydration can hurt your performance in the gym and on the stage. To prevent dehydration, you should drink the proper amount of liquid before, during, and after physical exertion.

During intense training, it is a good idea to weigh yourself before and after the workout to see how much water you are actually losing through perspiration. If you find that a large amount of body water is lost, replace it immediately to prevent dehydration. Dehydration increases your risk for heat illness during hot weather. Stop exercising if you have signs or symptoms of heat illness. Signs to watch for include; dry feel to tongue and mouth, extreme thirst, pass little or no urine, eyes look sunken, wrinkled skin, dizziness, confusion, muscle cramps, nausea, vomiting, headache, fast heartbeat, and breathing. If you think you are dehydrating, rest in a cool place and drink liquids.

On the opposite side of the coin, some bodybuilders may drink too much water. A bodybuilder may feel tired, experience nausea, or get a headache if he drank too much water. Many times bodybuilders who drink too much water also have low levels of sodium in their blood. If a bodybuilder's blood levels of sodium are low, he may also become confused and feel light-headed.

FOOD COMBINING

The associations of foods that are compatible with each other in terms of digestive chemistry are referred to as food combining. Proper food combining is a basic rule for optimal nutrition because it allows the body to digest and utilize the nutrients in our foods to their full potential. Proper food combining is important to help ensure effective digestion, utilization, and assimilation of the nutrients in our diet. Since different food types vary in the way they are digested, it is imperative to understand the body's digestive chemistry as it relates to the principles of food combining. To avoid stressing the digestive system it is important to follow the basic physiological principles for eating foods in compatible combinations. Two of the most important factors in the science of food combining are what foods are eaten together and which are kept separate. This is because when two or more foods are eaten at the same time, and those foods require different digestive conditions, the digestive process may be somewhat compromised, possibly resulting in less nutrients being absorbed.

Acid and alkaline foods require different digestive enzymes to aid in the digestion process. A basic rule in chemistry is that when acid and alkaline foods come in contact, they neutralize each other and this slows down digestion. For example, if you eat a starch with a protein, digestion is likely to be disrupted. Protein foods require an acid medium such as hydrochloric acid for digestion. Carbohydrates such as starches and sugars require a more alkaline digestive medium, which is supplied initially in the mouth by the enzyme ptyalin. Fats also require an alkaline medium for proper digestion.

Various kinds of digestive disorders can occur from the undigested foods within your internal system. Such conditions may lead to bacteria fermenting and decomposing these materials. This situation often leads to indigestion, bloating, gas, abdominal discomfort, and poor absorption of nutrients. It also creates havoc on the nerves of the digestive tract by suspending their vital action and causing constipation. For example, simple sugars from fruit must wait until the slower digesting foods leave the stomach before they can be properly digested, a process that can take several hours. While waiting, the simple sugars undergo some decomposition and fermentation, which in turn produce gas, acid, alcohol, and indigestion. The discomforts of indigestion are so common in today's modern society that indigestion is almost considered normal. The statistic that Americans spend millions of dollars each year on antacids is clear proof of this fact.

During my high school days, I purchased *Food Combining Made Easy*, a book written by Dr. Herbert Shelton. In his book, Dr. Shelton outlined the following basic rules for proper food combining:

A. To avoid the indigestion and fermentation that acids can cause be sure to not consume them with starches at the same meal.

B. Protein foods require an acid base for proper digestion. Eat them and carbohydrates at separate meals.

C. Consume only one source of protein during a meal.

D. Since the acids of acid foods inhibit the secretion of the digestive acids required for protein digestion they should be eaten separately from protein. Protein that remains undigested putrefies in bacterial decomposition and produces some potent poisons.

E. Fats and proteins should be eaten at separate meals. Some foods, especially nuts, are over 50% fat and require hours for digestion.

F. Eat fruits and proteins at separate meals.

G. Avoid combining fruits and starches in the same meal. Since starches take longer to digest than fruits, they might hold up the digestion of these simple sugars and cause indigestion.

H. Eat melons alone. They do not go well with other foods.

I. Eliminate the desserts. Sugary foods require little digestion and ferment while waiting for other foods to be digested. A bacterium turns them into alcohols, vinegars, and acetic acids.

These rules helped to form some of the guidelines I followed when I began to experiment with food combining. In reality, bodybuilders can find the strict practice of proper food combining, as outlined above, nearly impossible. Even I have had to modify the rules to meet my current needs. Intensely training muscle builders need more than average amounts of calories and nutrients, not only to sustain their health but also to help guarantee further gains. However, as difficult as proper food combining may be for some bodybuilders, they still should make every effort to simplify their diets in order to minimize the chances of indigestion and discomfort. The important thing is to eat several small meals throughout the day so you can maximize the absorption of every muscle-building nutrient. The more efficient your digestive system becomes, the less food you will need to make your body run like a finely-tuned machine. Give proper food combining a chance and see how much better you look and feel.

ADDITIVES IN YOUR FOODS

For centuries, people have relied on food additives. Preservatives such as salt, sugar, and vinegar were among the first to be used. However, since the arrival of processed foods in the 1970s, there has been a massive explosion in the chemical adulteration of foods with additives. Considerable controversy has been associated with the potential side effects and possible benefits of food additives. Most food additives are considered safe. However, some are known to be carcinogenic or toxic. For the purposes of this book, let us look at two of the more popular food additives that are consumed by the average American each day.

SALT

Bodybuilders need salt for their physical systems to function properly. Sodium is the main component of the body's extra cellular fluids and it helps carry nutrients into the cells. Without sodium, the human body would not be able to regulate bodily functions such as blood pressure and fluid volume. Sodium also works on the lining of blood vessels to keep the pressure balance normal and it is one of the primary electrolytes in the body. All four cationic electrolytes, sodium, potassium, magnesium, and calcium as well as other vital minerals needed for optimal bodily function are found in salt. An imbalance of salt in the diet can lead to muscle cramps, dizziness, or even an electrolyte disturbance, which can cause severe and even fatal neurological problems. Drinking too much water with insufficient salt intake puts a person at risk of water intoxication or hyponatremia. Any excess amount of salt added to food, outside of what is contained in natural foods, may increase the risk of disease. Excess salt consumption has been linked to stomach cancer, hypertension, and cardiovascular disease. For optimal health, I believe that table salt should never be added to any food or meal. The famous DASH study found that Americans consume five to ten times more salt than they normally need and that high sodium levels over the years has a predictable effect on raising blood pressure. The National Research Council of the National Academy of Sciences in Washington, D.C., has determined that the recommended safe minimum daily amount is about 500 milligrams of sodium, with an upper limit of 2,400 milligrams. However, the council has stated that lowering the upper limit of sodium to 1,800 milligrams daily would probably be healthier.

Just because you don't have high blood pressure now doesn't mean that you will not develop it in the future. The last time I added table salt or any other forms of sodium to my foods was way back in 1969, the same year the New York Mets won their first World Series! That's quite a long time ago and yet, miraculously according to some health journals I've read, and contrary to what some doctors that I have conferred with believe (regarding the human body's need for additional salt outside of what nature provides in its foods), I am living proof that a healthy, normal man, does not need additional salt added to his diet. I train feverously, sweating away pounds of electrolytes each year, and my pulse, blood pressure, and health are perfect, with no medical problems pestering me. I think somebody better get back to the drawing board on this one.

SUGAR

Like salt, I have not consumed a gram of the sweet stuff since the great year of 1969. Before that time, I use to eat sweets and drink soft drinks. Along with the goodies came cavities and the occasional colds. It has been decades since I have consumed any sugary sweets and not only do I not miss them, but I am glad I rid them from my diet when I was a teenager. In large part, it is because of my sugar-free diet that I have not had a cavity in decades. Whenever I go to a dental office for a checkup the dentist says, "No problems as usual, Mario," and knowing me the way he does, tells me to come back in another five years.

Unfortunately, it is not the same for the average American, who consumes an astounding 2 to 3 pounds of sugar each week. This is not surprising considering that highly refined sugars in the forms of sucrose (table sugar), dextrose (corn sugar), and high-fructose corn syrup are being processed into so many foods such as bread, breakfast cereal, mayonnaise, peanut butter, ketchup, spaghetti sauce, and soft drinks. In the last twenty years, we have annually increased sugar consumption in the United States from 26 to 135 pounds of sugar per person! Prior to the turn of the 20th century, the average consumption was only 5 pounds per person per year! Cardiovascular disease and cancer was virtually unknown in the early 1900s, but not any more!

Sugar's Effects on the Immune System

A major problem with sugar is that it raises the body's insulin level. An influx of sugar into the bloodstream triggers the release of insulin, which the body uses to keep blood sugar at a constant and safe level.

As insulin rises, it inhibits the release of growth hormones, which in turn depresses the immune system. This can result in unwanted illnesses and disease. Insulin can also promote the storage of fat. This occurs when you eat sweets high in sugar, causing your body to gain weight rapidly and elevate triglyceride levels, both of which have been linked to cardiovascular disease. Complex carbohydrates tend to be absorbed more slowly, lessening the impact on blood sugar levels.

The health dangers associated with consuming too much sugar on a daily basis are well documented. Simple sugars are known to aggravate asthma and increase the possibilities of mood swings, personality changes, mental illness, nervous disorders, diabetes, heart disease, gallstones, hypertension, and arthritis. Refined sugars lack minerals and vitamins, therefore drawing upon the body's micronutrient in order to be metabolized into the system. When the body's micronutrient stores are depleted, the metabolism of both cholesterol and fatty acids are impeded. This can result in higher blood serum triglycerides and obesity, due to the higher fatty acids stored around organs and in sub-cutaneous tissue folds. Since table sugar is devoid of minerals, vitamins, fiber, and has such a deteriorating effect on the endocrine system, researchers and health organizations such as the American Dietetic Association agree that America's sugar consumption is one of the three major causes of degenerative disease.

INSULIN
Insulin is a vital hormone secreted by specific cells in the pancreas, which release it into your bloodstream every time you have a meal. After a meal, insulin stimulates the muscles to absorb the glucose surging through the bloodstream. An indication that you have more sugar than you need at that moment is when your body notices that the sugar level is elevated. This means that your body is not burning the sugar and therefore it is accumulating in your blood. At this moment, insulin is released to take that sugar and store it. All the glycogen stored in your liver and muscles cannot provide you with enough energy to last through one active day. Once your glycogen reserves are maximized, the remaining sugar is stored as body fat.

High levels of insulin have been associated with several medical problems, one of which is high blood pressure. A main function of insulin is to assist with the storing of excess nutrients. As an example, insulin plays a role in storing magnesium, which is an intra-cellular mineral that relaxes muscles. However, if your cells become resistant to insulin, you will not be able to store magnesium and you will excrete it through urination, thus causing blood vessels to constrict and blood pressure to rise. Many anabolic hormones such as growth hormones, testosterone, and progesterone are controlled by insulin, which is a master hormone. In insulin resistance, the anabolic process is reduced. Bone is built upon the command of such hormones. When these hormones are reduced, the amount of bone building is reduced, and the amount of calcium excreted is increased.

An interesting tool to measure how a given food affects the blood-glucose levels of another food is the Glycemic Index. The Glycemic Index assigns each food a number rating. The lower the rating, the slower the absorption and digestion process, which provides a more gradual, healthier infusion of sugars into the bloodstream. A high rating means that blood-glucose levels are increased quickly, which stimulates the pancreas to secrete insulin to drop blood-sugar levels. The stress placed on the body because of this rapid fluctuation in blood-sugar levels can be dangerous to your health.

Many in the medical field believe that an increasing number of bodybuilders are putting themselves at risk by injecting themselves with insulin. Medically, diabetics take insulin to help control their blood sugar levels. It is also highly effective in helping bodybuilders build muscle mass. However, this practice has proven to be detrimental for some non-diabetics. Careless use of this drug can drop a bodybuilder's blood sugar to levels where his brain is deprived of oxygen, causing severe cerebrum damage, coma, or even death. Over a period of time, the ill-taken insulin could cause irreversible damage. As a result, healthy bodybuilders, who take insulin for muscle building purposes, could end up becoming diabetic themselves as their body's natural mechanism for producing the hormone stops working properly. This is a dangerous practice that bodybuilders and anyone in training should avoid.

GO ORGANIC
The last few decades have witnessed an enormous concern over chemicals being used on fruits, vegetables, seeds, and grains. It is estimated that, worldwide, the agricultural chemical industry is producing about 50,000 different pesticides based on approximately 600 active ingredients. For example, cereal crops receive several applications of chemicals between the times when they are planted and eaten. It is also not unusual for fruit and vegetables to be sprayed

several times before being consumed. The classes of pesticides used include Insecticides, Herbicides, Rodentcides, and Fungicides. Some pesticides are carcinogenic in nature and may be responsible for a host of illnesses ranging from impotency and birth defects to mutated genes and cancer. Another problem with the use of pesticides is that their residues find their way into our rivers, streams, and oceans, eventually being consumed from the livestock taken from these waters. Organically grown foods are grown without pesticides and artificial fertilizers. They are grown in soil whose humus content is increased with applications of natural mineral fertilizers and has not been treated with preservatives, hormones, antibiotics, etc. In reality, it is difficult to avoid pesticides in the diet. If humankind is to survive, we need to reverse the destruction of the planet on which we live and reclaim our health. The choices we make as consumers not only affect our health today, but more importantly, will have a profound impact on the health of future generations.

OBESITY

The World Health Organization considers the problem of overweight and obesity as a matter of priority. Since 1960, the number of overweight and obese Americans has grown on an annual basis to today, where nearly 65 percent of adult Americans (about 127 million) are now categorized as being overweight or obese. Each year, obesity is believed to be responsible for at least 300,000 deaths in the United States, while the healthcare cost of treating such a serious condition has risen to approximately $100 billion.

Our bodies are made up of water, protein, carbohydrate, fat, vitamins, and minerals. If we have an excess amount of body fat we are considered obese, especially if the fat is stored in the waist area, which makes us vulnerable to various health issues including; high blood pressure, high blood cholesterol, diabetes, coronary heart disease, and stroke. Coronary heart disease is a leading cause of heart attacks. Aside from increasing the risk of heart disease and harming the heart and blood vessel system, obesity is also a major cause of gallstones and can worsen degenerative joint disease. One simple fact as to the cause of obesity is that many people eat too many excess calories. In other words, they are consuming more calories than they are expending and the surplus is being stored as fat. Another factor in heart disease is the excess consumption of saturated fats and cholesterol in the diet. This practice has been shown to raise blood cholesterol levels.

For example:
A. Obesity raises blood cholesterol and triglyceride levels.
B. Obesity lowers HDL (good) cholesterol. HDL cholesterol is linked with lower heart disease and stroke risk, so reducing it tends to raise the risk.
C. Obesity raises blood pressure levels.
D. Obesity can induce diabetes. In some people, diabetes makes these other risk factors much worse. The danger of heart attack is especially high for these people.

Obesity and the Sexes

The sedentary and overindulging lifestyle of the average American is the main factor why this country has become a nation of the obese. A recent study followed the physical conditioning progress of dozens of severely obese men and women. The researchers wanted to learn the effects of physical exercise on the participants, who had body mass indexes (BMI) of at least 40. They found that the obese women had better fitness levels than the obese men. They also learned that the obese men were not able to process carbohydrates as efficiently and were less physically fit than their female counterparts. As a result, they had less physical endurance. Furthermore, while an obese person is already at an increased risk of developing diabetes, the combination of being obese and unfit meant that the male participants were at an even greater risk of developing diabetes than the female participants. The researchers believe that the results may be explained by the way in which fat is distributed throughout the body. In men, fat tends to be stored in the upper half of the body, while in women; it is stored in the lower half. This is because women are better equipped for energy storage due to their inherent need to feed their offspring. When food is abundant, such as in our modern society, both genders may become obese, but men simply do not have the reserve capacity to handle excess food, which puts extra stress on their bodies, causing decreased performance and possible illness.

Health Effects of Obesity

Persons with obesity are at risk of developing serious medical conditions, which can result in poor health and premature death. Obesity is associated with more than 30 medical conditions, and scientific evidence has established a strong relationship with at least 15 of those conditions. Preliminary data also shows the impact of obesity on various other conditions. Overweight persons losing ten percent bodyweight can help reduce the risk of some obesity-related medical conditions like diabetes and hypertension.

The following are medical conditions related to obesity:
Osteoarthritis, Rheumatoid Arthritis, Birth Defects, Body and Musculoskeletal Pain, Breast Cancer, Cancer of the Esophagus and Gastric Cardia, Carpal Tunnel Syndrome, Colorectal Cancer, Endometrial Cancer, Renal Cell Cancer, Cardiovascular Disease, Deep Vein Thrombosis, Diabetes, End Stage Renal Disease, Gallbladder Disease, Gout, Hypertension, Impaired Immune Response, Impaired Respiratory Function, Infection Following Wounds, Infertility, Liver Disease, Low Back Pain, Obstetric and Gynecologic, Complications, Pancreatitis, Sleep Apnea, Stroke, and Urinary Stress Incontinence.

Final Thoughts on Nutrition

No matter who you are, what you do, or what your goals may be, you can always do it better with nature. Nature provides us with all the nutritious substances we need to manufacture our bodies into Herculean form. When planning your nutritional program, stay as close to nature as possible to help ensure maximum gains in muscle, fitness, health, strength, and vitality. Remember, if we stuff ourselves with all kinds of manufactured foods, we not only run the risk of impairing our muscular growth, but also depleting our body of its natural reserves of health. While we are building a championship physique, we are also building long lasting health. It is possible and actually easy to stay in shape all your years. All you need do is apply an intelligent, well-planned, instinctive, natural bodybuilding program to your life.

With proper nutrition to fuel your starship, you, the natural bodybuilder, are on your *JOURNEY TO THE OLYMPIAN ZONE*!

MIND INTO MUSCLE

THE TRIUMPH OF THE MAN WHO ACTS

Our society is filled with couch potatoes that spend their evenings watching meaningless shows on their plasma TVs. We have become a nation of remote controls, joysticks, and keyboards. While some entertainment is welcome, for many it has become the only form of stimulation they receive throughout the day. I say, "It's time to pull the plug and get motivated in becoming a better you, both physically and mentally." By following a natural bodybuilding program, you cannot help but look better and feel stronger. Training with resistant type exercises is the best way in achieving a sculpt physique that will set you apart. As you train through the weeks, months, and years, you will find yourself becoming more confident as your attitude towards life becomes increasingly positive.

Because we are athletes, our mental attitude plays a large role in the outcome of our success. The more positive a thinker you are, the better your chances of realizing your goals. Before a bodybuilder can ever begin to plan his or her exercise routine, they must first have the proper mental attitude towards their training and life in general. Every bodybuilder should look towards their workouts with renewed enthusiasm for maximum gains. Too many men dread the thought of lifting weights and psyche themselves out even before they touch a barbell. In order for your dreams to be realized, you must learn to conquer your fears and believe that you can accomplish anything you desire. Let us look at how this is done.

PROCRASTINATION

What a strange word. Its letters are many, but its meaning amounts to very little. Those who procrastinate often find themselves falling behind with their lives, sinking deeper in despair with each new sun that sets. In these busy times, it's easy and more often desirable to delay things that require some effort in exchange for ones that are simpler and more enjoyable to do. However, eventually time runs out and you find yourself with a much bigger problem to solve.

Sadly, many of us suffer because we often procrastinate with our health. How often have you made plans to quit smoking, or start exercising; maybe even improve your diet, just to put it off for another day? Probably, more often than you realize. All the knowledge and tools in the world are useless if they are not put to proper use. Every new day arrives with new opportunities. So, why not make the best of it? Starting right now!

Make this day the most important day of your life and stop procrastinating! Take a good look in the mirror and see if you like what you see. If you do, more power to you. Nevertheless, chances are you will only be fooling yourself. No one is perfect! We all have our faults and realizing them is the first step towards a new you. Americans have many reasons to be thankful. Throughout our land, we have some of the most advanced health related facilities in the world that are ready and able to meet the medical demands of our stressful times. In just about every county, you will also find a health food store stacked with natural foods, supplement products, and informative materials that can help you improve your health. The Internet has also become popular with the fitness minded individuals seeking knowledge on nutrition and exercise. My very own Web site, MarioStrong.com, is loaded with tons of advice, ranging from weight loss to muscle building, and calorie charts to strength training. Be sure to check it all out. As our society and world evolve, we all must learn to adapt to the changes. Keeping up with the latest technology and advances of the 21st century will help raise our nation's health to optimum levels.

Another evolution has taken place in this country. Throughout this great land, you can find several fitness centers in just about any town or city. Unlike the beginning of the last century, these well equipped, state-of-the-art training centers are popular with today's generation and are designed for maximum gains in the shortest time possible. From the early days of physical culture, where muscle display was a show attraction, to modern day bodybuilding, where the fitness industry has grown into a billion dollar business, those that have made fitness a priority in their lives have benefitted in a big way. In today's society just about everyone – from teenage athletes to never-say-die grandparents – are getting in on the fitness revolution.

Aside of this revolution, a battle has been raging between the true natural bodybuilding athletes and the android freaks who risk their health for a few pounds of muscle and some cheap glory. It is important that you not be swayed down the wrong path, for you could easily find yourself at a permanent dead end, where so many other bodybuilders have found themselves.

BE SMART

As important as nutrition and exercise are to our health, so to is the factor of unhealthy habits. For example, smoking is a leading cause of many illnesses including heart disease, cancer, and emphysema; yet millions of Americans practice this stupid habit daily. If only they would stop, how much better they would feel. Unfortunately, smoking is just one of the many unhealthy habits practiced daily by many of our neighbors, friends, and family members. Such bad habits have sent the cost of medical care soaring, while depleting the health of our country to an alarming level. If we are to survive as a nation, we must learn to focus on the big picture while we still have a chance.

Read, listen, and learn. There are many facts and theories on health related topics going around these days and it is up to each individual to find out what works best for themselves. Several ways to educate yourself about exercise and nutrition are to read as much fitness oriented material as possible. Try to grasp onto what each piece of literature offers. Take notes as if you were in school; draw some conclusions of your own. Learn to listen to those who are knowledgeable in the field of physical culture and apply what you believe will work best for you and your lifestyle.

Also learn from your mistakes. In my twenties, I use to tan quite frequently. Although I enjoyed my time at the beach, it didn't compensate for the severe sunburns I would occasionally experience. The burns were so bad that I couldn't sleep with sheets at night, but nevertheless, when it came time for my morning workout I was at the gym to give it my all, no matter how much suffering I pained through. Eventually, I got smart and reduced my exposure to the sun. This bit of common sense thinking applies to everything we do in life.

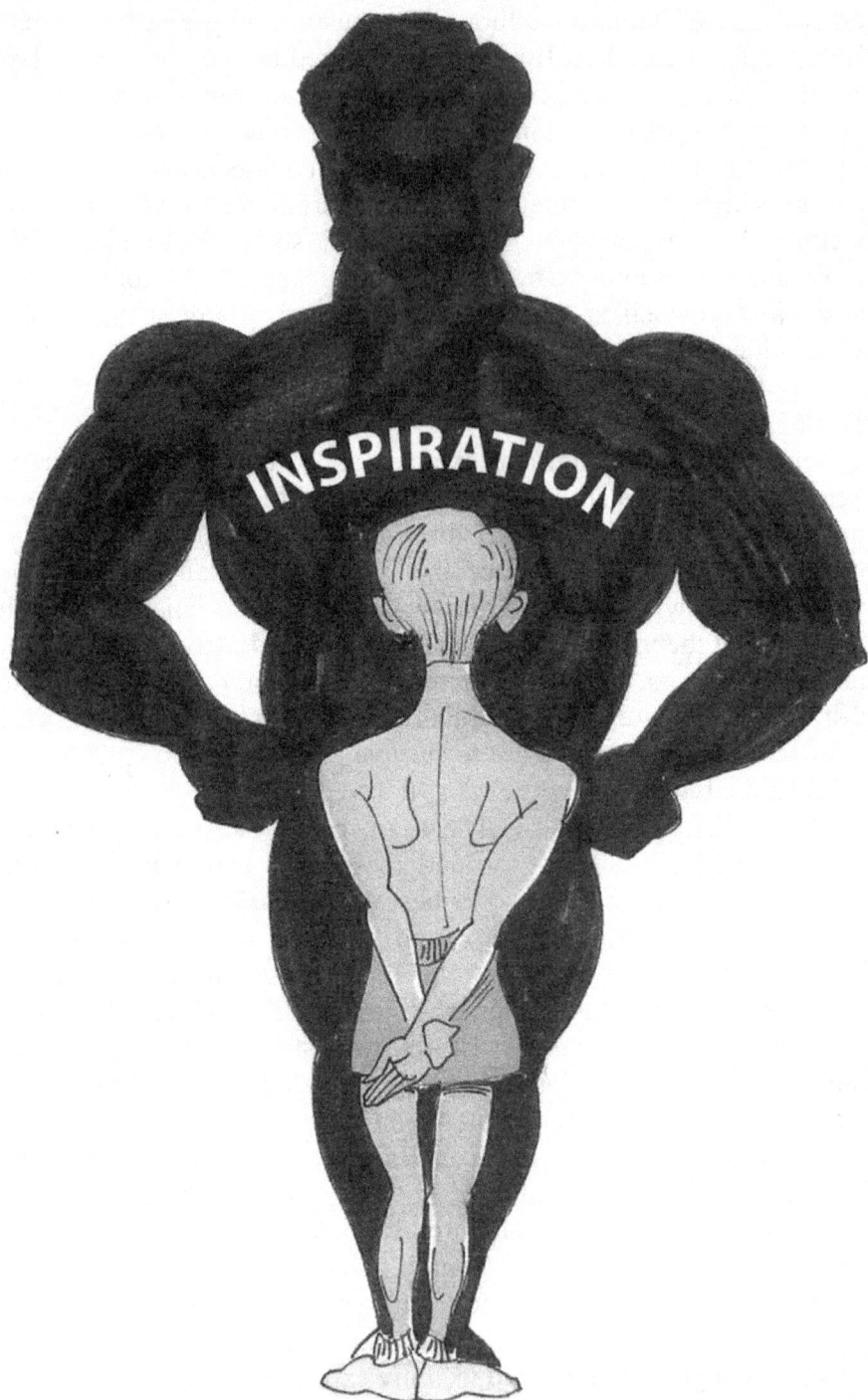

Believe that you can achieve your goals

VISUALIZE

Setting a goal is the first step towards a new you. Believe in your ability to make your dreams a reality. Visualize yourself with slabs of new muscle throughout your body and create a plan of action to accomplish this. Make a mental note of what you desire and go forward with your plan. When I train, I visualize myself as having endless power and mass. For example, when maxing out on a set of Full Squats, I will tell myself the weight on the barbell is puny when compared to what some world powerlifting champions have done. This brings my ego into play, which in turn pushes me to break my previous records. In my mind, if they can do it so can I, and soon I find myself reaching higher levels of power. The same principle applies when I am training to increase muscle mass. As an example, when performing the Barbell Curl, I will imagine my arms expanding as blood gorges into them. I mentally visualize my biceps becoming the size of softballs, with high mountainous peaks, flowing with streams of rippling muscle pouring down their sides. Remember, it is a simple game of mind over muscle, and when you conquer the act of visualization, you will realize gains in both size and strength you never thought possible before.

HAVE PATIENCE

When applying a new exercise or nutritional idea to your bodybuilding lifestyle give it time to see if it works for you. Sometimes great results take a bit of time and jumping ahead of the effort may make you miss a potential gain. Most importantly, never be satisfied and always strive to improve yourself a little bit more each and every day. Patience is a great virtue when striving towards any worthy goal. It takes time to become what your dreams are made of, and it is important to take each new day as it comes. Wanting everything to happen overnight will only result in disappointment and anguish. Let the flame of desire burn strong, but watch closely or it may burn out of control, stopping you in your tracks long before you realize the results you seek. Be thankful for what you have and give each new day a little bit extra. Before you know it, you will have climbed the mountain. Remember, time has no limits and neither shall you.

DON'T OVERWORK

Overwork is one of the bodybuilder's biggest mistakes. I have seen hundreds of bodybuilders mistakenly increase the workload in their training routines until they reached the point where their gains stopped coming and actually began to diminish, all because they were burning themselves out in the gym. Instead of cutting back on their training, these overzealous bodybuilders would continue to keep it up at the same pace for fear that if they were to shorten their workouts by even one set, they would be cheating themselves out of the gains they so readily deserve. Sometimes we need to sit back and rationalize our training philosophy. For most of us, eliminating an exercise or reducing the workload may not seem to make sense. However, what really counts is the muscle gains that we pour gallons of sweat for, each day at the gym. To get big and strong you must train smart. Advanced bodybuilders know this and perform just the right amount of work to stimulate their physiques, before they leave the gym for the day. Learn through trial and error how much training is best for you and be consistent in your efforts.

When you learn to train correctly, your workouts will produce more results, which in turn will give you energy that is more physical and create a mental desire rich in enthusiasm and motivation. Desire is important to the bodybuilder as it helps him create a positive attitude towards his training and goals. The stronger the desire, the better equipped the bodybuilder will become with knowledge in his chosen field. In his mind, he visualizes himself improving day by day. He envisions his legs becoming powerful, his torso becoming massive, his waist cubing, and his arms enlarging. He cannot wait to get to the gym and start the workout. He is burning with desire and his gains are going to show it.

I remember when I first began to train. My father put me on an exercise program that I followed religiously. I would workout three times a week on alternate days. Monday, Wednesday, and Friday were my training days. The other days I would rest and grow. By resting a full day between workouts my muscles would fully replenish as I burned with desire to return to the gym. Every workout day, before I hit the weights, I would check my physique in the mirror, just to see what kinds of improvements I had made since my last bombing session. Each individual training day my enthusiasm would soar to the stars. There was always some kind of noticeable improvement. One day it might have been my arms, another day my legs, sometimes it was everything. My motivation and desire grew quite strong from this. Every workout became an all out effort. It was like setting off a chain reaction inside of me. I improved day by day and it was great!

MOTIVATION

Today's novice bodybuilders need to be continuously motivated. With all the mass monsters around these days, it is easy for beginners to become discouraged and quit. A great way to add interest to your training is to use a variety of equipment and exercise systems. Muscle tissues become accustomed to the same type of routine day in and day out. This is one of the reasons why every beginner should train at a professional gym. The first few months of training can either make or break a newcomer. By training around other muscle builders, the new trainee will see and learn about all sorts of exercises and routines.

With time, the novice absorbs this new knowledge into his mind's data bank for future reference. When a particular exercise does not feel right to him, he tries another in its place, learning through trial and error what works best for him. Because of this, his gains are better, giving him a more positive outlook on his training and hopefully a more successful hobby or career choice.

A workout partner is another excellent way of keeping your training enthusiasm at an optimum level. On days when you find yourself lagging behind, a partner could be just the thing you need to help get you out of your slump. He could challenge you at a certain exercise to see how many reps or pounds you could handle. You could even have a contest to see who trained with the most intensity. Best of all, you will know that he will be there to help and encourage you with your training in much the same way as you would be there for him.

Another way to keep your motivation up is to have some sensible goals. Let's say your chest is forty inches and you want to increase its size to forty-six. Instead of making your goal a full six inches, try breaking it up into smaller parts. Strive to add one inch to your chest every few months. Work as hard as you can to make these inches a reality. Each time you gain an inch, you will be one-step closer to your goal. This will raise your motivation up so high that your training will become harder and with a greater intensity than ever before. Soon all your goals will mesh into one.

Motivation is an important factor in helping us strive towards our desired goals. For bodybuilders, seeing the poundage of the weights increase, along with new muscular size and shape, is not only satisfying, but also self-motivating. The key is not to set unrealistic goals. Wanting to be the strongest, most muscular person that ever lived just might be out of your reach. Be realistic and conquer your goals one step at a time. Stay motivated!

INSPIRATION

While training at home during the early 1970s, I would turn on the radio and listen to talk-show host such as Bob Grant to stimulate my intellectual mind. Although I found such opinionated programs very informative, I needed something more to inspire my 'training mind' to a higher level. When I opened my gym in 1976, I discovered what that something was. It was music! In much the same way as it invigorated me; music can add a new dimension to your bomb and blitz routines. Whether you enjoy rock, disco, jazz, or country, get a group of your favorite selections together on a CD or iPod to help push you through the pain barrier and keep you psyched throughout your entire workout. After several years of watching gym members listen to iPods to motivate themselves, I decided to try it. I got tired of listening to the sound system of whatever gym I was training at, so I purchased a small iPod and loaded about two dozen of my favorite tunes from the movies *Rocky*, *Superman*, *Conan the Barbarian*, *Gladiator*, *Pumping Iron*, etc. into it. I have to say, "The iPod is the greatest invention since the barbell." In the old days, when I owned my own health club I was able to blast my favorite tunes on its sound system. These days I am at the mercy of whatever club I am training at, and being able to block out the static while listening to my own musical selections helps me keep the fire burning within my blood as I strive for further gains.

If you prefer complete silence during your training, you may want to add some inspirational bodybuilding posters to your workout area. On days when your training is not going so well, a look over to your favorite muscle builder can be just the thing needed to turn your workout from a flop and into a championship bombing session. At my Staten Island Bodybuilding Club, we had dozens of such posters displaying the champions at their best. This helped to create an atmosphere at the gym, which continuously served to motivate the members towards success.

Another way to get inspired is to train alongside some advanced bodybuilders. In 1983, I had the pleasure of training at both Gold's and World Gyms in Venice, California. While there, I watched many well-known physique champions go through their heavy-duty bombing sessions. It was very motivating to observe how their muscles gorged with blood as they flawlessly performed their exercises beyond normal limits. I even had the good fortune to train with quite a few legends, including Arnold Schwarzenegger. Arnold was true to form in both quality of physique and exercise technique. During my stay in

California, I was able to train several times with the Austrian Oak and was inspired every time I pumped the iron with him. We both trained with moderate weights and focused on exercise style for maximum benefit. Watching Arnold pump his muscles while we trained was overwhelming. His physique actually transformed right before my eyes as he gorged endless amounts of blood into the muscle group he willed to grow. Naturally, training with Arnold and being in such a motivating environment for bodybuilding was extremely inspiring to someone as hard-core as I was. The same can apply to you. Although you may not be fortunate enough to train alongside the Terminator, you can nevertheless find some advanced muscle builders in just about any gym in the country to guide you and motivate you. When approached correctly, these muscle artists will be more than delighted to help and inspire you with your training. Give it a try.

THE HARMONY WITHIN
Probably the most important aspect of developing a sound mind in a sound body is to find inner peace within yourself. As a teenager, I remember watching the hit TV show, *Kung Fu*, which stared David Carradine as Kwai Chang Caine. Kwai was a Shaolin Temple priest who lived a life of simplicity, wanting little for himself but capable of accomplishing so much. He was a master of not only his physical being but of his mental state as well. Kwai Chang Caine had the ability to focus on the task and look at things in simple terms in order to solve the problem. The same applies to you. Life is full of distractions and sometimes you might find yourself just drifting along like a heavy log in a fast stream. Slow down, look around, and smell the roses. Worrying about every little thing in life will only clog your thoughts and keep you from finding harmony within yourself. Forget about the bills, or that bumper-to-bumper traffic. Just take each day in stride and enjoy the fruits of life. I know that life can sometimes throw a fastball that will hit you hard if you let it. You must try to be mentally prepared for the unexpected when hardships or disasters strike. Absorb the pain and focus on how to best work out the problems. Sometimes there are no perfect solutions and we find ourselves limited in our abilities. That's life. Do the best you can for yourself and others, and be able to accept the limits of being a human being. Understanding your capabilities and limits is necessary in the ability to accept life for what it is and to find harmony within yourself. "Which way young grasshopper?"

STAY FOCUSED

When you enter the gym, leave the problems of the world outside its doors. You have to forget about the bills, the job, and perhaps the nagging spouse. You have to block negativity from all your thoughts and have a clear focus on what you are about to encounter. Bodybuilding is tough business. It takes a great deal of concentration to lift heavy steel, and the last thing you want is a serious injury because your thoughts and worries were still at the office.

I can remember going to my gym early one summer morning in 1979. It was a bright, sunny day, and I arrived for my workout at 7 AM so I could get my training in before the mad rush of muscle builders took over the club. I was psyched and ready for a heavy bombing session when suddenly, after opening the club, I noticed an unusual light coming from the back of my gym. Upon closer inspection, I was angered to see that someone had attempted to burglarize my establishment overnight by breaking its back window and bending the steel theft proof bars inward. There was shattered glass everywhere, but luckily, the perpetrator was unable to gain access and do more damage or commit a theft. Now, I could have gotten upset and let the incident ruin my workout or I could have put the incident on the back burner to be taken care of later in the day. I chose the latter and had a great thigh workout. Afterwards, I made several phone calls and had the area where the window was broken sealed with cement so I would not have any more unwelcome surprises in the future.

I have been through many similar scenarios in my life where incidents or people have caused great aggravation before my scheduled workouts and for the most part, have never let these unwelcome moments stop me from getting my training in. The same applies to you. To get big and strong, you have to focus on the task and not let any negative roadblocks prevent you from achieving your desired goals. You have got to zone in and stay locked onto why you are sweating blood and giving your maximum effort. Don't worry, the world will be waiting to smack you hard with reality when you leave the gym, but at least you will know that you accomplished what you came for and feel satisfied with that.

CHART YOUR PROGRESS

From my first workout in 1965 to the present day, I have maintained bodybuilding journals to record every workout I've performed. A bodybuilding journal is a great way to monitor your progress and keep track of what worked or didn't work for you. Each year, I add a completed journal to my annual collection. On occasion, I will look through several pages of some of my old bodybuilding journals and muse at the thousands of workouts I've endured. Each journal entry reflects sweat and pain. Each recorded set and rep represents new muscle. Each documented workout brings me a step closer to a goal. Every bodybuilder should keep a journal of his or her workouts. A bodybuilding journal can also tell you if a certain routine or time of day is or isn't working for you. It is also interesting to look back on your old logs and study the progress you made over the years. Keeping track of your workouts is easier than you might think. A well-documented journal will show you what worked and what did not. Go back several months and see if you made any specific changes for any particular muscle group. What did you do to add muscle mass last year, and what are you doing now that has not given you any muscular gains for the past three months? What can you do to improve your diet to get that six-pack? I think you get the idea. Again, the bodybuilding journal is a record of your success!

Keeping a bodybuilding journal can be quite a confidence booster. Looking back through its pages can put a smile on your face as you notice the progress recorded over time. Of course, you might also notice that your gains have not improved that much and that you may have even hit a plateau. By reviewing your bodybuilding journal, you should be able to find out why. The bodybuilding journal is a tool that will help you gain motivation and confidence as well as keep you focused on your training momentum. However, even if you are self-motivated, you can still gain some great insight. Keeping a journal of your muscle building efforts can make or break your progress. Think of it as a road map. The journal is going to show you the correct route and help you get there in the shortest time possible. The best thing about a bodybuilding journal is that it is firsthand knowledge to use as a reference in helping you avoid unnecessary pitfalls and perhaps find shortcuts to help you realize your goals sooner, rather than later. Without a journal, it is easy to lose focus and give up. If you do not record it, it can become easier to forget the whole point of what the plan was. Good intentions and great ideas become just a passing thought if you fail to document them.

I have seen many bodybuilders who are overly analytical about their training and clutter their journals with too much analysis and detail, so be careful of this. Beware of the old proverb, "Paralysis by analysis." Remember, the primary reasons you are working out are for quality size, strength, health, and longevity. Your bodybuilding journal should contain the following elements:

The Exercise Log

In the exercise portion of your bodybuilding journal write down the exercises, the weights, and the number of sets and reps. Write down the total time spent on each muscle group and give yourself a grade, from good to bad, on how intense your workout was. Do not forget to record all cardio work performed during your training session. Also, chart your pulse rate and the approximate amount of calories burned. It all adds up!

The Nutritional Log

In the nutritional portion of your journal, record the time of each meal and what you consumed. Be sure to chart the total amount of calories, protein, carbohydrates, fats, and supplements consumed. Make a note of everything! Learn the nutritional value of each portion of the food you consume and document it. Do not forget to write down fluids, such as spring water and fruit juices. If you consume something bad, make a note of it as well.

The Photo Library

Photos are an excellent way to monitor your progress throughout the months and years of training. Take some before shots in various poses; from the front, sides, and back; both flexed and standing relaxed. Then every couple of months take new photos and study the progress you have made. Create a photo library of yourself to use as a reference.

Record your Bodyweight, Strength, and Measurements

This is another great way to monitor your progress. Use a tailor's tape; measure your chest (expanded and normal), waist, hips, thighs, calves, and upper arms. Take these same measurements every few months and compare. Also, record your strength at various lifts to see how you are progressing. Seeing your physique become more muscular and your strength increasing will definitely help to motivate you to train harder and realize greater gains to come.

Remember, the bodybuilding journal is your tool for monitoring your progress. Use it wisely.

STRESS

Something that can bring your muscle building to a crashing halt is unwanted stress. Stress drains brainpower! People use to think stress-related health problems were 'all in their heads.' Now we know better. Stress is a mind/body event, and its physical effects are real. Excess stress can contribute to headaches, digestive problems, frequent colds, reduced immunity, and even heart disease. Natural bodybuilding is a great way to reduce feelings of stress. Ask those who weight train why they stick to their exercise programs. Many will tell you that it helps them relax and feel better about themselves. Exercise helps you work through the fight or flight response that is built into your genetic code. After exercise, you feel more relaxed and as if you don't have a care in the world. Exercise may also reduce feelings of stress by providing a diversion from sources of stress, such as your job or family. Getting to the gym and pumping the iron is a great way of relieving any stress that you may have. To me, there is no better tool to rid myself of unwanted stress than a well-designed training program. It gives you a sense of personal power and control that not only helps combat feelings of depression and anxiety but also makes you more optimistic about your life and your future. Try it!

DEVELOP A POSITIVE ATTITUDE

One of the more important aspects of bodybuilding is the amount of belief a bodybuilder has in himself. You have to believe! You have to want it so bad that you can taste it. The more you believe in yourself the better your workouts are going to be and the faster you are going to realize your goals. I know some bodybuilders who believe so much in themselves that all they have to do is look in a mirror to become psyched. There is no power greater than that of a positive attitude. Believe that you can and you shall. Those who believe in themselves are a step ahead of the game. The ability to look at each new day as a glorious challenge helps create an adventurous, strong desire to achieve any goal. If you believe that each new day will be better than the last, chances are, it will be.

A positive attitude is a giant steppingstone towards success. Obviously not everyone can look in the mirror for instant motivation, but you can look at yourself and believe that one day you will reach your goals and become whatever your dreams are made of. When you workout, train with confidence. Know that one day soon your goals will be achieved. Show your muscles no mercy; bomb them with every ounce of energy you have. The more you train like a champion, the sooner you will become one. Keep believing in yourself. Don't let negative thoughts sway you away from your dreams.

In 1952, the Reverend Norman Vincent Peale wrote the book *The Power of Positive Thinking*. During my high school years, I was fortunate enough to come across a copy and eagerly read its contents cover to cover. The book's positive message played a key part in my outlook towards life. Since those early years, I have remained highly motivated, full of confidence, and ready to take on any challenge that has come my way. Look at the following questions to see how positive or negative a person you might be:

A. Do you consistently think of yourself as a winner?

B. Do you have positive expectations for your training and everything you do in life?

C. Do you learn from your past successes to chart your life's course?

D. Do you put failures in the trash and look forward with optimism to the challenges of each new day?

E. Do you surround yourself with positive people and ideas? Negativity will drain the blood right out of your biceps!

F. Do you learn from your mistakes and move on? Only time stands between you and success!

Visualization techniques can also promote a positive attitude. Sometimes, while I am alone in a quiet room by myself, I will close my eyes, take a deep breath, and clear my mind. I then visualize myself succeeding at something I desire. As I focus on my goal, I add details to my thought. Gradually I add words, actions, and sensations to the image. When you have a moment, try practicing this same visualization technique. Keep your visualization handy in your mind and rehearse it from time to time. When properly used, visualization techniques can help give you a big boost in lifting steel you never imagined possible. Practice visualization often!

An affirmation, or positive statement, is another technique that I use to develop a winning attitude. This simple practice has helped me to realize my goals in a relatively short amount of time. To record an affirmation you wish to achieve in the nearby future, simply get a blank piece of paper, and complete the following:

I _____ _____ will _____
_____!

Hang the paper where you can see it and repeat your affirmation to yourself at least once a day. Believe in it and believe in yourself! Believe that you can and you will. Keep your desire burning strong; let your enthusiasm fly high and watch your motivation explode with power. The power necessary for you, the natural bodybuilder, to command your starship on its *JOURNEY TO THE OLYMPIAN ZONE*!

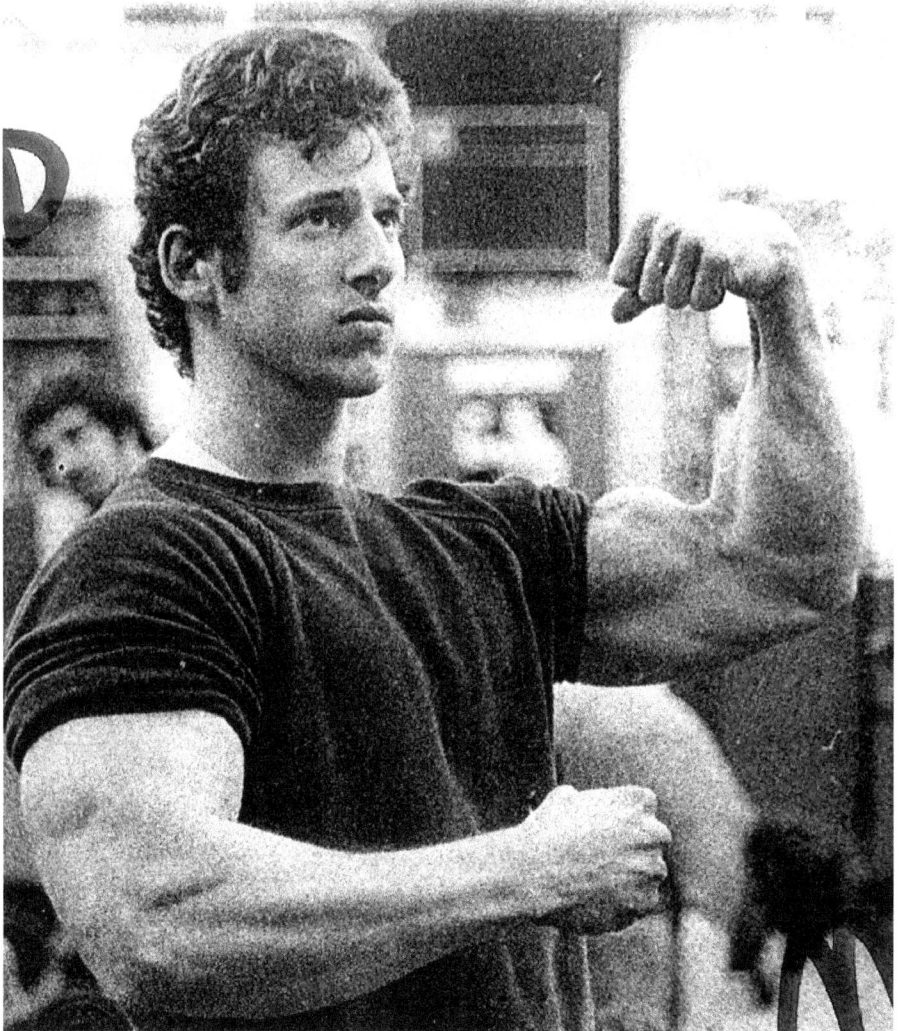

Mario Strong focuses on the future to come - 1978

REST & RECUPERATION

As important as diet and training are in building muscle and gaining strength, so too, is the importance of plenty of rest and recuperation to keep us healthy and feeling vibrant. After a heavy bombing session at the local gym, your body needs time to rebuild its worn muscles by replenishing them with nutrients lost during the workout. Our bodies and minds need rest and sleep to rejuvenate. Sleep is an evolutionary requirement. Through the process of evolution, human beings have evolved to perform actively throughout the day as their bodies produce adrenaline and steroids during their waking hours. At night, while sleeping, our body's vital systems recharge when growth hormones are released to rebuild the tired and impaired tissues caused by the day's earlier occurrences. Living on a twenty-four hour rotating earth, most people need eight hours of peaceful sleep to provide rejuvenated energy that can last for sixteen hours of sustained wakefulness. Those who sleep less, tend to become drowsy during the day and sometimes find themselves falling asleep at the wrong times. Individual sleep requirements and sleep patterns vary greatly. Studies have shown that infants and children require eight to ten hours of sleep nightly. By age twenty, the need is about seven hours, and most forty year olds seem to require only about six hours. Those older than forty spend more time in bed but less time actually sleeping, while those over sixty commonly experience repeated sleep interruptions.

If you find yourself overtired because of lack of sleep and suffer from some form of insomnia that is affecting your daily routine, consult your health care provider. Though prolonged spells of sleeplessness may not have immediate consequences on your health, they will with time.

There are two types of sleep that alternate at approximately ninety-minute intervals: REM (rapid eye movement) and non-REM. REM sleep occurs when a person is dreaming and the eyes move beneath the closed eyelids. During this stage of sleep, muscles stiffen and sometimes twitch. Following REM sleep there are four progressively deeper stages of non-REM sleep. On average, this cycle is repeated four to six times during an eight-hour period of sleep. The REM periods grow progressively longer and as morning approaches, sleep becomes gradually shallower until the body awakens. Another reason to get your quota of sleep is that long-term memory is programmed into your subconscious mind during this time through the process of replaying experiences and images of the day.

As natural bodybuilders, we train hard and break our muscles down in relatively short periods of time. To grow larger and get stronger, rest is just as important as how much steel we can lift or how often we bomb and blitz. However, many bodybuilders fail to realize the importance of proper rest and unintentionally hold back their potential gains. Rest gives our muscles a chance to recuperate to previous physical levels, while also helping us to gain progressively in mass and strength. Rest is a vital factor necessary to make continued gains in the gym.

When I sleep, my body's growth hormone levels are at their highest. It is also no coincidence that most of my physiological improvement occurs during this restful period. Heavy and intense training taxes my body's recuperative powers. It improves the efficiency of my muscular system and increases both the glycogen stores and mitochondrial enzyme systems within my body. After a heavy-duty workout, my body immediately begins to recuperate as these systems work together to improve my physical capabilities.

The same applies to you. Without the proper recovery time, your body will not be able to regenerate and it will store less of the glycogen needed for your Herculean workouts. When this happens, you will have less explosive power and your physique will begin to look smooth and flat. If your body lacks rest for an extended length of time, its health will begin to decline and the gains that you worked so hard for will begin to diminish. Not only will your performance levels decline but you will also run the risk of injury. There are other factors such as nutrition and exercise that contribute to how your body responds, but without proper rest, your keys to success will be lost. If your body needs rest, get it - if it is lazy, get to the gym!

TIPS FOR A RESTFUL SLEEP

A. For complete rest and recuperation, it is imperative that a regular bedtime and rising time be established.

B. Exercise vigorously each and every day so that your body feels the need for rest at bedtime. If you miss your weight training session, try performing a slow run a few hours before bedtime.

   * Regular active exercise during the day also helps since it stimulates the elimination of lactic acid from the body. Incidentally, the presence of lactic acid correlates with stress and muscular tension. Regular exercise also produces hormonal changes which are beneficial to the natural bodybuilder and which help fortify the sleep pattern.

C. Follow a well-balanced nutritional program. Research has proven that diets deficient in certain nutrients such as copper, iron, and aluminum, can cause disruptions in sleep patterns.

D. Enjoy your sleeping environment. The average person sleeps best when the room temperature is between 60-65 degrees Fahrenheit. The bedroom should provide maximum comfort and be free of distractions.

E. Learn to relax by using techniques such as yoga and deep breathing.

F. Gradually work towards obtaining the right amount of sleep each night by learning the optimal amount of rest you need.

G. If automobile horns or dogs barking constantly disrupt your sleep, try using a fan, sound machine or soothing classical music to block the intrusive noise.

Avoid the Following:

A. Taking a short nap before your scheduled bedtime.

B. Exercising vigorously right before bedtime.

C. Drinking caffeinated beverages (coffee, tea, soft drinks) before bedtime. Try a glass of spring water instead.

D. Eating heavy or spicy food before bedtime.

E. Consuming large meals or drinking large quantities of liquids right before your bedtime.

F. Watching TV, eating, reading, or working in bed for extended periods of time. Close your eyes and get to sleep!

G. Avoid lying awake in bed for long periods of time. If you cannot fall asleep within 30 minutes, get out of bed and do something to make you slightly fatigued. Then go back to bed and try to sleep again. Learn how to clear your mind of all negative thoughts!

* While lactic acid may play a role in fatigue, its supposed role in muscle soreness has been disproved and it is now being recognized as more of a positive player in metabolism. Muscles create lactic acid from glucose and then burn it to obtain energy. The reason advanced bodybuilders can workout hard for a long period of time is because their intense training causes their muscles to adapt so they more readily and efficiently absorb the lactic acid.

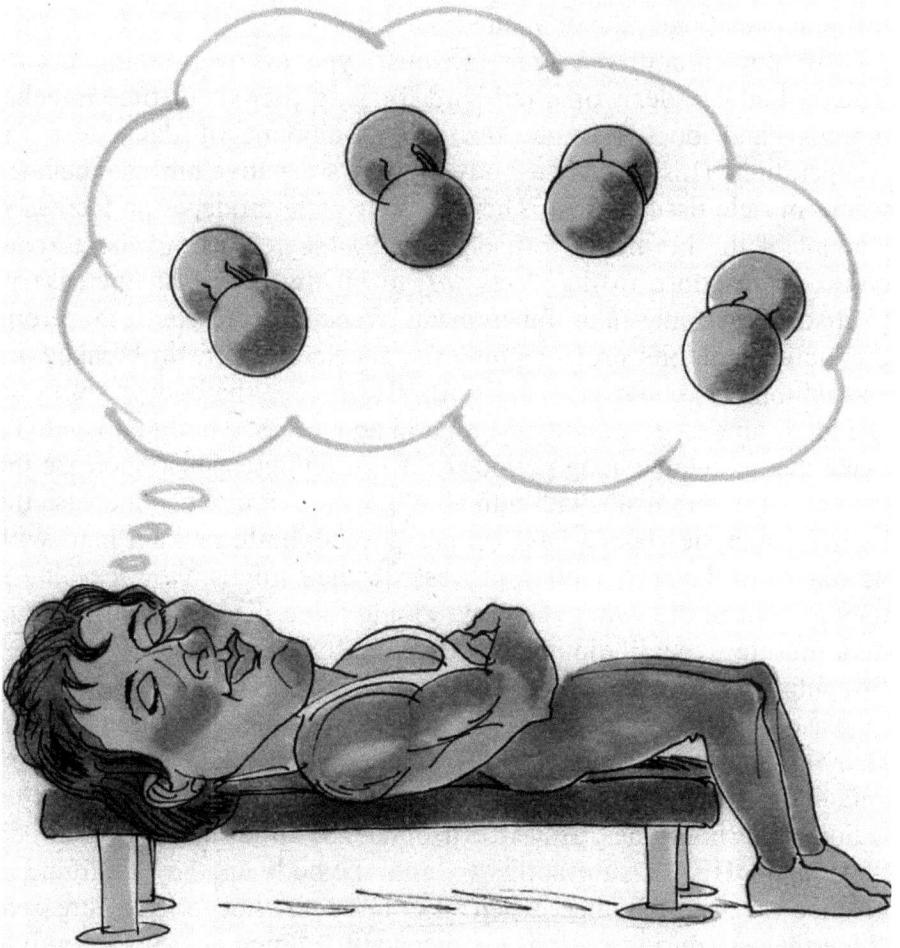

Try to focus on pleasant thoughts during periods of rest

OVERTRAINING

Probably the biggest mistake bodybuilders make while on their quest for size and strength is to over-train. Overtraining is like a dog chasing its tail, and those who continually partake in this foolish practice find themselves going nowhere in our sport. Unfortunately, thousands of bodybuilders waste tremendous amounts of time and energy every day as they pour gallons of sweat in gyms with nothing to show for their hard strained efforts. When you workout too much, eat poorly, and get insufficient amounts of rest, you are subject to a condition known as overtraining. The most common type of overtraining is when a bodybuilder trains too frequently, or works a particular muscle group directly or indirectly on consecutive days, thus preventing those muscles from fully recuperating. I am sure we have all been guilty of this practice at one time or another.

An uncommon, but more serious, type of overtraining occurs when a bodybuilder works out hard for long periods of time (weeks-months) and does not get the proper amount of daily rest for recuperation. This causes the body to enter a negative nitrogen balance where muscle tissue is lost. This catabolic state produces an increased amount of the hormone Cortisol, which is secreted from the adrenal cortex in response to the stress placed on the body. An increase in Cortisol slows muscular function and repair, decreases testosterone production, inhibits protein synthesis, accelerates protein breakdown, and inhibits muscular growth. It can also reduce the body's ability to use fat as an energy source, resulting in an increased body fat level. To make matters worse, long periods of overtraining can also increase the amount of free radicals within the body, which in turn can increase the body's catabolic state. I have witnessed bodybuilders train hard with no regard to the recuperation process. In their minds, they fear that if they are not in the gym every day, giving more than 100% effort, that their muscle size will diminish, when actually, the opposite is true.

Bodybuilders who over-train for extended periods of time not only increase their Cortisol level, but just as important, their Dehydroepiandrosterone (DHEA) level. DHEA and Cortisol are antagonistic to each other and both play a part with the body's long acting stress hormones. Since Cortisol has the ability to break the body down and DHEA has the ability to build the body up, they are found in balance to one another when the body is not overly stressed. Nevertheless, during periods of extended training, when the body's recuperative powers are taxed, these hormones become imbalanced.

This condition can only be corrected when the body is given adequate time for rest and recuperation, otherwise the body will continue to make increasingly greater amounts of Cortisol while reducing the amount of DHEA produced. Elevated levels of Cortisol have been shown to create a craving for carbohydrates and make the individual feel fatigued. It can also increase cholesterol and triglyceride production, decrease serotonin levels in the brain, and deplete certain vitamins and minerals from the body. Therefore, it should be clearly understood, that Cortisol and DHEA must be kept in proper balance for the prevention of the negative side effects of overtraining.

General Negative Effects of Overtraining

A. Possible reductions of growth hormones produced, resulting in increased levels of body fat, reduced muscle mass and strength, and a weakened immune system.
B. Reduced ability to synthesize protein.
C. The occurrence of muscle and bone loss increases; while the body's muscular system weakens from the breakdown of proteins.
D. The immune system is compromised, resulting in an increased risk to infections and disease.
E. The function of the thyroid is weakened, resulting in a decreased metabolism and an increase of unwanted body fat.
F. The ability to utilize glucose completely and the function of insulin are diminished, resulting in higher blood sugar levels.
G. Rise in blood pressure from salt and water retention.
H. The risk for heart disease increases as cholesterol and triglycerides levels rise.
I. Sleep patterns may be disrupted as reduced R.E.M. is experienced.

Short Term Effects of Overtraining

A. Morning pulse rate may be elevated.
B. Blood pressure remains elevated throughout day.
C. Muscular soreness lags for several days.
D. Increased frequency of common illnesses, decreased appetite.
E. Increased occurrence of injuries, muscle tissue loss.

In addition to the above, abnormal behavioral and emotional temperaments from short periods of overtraining can also occur. Typically, they are observed because of chronic overtraining (weeks to months) as listed below. This condition is called burnout.

Long Term Effects of Overtraining
A. Continuous state of irritability.
B. Behavioral changes throughout day.
C. Inability to sleep.
D. Feelings of depression.
E. No desire to workout.

As you can see, overtraining for long periods may create conditions that are different from the shorter term because fatigue and behavioral dispositions continue well into the recovery period. Many factors can affect your recuperative powers and put your body and mind into an over-trained state. Such factors include hormonal balance, sleep quality, nutrition, muscle fiber composition, enzymatic concentrations, and previous training experience. The real key to avoiding overtraining is to be able to detect the warning signs early and get the required rest needed. Throughout the decades, I too, have been guilty of occasionally overtraining. When I workout, I like to train until I have nothing left in the tank. This is okay as long as you don't go past the point of no return. There is a fine line between having a great workout and wasting everything you just trained so hard to accomplish. Advanced bodybuilders know their limits and train within their recuperative boundaries so as not to waste their time and hard-earned sweat. Unfortunately, only through trial and error will you learn the limits of your body's recuperative powers and then be able to safely train within its boundaries.

By letting your body re-energize for the workouts to come, you, the natural bodybuilder, are on your *JOURNEY TO THE OLYMPIAN ZONE*!

THE BASICS OF BODYBUILDING

What is your reason to body build? Perhaps it was an awakening to some of your physical deficiencies that made you realize it was time for a change. Do you desire larger muscles and greater strength, or is it the need for health and vitality that motivates you? Bodybuilding with weights is the fastest way to add on some needed muscle and build mountains of confidence. Regardless of one's age, sex, or present physical condition (provided the individual is in reasonably good health and there are no medical reasons why exercise cannot be undertaken), a well-planned weight-training program provides the safest, fastest, and most efficient way to improve one's health and build the body to improve one's personal appearance.

Resistance training improves coordination, balance, speed, reaction time, and control of most of our skeletal muscles. In addition, it builds muscle mass and is the fastest way known to build strength. Every bodybuilder that has ever championed a physique stage has used progressive resistance training to improve his or her physique. Resistance training with weights is also a great way to prevent or overcome injuries and physical deficiencies. It conditions the entire body to be more responsive to our mental processes and helps improve the body/mind connection so reaction times will be quicker when danger or stress occurs. Conditioned muscles often prevent accidents, possibly fatal ones. For our purposes, weight-training exercises are high intensity movements in which an oxygen debt is created and the glycogen stored in the muscles is used. When you body build with weights your body burns mainly glycogen, which is produced by the carbohydrates you consume. It is impossible to lift weights intensely for a half hour without at least 15-30 second rests between sets because your body would run out of energy. In comparison, you can do aerobic exercises for 30 minutes without resting because they are low intensity and there is an abundance of oxygen. Instead of burning a great deal of glycogen, aerobic exercises burn fat. They are not capable, however, of reshaping the body into he-man proportions. Only a well-designed, intense weight-training program can do that.

The combination of proper nutrition, exercise, and rest can transform your physique from a wreck into championship form. Now, when I say, "Fast," I do not mean you will have that he-man body in six weeks by training just several minutes a day, three times a week. I know you have seen and heard all the advertisements for overnight muscle gains and that is what Madison Avenue would like you to believe. These days, newsstands are stocked with magazines whose pages are full of muscle building knowledge. At least that is the way they are marketed. Gone are the days of pure hard-core bodybuilding info and training advice. Today's publications are loaded with tons of advertisements and more T&A than a porno rag. Your best bet in getting some sensible guidance is from those that have trained through the decades and passed the test of time. The reality of it all is that bodybuilding is hard work. It takes years to build a strong and vibrant physique that is worthy enough to step onto a posing dais. It doesn't sound quite as easy as those ads, does it?

Natural bodybuilding is not only a sport of building muscles, but also a healthy way of life that reaps many benefits for those willing to put in the effort and time. In this chapter, we will focus primarily on building muscle and gaining strength. One of the great things about bodybuilding is that you can achieve great results with very basic equipment and a few hours of training, several times per week. The key to becoming bigger and stronger is to progressively train with heavier resistance through the months and years. Results come from consistent regular training, eating properly, getting plenty of rest, and maintaining a positive outlook on life.

THE BENEFITS OF NATURAL BODYBUILDING
Natural bodybuilding has many benefits. Through the proper application of exercise, nutrition, rest, and positive thinking, those who take part in natural bodybuilding soon realize the many benefits the sport can bring. Natural bodybuilding is amazing! It is a way of life

that stays with you twenty-four hours a day. When practiced in its truest form it has the potential to add years of healthy living and radiant vigor to your life. It is a means to an end that is never reached and yet so very rewarding along its path. Here are a few benefits that the training aspect of natural bodybuilding can provide:

General Benefits of Physical Exercise
A. Shown to improve psychological well-being.
B. Enhances work, recreation, and sport performance.
C. Improves circulation and sexual performance.
D. Reduces body fat levels.
E. Reduces the risk of premature death.
F. Builds and maintains healthy muscles, bones, and joints.
G. Reduces the risk of developing heart disease.
H. May reduce high blood pressure or the risk of developing it.
I. May reduce high cholesterol or the risk of developing it.
J. Reduces the risk of developing diabetes.
K. Reduces depression and anxiety.

Benefits of Cardio Training
A. Increases blood supply to muscles and ability to use oxygen.
B. Lowers heart rate at sub-maximal exercise level.
C. Decreases blood triglycerides.
D. Improves cardiovascular and respiratory functions.
E. Lowers resting systolic and diastolic blood pressure.
F. Increases HDL Cholesterol.
G. Reduces body fat and improves weight control.
H. Maximizes oxygen consumption.
I. Increases threshold for lactic acid accumulation.
J. Improves glucose tolerance and reduced insulin resistance.

Benefits of Progressive Resistance Training
A. Increases muscular strength.
B. Reduces body fat and increases muscle mass.
C. Increases strength of tendons and ligaments.
D. Improvement of flexibility in the joints.
E. Improves strength, balance, and functional ability in elders.
F. May decrease resting systolic and diastolic blood pressure.
G. May improve blood cholesterol levels.
H. Improvement of glucose tolerance and insulin sensitivity.
I. Decreased risk of Osteoporosis.

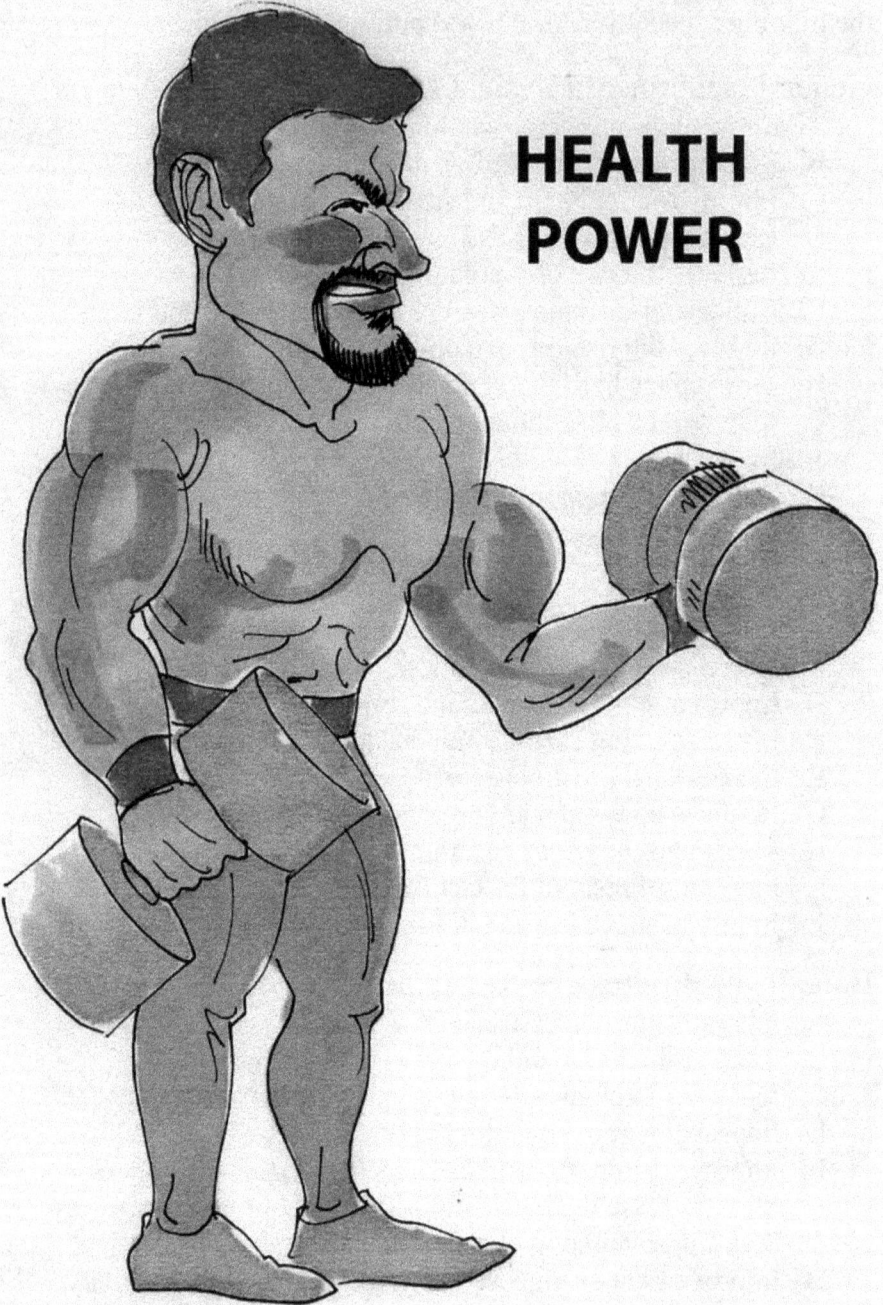

HEALTH POWER

One of the benefits of natural bodybuilding is radiant health

Natural bodybuilding has been my way of life since my teenage days. From those early times to today, I have been learning and applying its many concepts to my life on a daily basis. It has been many decades in the gym and thousands of healthy meals since my father first introduced me to the iron, and it has been worth every ounce of sweat that has dripped off my brow. One thing that is needed in this sport is patience. You have to want it so bad that you can taste it. However, you must keep the flame of desire at a low burn so it does not extinguish before its time. Another requirement is consistency. No champion every made it to the top with haphazard training or by missing regular workouts. Natural bodybuilding is the scientific application of exercise, nutrition, rest and a positive mental attitude. You have to be consistent in all these factors to succeed in our sport. At the very least, it takes all these ingredients to come together through the years for you to realize your goals. Do you think you have what it takes? Let's see!

If you are a beginner to bodybuilding, it is important to first check with your medical doctor before starting an exercise and nutritional program. When beginning to body build, remember to start slow and practice the proper form on each exercise. Through time, advanced bodybuilders have learned that exercise technique is one of the most important aspects in getting results from their workouts. To get you started on the correct path in bodybuilding try to schedule a workout or two with a personal trainer that has several years of experience in the sport. Other tools available to help guide you on your quest are the Internet, various fitness publications, and videos that instruct and teach self-improvement. Most importantly, take the time to learn the proper technique of each exercise performed.

Remember, to increase muscle size you will need to increase the resistance on weight training exercises progressively over time. Be patient. One of the biggest pitfalls among bodybuilders is overwork. I have also been guilty of this practice and on several occasions have wasted workouts because I was too enthusiastic. By maintaining a regular workout routine, coupled with proper nutrition and rest, you will begin to see great results in no time.

Bodybuilding is a war! To make constant gains in the sport you have to attack your muscles in ways they least expect it. Shock them with new exercises, sets, and rep schemes to hit them hard where they least expect it, thus forcing them to produce the results you desire. Natural bodybuilding is a constant battle that can reap glorious rewards to those who follow its true path. Those who are lucky enough to raise the flag on top of Muscle Hill have accomplished no easy task and can only smile while reflecting on the steep climb to the peak. Let's begin!

UNDERSTANDING YOUR PHYSIQUE
Have you ever looked into a crowd of people and noticed how many different body types there are? People come in many shapes and sizes, and bodybuilders are no different. When physique competitors lineup on stage they present to the judges an array of diverse physical structures for comparison. The bodybuilder who understands his own body type has the best possibility of developing his physique to its maximum potential. The physical differences in all of us dictate that different body types may respond differently to both training and nutrition. As a result, it is very important to be aware of what body type you have so that you can design a sensible diet and workout program to best suit your needs.

WHICH BODY TYPE ARE YOU
In the 1940s, American psychologist William Sheldon formed a theory, which connected body types with human temperament types. As a child, Sheldon was an avid observer of animals and birds, and as he grew up, his hobby turned into a focused study on observing the human body. This study helped him to form his much recognized body type classifications, which today are known as the samato types. The samato types consisted of three basic classifications of animal body types according to the prominence of different basic tissue types, roughly: digestive, muscular, and nervous tissues. They were labeled the endomorph, mesomorph, and ectomorph.

Because of the many different variables that can exist in any of the three main body types it is often difficult to classify most individuals. Although there are some people who are purely ectomorphs, endomorphs, or mesomorphs, most people fall into mixed categories with traits from more than one body type. For instance, it is not unusual to find persons who are classified as ecto-mesomorphs, or endo-mesomorphs, where largely, they are like the mesomorph, but with traits of the ectomorph (small joints or a trim waist), or traits of the endomorph (tendency to gain fat easily). Everyone is unique and it is up to the individual to learn what body type classification they fall into, to better understand his or her full potential.

The following are Sheldon's three basic body type classifications:

ECTOMORPH CHARACTERISTICS
A. Muscles Are Slight
B. Takes Long To Build Muscles
C. Chest Is Underdeveloped
D. Extreme Hard Gainer
E. Thin Skeletal Structure
F. Delicately Built Body
G. Fragile
H. Lean
I. Small Shoulder Structure

The Ectomorph Body
The ectomorph physique is fragile and linear in nature. It is somewhat delicate with bones that are light, joints that are small, and muscles that are slight. Ectomorphs have relatively long limbs and shoulders that appear to droop. Their fingers, toes, and neck may also appear to be longer than average. The features of the face are sharp and its shape may appear triangular, with a lower jaw that can be somewhat receding. Because of the length of the limbs and the lack of muscle mass supported on them, the ectomorph appears to be taller than he is or she actually is. Because of the ectomorph's large body area in relation to his muscle mass, he may suffer from excessive heat or extreme cold because of his low body fat content. The ectomorph's skin tends to burn easily in the sun and his hair may be fine, grow quickly, and become unmanageable.

Since ectomorhs have extremely high metabolisms it is imperative that they consume more calories than the other body type classifications, especially if their goal is to gain weight. The ectomorph is not naturally strong and has to work very hard to increase muscle mass and strength. When training to gain muscle mass he needs to increase the number of calories consumed daily as well as ensure that his diet is sufficient in carbohydrates. A nutritional plan for an ectomorph training to increase muscle mass would consist of approximately 35% protein, 50% carbohydrates, and 15% fat.

MESOMORPH CHARACTERISTICS
A. Builds Quality Muscle Mass
B. Body Is Hard
C. Athletic Abilities
D. Females Are Well Proportioned
E. Builds Muscle More Easily Than Ectomorph
F. Males Build Balanced Physiques
G. Skin Is Thick
H. Body Is Muscular
I. Posture Is Excellent
J. Gains Fat More Easily Than Ectomorph

The Mesomorph Body
The mesomorph physique displays a body type that has toned muscles and large bones. The torso appears symmetrical, as the upper shoulder region tapers down to a relatively narrow waist to create the V-look. The mesomorph's skeletal structure and muscles of the head are prominent. His facial features are long and broad, with clearly defined cheekbones and a heavy jaw that appears squared. The hair may be heavy in texture. Both sets of limbs on the mesomorph are well developed; even the digits of the hands appear to be muscled. The mesomorph's skin tends to be thick and tans well, giving physique competitors a visual edge on the stage. The majority of bodybuilding champions fall into this category.

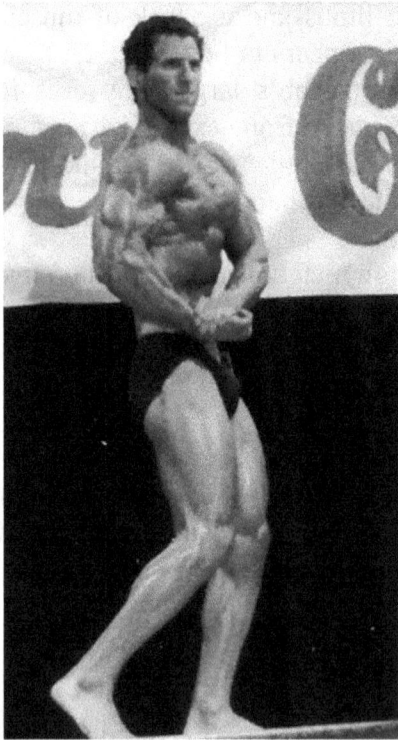

Mesomorphs have highly efficient metabolisms and are able to absorb moderately high amounts of protein and carbohydrates without fear of adding body fat. Generally, mesomorphs find it easier to build greater muscle mass than ectomorphs do. A nutritional plan for an average mesomorph would consist of approximately 40% protein, 45% carbohydrates, and 15% fat.

ENDOMORPH CHARACTERISTICS
A. Difficulty In Losing Weight
B. Body Is Soft
C. Can Easily Build Muscle
D. Muscles Are Undeveloped
E. Physique Is Round

The Endomorph Body

The endomorph physique is round and soft in nature. The waist appears high and gives the illusion that much of the body's mass is concentrated in the abdominal area. Both the arms and legs may be short in length and taper, with the upper arms and thighs more developed than the lower parts of the limbs. The hands and feet of the endomorph may be small in comparison. The skin of the endomorph is soft and smooth, and the hair is fine. The head is large, spherical, and the face broad.

Because the metabolism of the endomorph is slower than either the ectomorph or mesomorph, he finds it easier to gain body fat. He can also gain muscle mass quickly, but should be careful not to gain unwanted bodyweight while in the process of doing so. To avoid excess body fat, endomorphs should follow a natural diet while carefully monitoring their fat and calorie consumption to help insure that their weight gains are mostly muscle. Because endomorphs tend to eat fewer carbohydrates than the other body types, they must balance their diets with more protein. A nutritional plan for an endomorph wanting to lose a few excess pounds would consist of approximately 50% protein, 30% carbohydrates, and 20% fat.

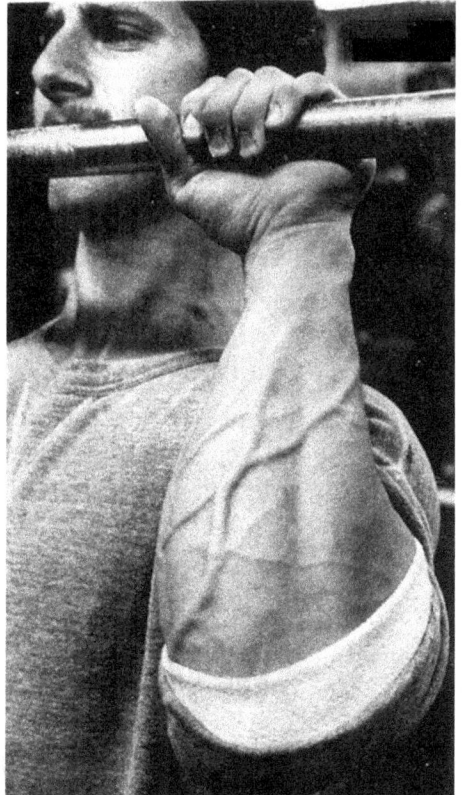

METABOLIC RATE

The rate at which bodybuilders metabolize their food helps to determine the level of success they will realize on the physique stage. This important factor is a main reason why some bodybuilders are able to get harder and more ripped than others are in competition. However, as helpful as an efficient metabolism is, it can nevertheless derail one's muscle gains as some ectomorphs have learned. More important than being ripped on stage is the amount of actual muscle mass a bodybuilder displays. This balancing act requires a metabolism that processes food at a slower speed so that the maximum amount of nutrients can be absorbed.

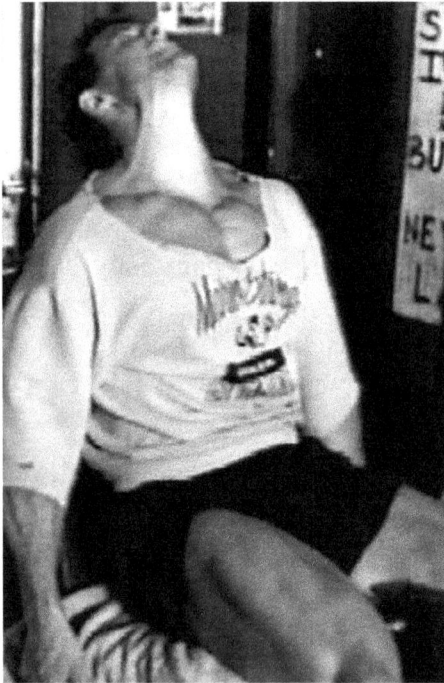

The more muscle a bodybuilder develops on his body, the more change he will see in his metabolic rate, and the more calories he will need to sustain his level of development. Some forms of exercise can also change our metabolic rates. For example, cardio type exercises (aerobic) are the preferred method to burn calorie and fat stores within our bodies. This method is far superior to anaerobic exercises, which build muscle tissue but do not use the excess bodyweight as readily as aerobic exercises.

As we age, our metabolic rate decreases and those who once found it hard to put on a pound or two, now gain weight easily. When the aging process is coupled with the lazy lifestyle and slow metabolism of a couch potato, a condition is created where unwanted body fat is accumulated at an exaggerated rate. As mentioned previously, mesomorphs have the best possible metabolic rate for gaining muscle while keeping their fat stores low.

SOME WIN, SOME LOSE, NOT TRYING IS THE GREATEST SIN

MUSCLE FIBERS

When bodybuilders train, they impair a substantial number of the hundreds of thousands of muscle fibers within their bodies. Muscle fibers come bundled together to create fasciculi, which are encased in sheaths called perimysium. Many bundles of fasciculi come together to form a complete muscle (bicep), which is then enclosed in another sheath called the fascia. The cells within every once of muscle contain several thousand rod-like structures known as myofibrils, which are the fibers within the cell. Both myosin and actin filaments (proteins) form together to make a sacromere, which is a chain of contractile units that creates a myofibril. Myosin filaments are temporary cross-bridges that connect to certain parts of the actin-filaments to form the basic components for a muscular constriction. During periods of rest, our muscles recuperate by inevitably becoming larger and stronger. Rest is an important and yet neglected factor that many bodybuilders wishing to gain both size and strength often overlook. Different types of muscle fibers require different rep and set schemes to make them respond to the stimulation provided. To accomplish this, a bodybuilder must first learn about the different types of muscle fibers there are and then determine which ones proportionally exist within him. Let's look at the different types of muscle fibers.

Slow-Twitch Red Muscle Fibers

Slow-twitch red muscle fibers consist of myofibrils that enlarge as a response to resistance training and therefore expand in width. Unlike the other two types of muscle fibers, slow-twitch red muscle fibers have access to a great deal of mitochondria and myoglobin, causing them to be used more often. Through evolution, our legs have become loaded with slow-twitch red muscle fibers to meet the endurance demands placed on them. These muscle fibers have the highest endurance of all three types of muscle fibers because of the perfusion and increasing number of capillaries within the cell. This can be observed in bodybuilders who have very demanding training schedules as opposed to people whose lifestyles are more sedentary. The more physically active a person is the more slow-twitch red muscle fibers they will have. Another factor that also determines the rate at which a muscle will grow is genetics. An example of genetics being a hindrance would be a bodybuilder who trains his back intensely but mostly makes gains in his biceps and forearms, no matter how hard he works on this muscle group. This is because his body is designed in such a way that it is very hard for him to add new muscle mass to his back. With slow-twitch red muscle fibers, the resistance used is secondary since these fibers seem to respond best to high repetitions (twelve or more) and constant muscle tension. Preferably, the repetitions should be performed in a slow, concentrated, and steady pace; with little to no pause between reps and followed through until muscle failure. The pump in the muscle group being trained is tremendous.

Fast-Twitch White Muscle Fibers

Fast-twitch white muscle fibers primarily consist of myofibrils and contain a great number of nerve bundles. They quickly respond to muscle stimulation and grow easier than the other two types of muscle fibers because they are used less. When a bodybuilder first begins to train, he greatly stimulates the fast-twitch white muscle fibers and enjoys the results in size that come from his efforts. Fast-twitch white muscle fibers seem to respond well to lower repetitions per set than either the slow-twitch red muscle fiber or intermediate muscle fiber. This type of training is heavy, quick, and explosive with a maximum of five to six repetitions per set and with the muscle brought to the point of failure. Because of the energy expended, a three to five minute rest between sets is appropriate to help ensure that the fast-twitch white muscle fibers recover and are ready for another set with maximum poundage. The pump is of secondary importance here.

Intermediate-Twitch Muscle Fibers

Intermediate-twitch muscle fibers have less myofibrils and nerve bundles than fast-twitch white muscle fibers but have more mitochondria, which are responsible for cell respiration and ATP production. Although the strength potential of intermediate-twitch muscle fibers is lower than fast-twitch white muscle fibers, they nevertheless have a substantially greater endurance factor. Resistance exercises performed in the range of ten repetitions per set and brought to the point of failure are sufficient for results with intermediate-twitch muscle fibers. Repetitions should be performed at a normal speed and through a full range of motion. A one to three minute-rest between sets is adequate.

THE SKELETAL SYSTEM

For bodybuilders, learning about the skeletal system is just as important as being knowledgeable about the muscles that surround them. The skeleton of an adult human is comprised of 206 bones and two systems, the axial skeleton (torso) and the appendicular skeleton (limbs). Aside from providing the rigid framework for our muscles to develop on, the skeleton also supports, protects, allows bodily movement, produces blood for the body, and stores essential minerals. A number of factors, such as nutrition, exposure to sunlight, hormonal secretions, and physical exercise influence bone development. Bone is deposited in proportion to the compression load that it must carry. For example, the bones of a bodybuilder are considerably heavier than those of a tennis player. Bones have relatively high compressive strength but poor tensile strength, which means they resist pushing forces well, but not pulling forces. The interaction of our muscular and skeletal systems determines the range of motion our limbs, neck, and torso can perform. Muscles are connected to bones by tendons. Ligaments connect bones to each other. Where bones meet one another is typically called a joint. Muscles that cause movement of a joint are connected to two different bones and constrict to pull them together. Two examples are the contraction of the biceps during a curling motion (while the triceps relax) to produce a bend at the elbow, and the contraction of the triceps during an extension motion (while the biceps relax) to produce the effect of straightening the arm.

WHAT ARE YOU MADE OF?

After looking at the different types of muscular tissue and skeletal structures, I find myself somewhere in the category of being a mesomorph with a genetic predisposition towards having many fast-twitch white muscle fibers. In the gym, my body responds best to super heavy weights and low repetitions. Even on the track, I am a much more explosive runner than a marathoner is. I enjoy this type of intense training by always pushing my body to the limit in a relatively short period. Personally, whenever I try high repetitions with the weights I get little out of it and feel as if I wasted my time. I need the heavy stuff and when I train with the big plates I leave the gym feeling satisfied, knowing that my body received the work it needed to make continued gains. Learn about your own body. See which category you best fit under and design your training and nutritional needs to best compliment your own genetic predisposition.

BEGINNING BODYBUILDING

So, you decide that weight training is the best way to build he-man physique. You purchase some exercise equipment for the home and proceed to pump iron. Many guys who have started this way have gone on to make tremendous gains; others are continuously distracted and go nowhere. With television, cell phones, your personnel computer, and the family, it can become quite a challenge to have a great workout. Just lifting steel any old fashion is definitely not the best way to go. Besides wasting energy, you also run the risk of serious injury or worse. Rare and exotic workout routines often produce rare and exotic results, that is, if you consider pulled muscles, strained backs, hernias, and broken bones exotic. Try to keep your workouts basic and intense for maximum gains.

The idea of joining a health club can be intimating to the beginner. After all, isn't everyone going to be extraordinarily built and strong? Not necessarily, you see, most gyms are stocked with members trying to either lose unwanted body fat or add some muscle to their frame. Luckily, these days there are plenty of clubs from which to choose. Try to find one that is well equipped and staffed with professionally-certified instructors. Look around the gym and get a feel for its atmosphere. A good club will have an energetic vibe that is conducive to the progress of its members.

Guys train with weights for lots of reasons. Today, before I ever begin to design a workout program for any of my new students, I first learn what kind of person I am dealing with. I learn about their athletic background, asking them if they have ever trained with weights before, and if so, what principles they used and for how long. I check to see if they ever participated in any sports such as gymnastics, football, swimming, etc. I ask them if they have a history of injuries, and I learn about their goals, as I try to find out just what they seek in our sport. In general, I try to educate myself on the person to which I will be offering training advice. Through my experience, learning about the type of person I am dealing with saves the both of us time and energy. As soon as I begin understanding my new student's goals, I start to explain what natural bodybuilding is all about.

I teach them about some of the basic benefits derived from our sport such as improved overall physique, increased physical strength, the ability to rid unwanted stress, added personal confidence, improved athletic capabilities, a better general appearance with a more positive outlook on life, and of course, (starting right with the first

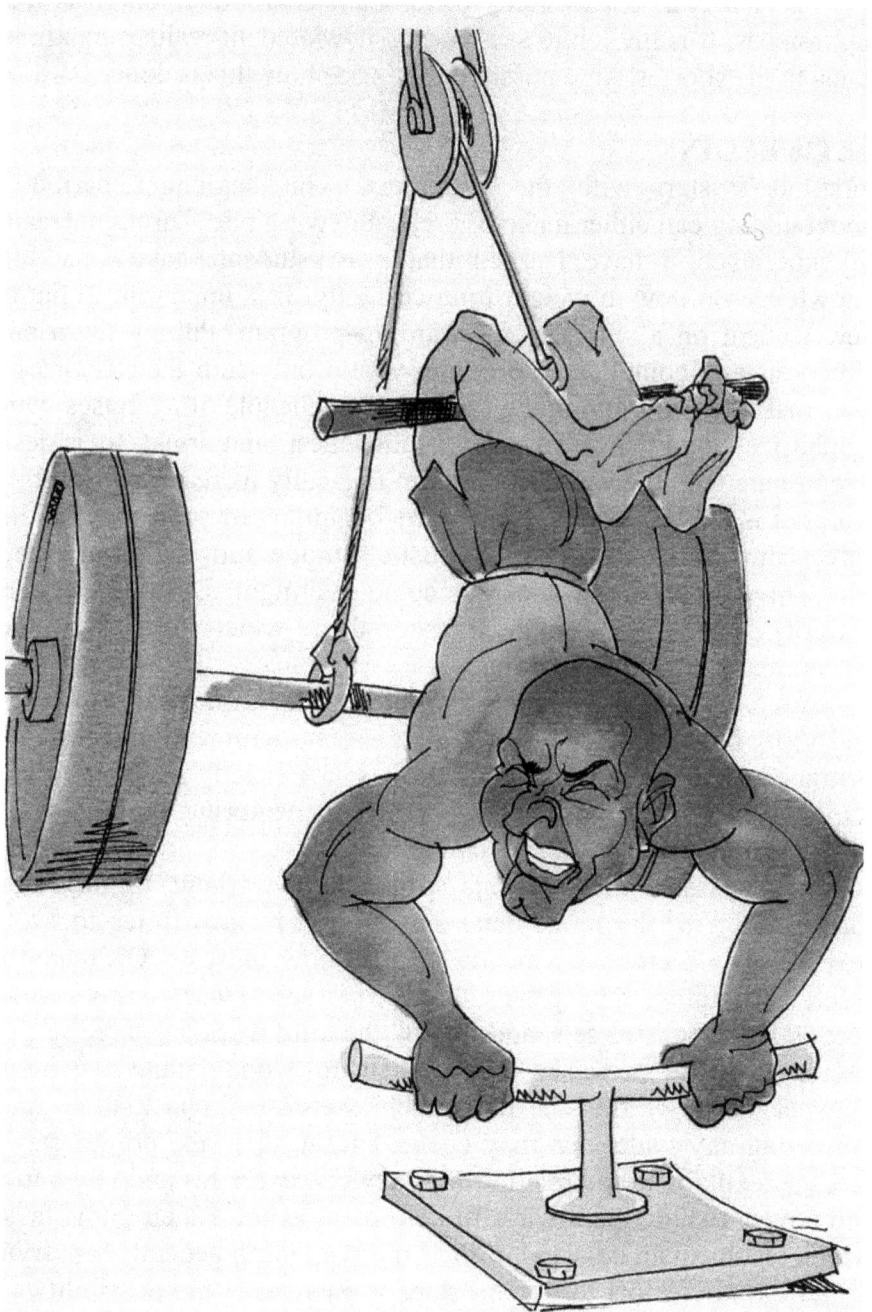

Exotic workouts produce strains and sprains

workout) a substantial increase in one's health. After the novice begins to understand what natural bodybuilding is all about I then proceed to lay out an exercise program designed to meet his or her needs.

There are almost as many different reasons for training as there are trainees. It is my job to see that my new student realizes maximum gains in the shortest time possible. Let's see how this is done.

LET'S BEGIN!

First, let's start with the beginners. The beginning period of bodybuilding can either make or break a new trainee. Through decades of experience, I have learned that most students have very little knowledge on how to weight train correctly. It is important to put the new student on a simple yet rewarding program. Putting them on a strenuous and complicated program would only ruin their chances of ever making it. By giving the beginners a schedule of exercises which emphasizes their "show muscles," (abs, chest, and arms), their desire to continue with the workout program is greatly increased. A full body workout is the best way to train at the beginning of your bodybuilding career. Just be sure to have a realistic attitude and understand that a Mr. Universe physique does not come overnight. Unfortunately, the majority of guys cannot foresee this, which leads to their discouragement and lack of interest.

Natural bodybuilding takes a lot of guts, determination, willpower, and years before one can ever realize their true potential. Getting the beginner to make it through all this is not exactly an easy task. It requires knowledge, experience, and good mentoring skills to take a beginner and turn him into a champion.

I always start new students with a basic workout, training them three times a week, on alternate days. I start them with ten to twelve exercises, with emphasis mostly on the show muscles. On their first week of training, they perform only one set of each exercise. The second week has two sets, and finally, the third week has three sets per exercise. On all exercises, I time them to a one-minute rest period between sets. As they perform each exercise, I check their form, correcting any faults that may occur. I teach them the proper way to breathe, explaining the relationship between exercises and respiration. Moreover, I show them ways to help them achieve their gains faster, which results in an upswing of their motivation. In general, I am trying to get the novice off to a good start by increasing the possibilities of them making it through this first and most difficult stage.

The following is a sample exercise routine, which I have successfully prescribed to many of my students:

BASIC WORKOUT #1

EXERCISES	SETS	REPS
Abdominal Crunch	1-3	15-25
Barbell Front Lunge	1-3	15-25
Front Pull-Down	1-3	12-15
Bench Press	1-3	12-15
Dumbbell Pullover	1-3	12-15
Overhead Shoulder Press	1-3	12-15
Triceps Push-Down	1-3	12-15
Barbell Curl	1-3	12-15
Reverse Curl	1-3	12-15
Incline Knee Pull-In	1-3	15-25

(See ANATOMY OF A BODYBUILDER chapter for technique details)

I start the routine with the Abdominal Crunch for two reasons. The first and most important is that it helps the trainee warm up and gets his blood pumping, thus preventing injuries. The second is to help firm up the abdominal region. Working the abs at the beginning insures that this area will not be neglected by forgetting it at the end of the workout.

From here on, the new student trains his largest body parts first, working down to the smaller ones. For thighs, I usually give the Barbell Front Lunge as the novice's first leg exercise. In earlier days, I use to start beginners off with several sets of regular Barbell Squats but found that they became discouraged with their training as the recovery and pain was too much for them to bear. I even had one trainee tell me that his first workout with squats resulted in more pain than his four years in Vietnam.

Therefore, experience has taught me that most beginners lack conditioning, motivation, and interest when it comes to training the lower body too intensely. By giving the beginner a light thigh workout, it increases the possibility of him completing this vital part of his muscle-building program, thus ensuring a desire for more later on.

Pain is one thing the beginner dreads. Giving him a simple exercise routine will do a lot to insure his continued interest in the sport. The rest of the workout is self-explanatory. Each muscle group is thoroughly stimulated for the new trainee to grow and progress at this first stage. Special emphasis is given to the arms and chest for the specific reasons already detailed. The routine is completed with the Incline Knee Pull-In because most beginners do not have the midsection endurance to perform two abdominal exercises in a row correctly. The novice follows this routine for about six to eight weeks. In that time, he begins to get a sense of what bodybuilding is all about.

FEELING STRONGER

After the first conditioning period, I outline a second routine, which is also followed three days per week. I want my new students to start feeling stronger and to be able to look in the mirror each day and smile as they see some form of continued progress. By designing a weight training routine that emphasizes increasing muscle mass and power throughout the physique, I am assured of the continued interest and desire of my students in achieving their goals. Because of this, many of my new students become infected with the *iron bug*, and for them, the only cure is to hit the gym with a vengeance.

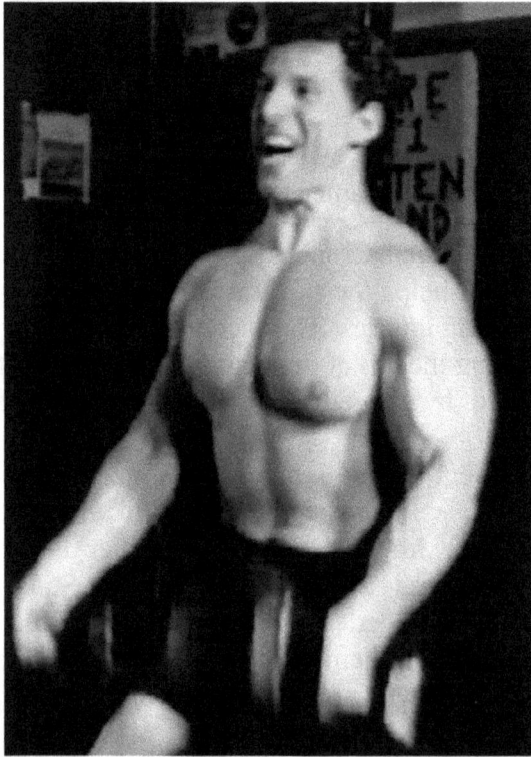

The following is such a program:

BASIC WORKOUT #2		
EXERCISES	SETS	REPS
Hyperextension	1-3	15-25
Incline Bent Knee Sit-Up	1-3	15-25
Full Squat	1-3	12-15
Standing Calf Raise	1-3	15-25
Bench Press	1-3	12-15
Incline Dumbbell Press	1-3	12-15
Dumbbell Row	1-3	12-15
Front Pull-Down	1-3	12-15
Triceps Push Down	1-3	12-15
Barbell Curl	1-3	12-15
Leg And Body Raise	1-3	15-25

(See ANATOMY OF A BODYBUILDER chapter for technique details)

Guidelines for Basic Workouts #1 and #2

A. For maximum results, perform these routines three times a week on Monday, Wednesday and Friday, or Tuesday, Thursday and Saturday. Use your off days for rest and recuperation. This is especially important if you are new to weight training.

B. Your weekly progression should be as follows:
  o Week 1: Complete one set with minimum repetitions.
  o Week 2: Complete two sets within a moderate range.
  o Week 3: Complete all three sets with maximum reps.

C. Use as much weight as is comfortable for the reps indicated. The last rep should feel difficult, but should not be an all-out effort during your beginning period of weight training.

D. As you continue weight training and your strength improves, the poundage you were using will begin to feel easier. Whenever you reach that point, increase the poundage until the last rep becomes difficult again. Document your training in a journal and keep accurate records of the exercises, sets, and reps you perform from each workout. Also, chart the foods you eat and count the calories, protein, carbohydrates, and fats of each food. This will enable you, among other things, to keep track of your progress from one workout to the next, rather than making the whole process haphazard.

E. Concentrate on correct form when performing each exercise and mentally focus on the body part you are working.

F. Correct breathing is necessary for most exercises, so be sure to follow the proper technique.

G. Unless stated otherwise, rest for sixty seconds to two minutes between sets. If you feel pain or need any kind of help during your workout, stop immediately and seek assistance. Remember, safety comes first when it comes to lifting steel.

H. Consult with a physician before and during a training program to ensure that you have no medical conditions that could put you at risk.

Should any exercises in these routines be uncomfortable or dangerous to perform, because of some sort of physical impairment you have, please substitute another exercise for the same body part, which will not aggravate the condition.

At this stage of the novice's training, I find that his understanding and desire to make it in bodybuilding has increased to where he actually wants to work harder and is ready to accept new challenges. He hungers to have strength and size equal to that of the bodybuilders he learns about through the media and in the gym. His motivation is like dynamite and this program is just the thing he needs to explode his gains into Muscledom.

Here are a few notes about the program: Since the new trainee will now be working out heavier, I schedule Hyperextensions as his first exercise. Through my observations in the gym, I have noticed that guys who never warm up before a workout eventually wished they had. The lower back can very easily be injured, discontinuing your training for months or longer. Performing Hyperextensions before every workout can and usually does save a lot of pain, tears, and sorrow. Besides, they are great for striations across the lower spinal erectors. When used in conjunction with sit-up and leg raise type movements, they help to firm the middle portion of the body.

For the first time the thighs are given a good workout. Remember not to go heavy while performing the Barbell Squat movement at this early stage. Just try to keep your form and breathing in a smooth and steady pattern.

Let's move on to the Standing Calf Raise. On some days (but not all), try going heavy. The idea is to keep the calves responding by not allowing them to become accustomed to any one type of stimulation. By working your calves right after completing Barbell Squats, you'll find that they pump easier, resulting in a faster growth rate.

Instead of prescribing the Barbell Row, which is a great overall back developer, I substitute it with the Dumbbell Row for some good reasons. One important reason is that most novice bodybuilders suffer some type of lower back injury while performing the barbell version rowing. In addition, there is a more complete range of movement while using the dumbbells. With dumbbells you have the ability to pull your arms higher and stretch out further, while also having the option of which way to face your palms. In my opinion, this does a lot more for complete back development than the Barbell Row could ever do. Why break your back if you don't have to?

Another exercise I like to mention is the Bench Press. For some reason the Bench Press has become the standard that we measure our upper body strength by. The Bench Press, although a valuable exercise, is no more important than the Chin, Row, Shoulder Press, Squat, or other basic movements that you perform in your routine. If you want to be able to Bench Press your whole life, then you must take steps to ensure that you do not blow out your shoulders early in the game. I know of countless guys who were huge benchers in their twenties whose shoulders are now ruined in their forties. One of the most important tips I can give you is to keep your form strict and not to use poundage that you cannot handle correctly. Do not bounce the bar off your chest and keep your butt on the bench! If you need a spotter to pull the weight off you on every rep, it's probably a good idea to lower the poundage and handle a weight within your normal limits. Be smart and leave the ego at home.

LET'S SEE THOSE MUSCLES!

For complete biceps development, *FORM* is the most important factor! Whenever someone asks you to show them your muscle, they are naturally referring to your upper arm, or more specifically, your biceps. In the gym, whenever I see a new trainee performing any type of curling movement incorrectly, I walk over to him or her and demonstrate the proper technique needed for maximum stimulation. I have seen too many bodybuilders waste time and sweat training their biceps incorrectly, with little to show for it. The reason their gains are minimal is not that they are not training hard enough, but that they are not training properly. I have also observed bodybuilders that have packed on slabs of muscle towards the center (medial) of the biceps while the lower (brachialis) part of the muscle remained shallow and weak.

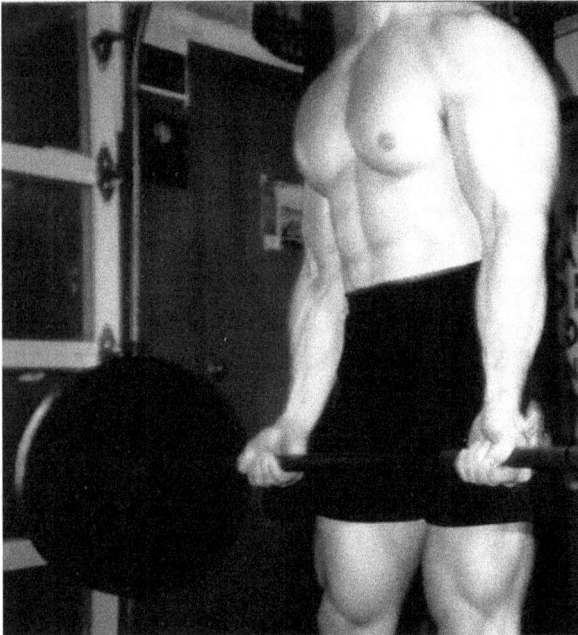

During my earlier training years, back when I was a young lad in high school (many moons ago), I trained my arms hard and heavy, seemingly as intense as any of my favorite muscle artist of the day. I tried all the exercises and systems I knew. Still my biceps' development did not equal the amount of work that was being spent on them. I was beginning to get discouraged. After all, here I was spending pain-soaked hours bombing my biceps endlessly and with little to show for it.

Then I remembered what my father told me when I first began to workout. "Son," he said, "When training your biceps, make sure you perform the curling movement through a full range of motion." I started to do just that. I would use a straight bar, gripping it with hands shoulder width apart and palms facing up. Before I would even begin to curl, I made sure my knees were slightly bent while sucking in my abs and extending my elbows in front of me. This leveraged my body in such a way that I received *100%* stimulation from all parts of the movement. Now, while remaining in this position I would begin to curl, raising the barbell up slowly while keeping my wrist straight and elbows stationary, to place constant tension on my biceps. As the bar reached my chin, I began to extend my elbows even further in front of me to the point where they were almost facing forward. This contracted my biceps fully, gorging blood into them for a super pump. At this point, I begin to lower the barbell slowly while forcing my elbows to remain extended in front of me. Most bodybuilders fail by stopping short of locking their elbows out at the extension part of the movement. I see this mistake all too often. Bodybuilders should focus not only on locking out the elbows, but on continuing the movement even further by trying to extend their arms straighter with an exaggerated effort to lower the bar down to the knees, thus stretching and pumping their lower biceps tremendously.

After a period of training with the above-prescribed technique, I began to notice changes in my upper arm development. My biceps became fuller and longer with a higher peak than ever before, making them one of my most outstanding body parts. This style of curling can be incorporated into most types of curling movements. The important thing to remember is to perform your curls through a complete range of motion while using correct form and exercise style.

The same range of motion principle also applies to the Reverse Curl. The Reverse Curl is a basic lower arm exercise that packs on slabs of muscle all across the forearms, especially the top area. In my opinion, the exercise is best performed with a straight bar while using a thumb-less grip and with your hands about shoulder width apart. While keeping your knees bent and upper body straight begin to move the barbell up slowly, focusing on keeping your elbows close to your sides and not allowing them to sway. A slight extension forward is permissible. Curl the barbell as far up to the chin as possible. Now squeeze the bar tight and feel the blood being pumped through your forearms veins. After completing the repetition, begin to lower the barbell, making sure that the elbows remain stationary at the sides. As you reach the bottom of the movement push down on the bar. This will help to create new shape and symmetry throughout your forearms, developing the big brachioradialis muscle to its maximum.

The other body part I like to discuss is the triceps. I see too many bodybuilders walking around with elbows that seem to protrude an inch or two abnormally away from the joints. I am amazed at the amount of elbow injuries reported each year. It is a shame, because many of these injuries could easily be avoided by eliminating, or at least using caution, while performing the Overhead Triceps Extension. For most trainees, this exercise is an unnatural movement, creating unwanted stress in the wrong areas.

Through time, I have learned that bodybuilders could easily develop complete triceps development by employing a variety of pushdown movements in their routine. I've even known men who do Triceps Extensions strict, light and heavy, with little to show for their efforts. After putting them on a routine consisting of Regular, Reverse, and Rope Pushdown type movements, their triceps responded like never before. Training them actually became a joy instead of being a dreaded dull experience, resulting in gains for them that were once believed to take years. While overhead triceps movements have their place in bodybuilding, the beginning stages of muscular development are not when to incorporate theses exercises.

I would like to emphasize once again that beginners should do all their exercises in a complete and strict form by using a weight that is comfortable for them. Forget about half movements and cheating principles for now. First, learn to build a solid foundation with no weak links. Be confident in what you do, believe that your workout is the best. The more trust you have in what you are doing, the better your chances at becoming successful. This does not just apply to bodybuilding either. It applies to everything you do in life. A positive attitude knows no limits.

SUPPLEMENTATION

As you have probably figured out by now, I am not a big supporter of supplements for the purposes of building muscle or gaining strength. I believe trainees should get all their nutritional needs from a well-designed nutritional program. I have not taken any form of supplements since my high school days and have not had the need for them because of my natural bodybuilding lifestyle. Whenever I stroll through a health food store or read an ad in a muscle publication, I become amazed at the ever-increasing variety of designer supplements created for the consumer. Most bodybuilding supplements are marketed with the promise of turning the user into a Herculean specimen that women cannot resist and men admire with great envy. It is all legal marketing but a bunch of hogwash in my book. For the

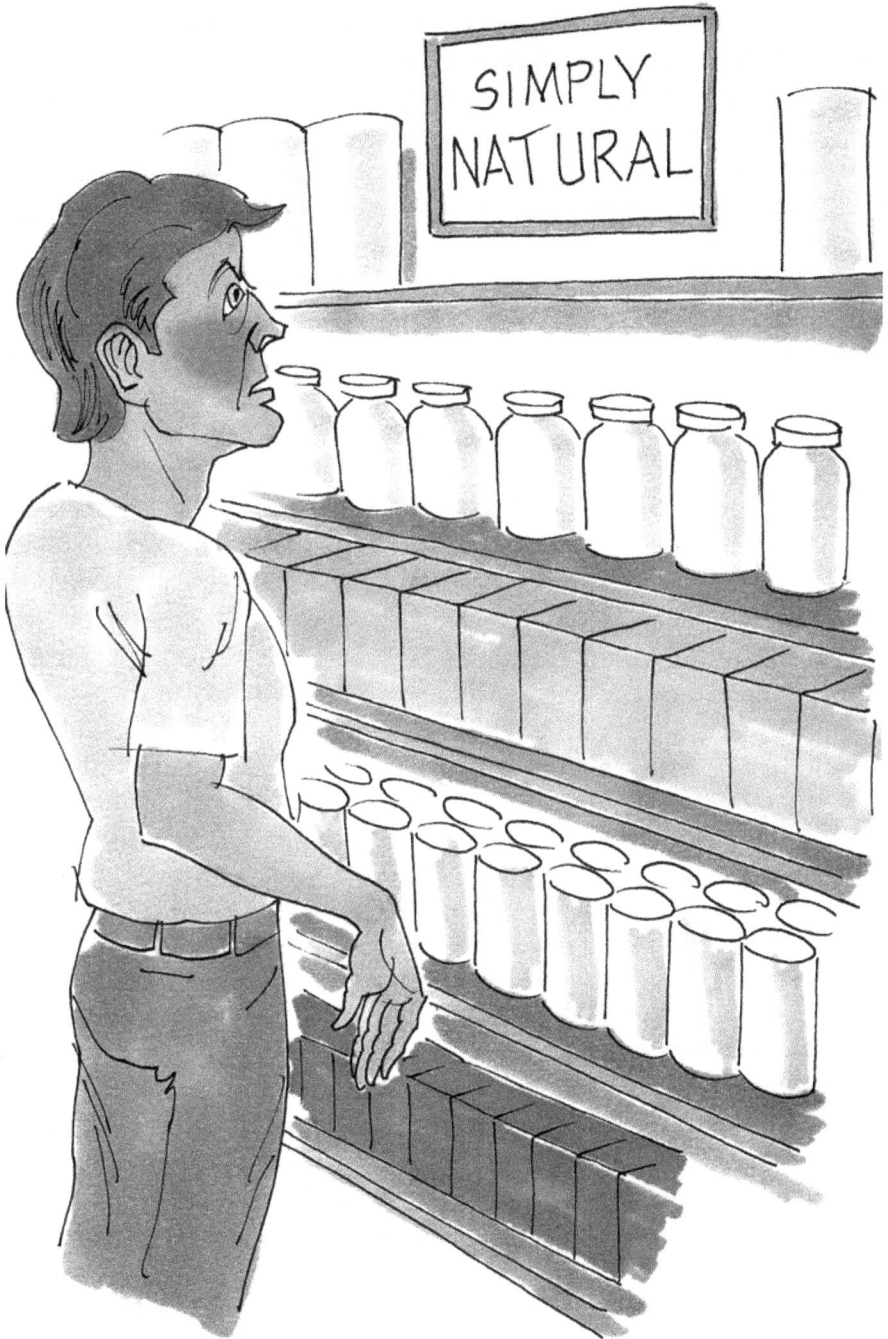

Supplements are a billion dollar industry

most part, these ads are misleading and the only ones making any gains from this marketing ploy are those who financially profit from the sale of these supplements.

Being a realist, I understand most bodybuilders do not practice sound nutrition and rely somewhat on supplements to help them meet their dietary requirements. If you feel the need for supplementation then stay with the basics such as a good vitamin/mineral supplement and perhaps a protein powder derived from eggs. You do not have to pop twenty different pills a day unless you have a medical condition, and if that is the case, seek a doctor's advice. For the most part, bodybuilders should only take supplements to fill the void of substances that are missing from their diets, or which their bodies cannot manufacture or fully assimilate. Do not get into the habit of solely relying on supplements to make gains. If you do, most of what you swallow will end up as waste and flushed down the bowl, along with the hard-earned money you spent on them. Look at it this way. Let us say you have a small houseplant that requires occasional watering and sunlight to grow. Do you think overdosing it with water every hour or exposing it to sunlight twenty-four hours a day is going to make it grow at a faster rate? The answer is no, and you will probably wind up killing the plant. The same rule of nature applies to people. Our bodies can only assimilate so much of any nutrient at any given time. It is a fact of life that too much of anything, no matter how good it may be for you at the proper amount, might bring you ill health and end your bodybuilding days with a crashing halt. If I can eat naturally for decades without any form of supplementation to sustain my size or strength, then you too can eat in the same manner and make great gains from following a well-designed nutritional program. Let us look at a sample diet.

EATING TO BUILD NATURAL MUSCLE
When I first began to train with weights at the age of ten, the last thing on my mind was following a balanced nutritional program. As I continued to workout throughout my teenage years, I became more conscious of the importance of proper nutrition as it related to bodybuilding. I began reading every piece of literature I could on nutrition and started to develop some theories on what constituted a proper diet. While in high school, I relied heavily on supplements to further my muscle gains, not realizing that much of what I was consuming was not being assimilated by my system, but instead taxing

my bodily functions and putting undue stress on my organs. Since my first concern in bodybuilding was and is my health, I gradually moved towards an all-natural diet, void of supplementation.

When we develop our strength and physiques, we live a healthier and more normal way of life, filled with endless energy and drive. A properly designed nutritional program will bring you lasting gains, not only in bodybuilding but with your health and vitality as well. Intensely training bodybuilders know they need substantial amounts of nutrients to help guarantee gains in their chosen sport. As bodybuilders, we require sufficient calories, protein, carbohydrates, fats, vitamins, minerals, and water to help regenerate our muscles after we tear them down through our intense bombing sessions. Because of the need for these nutrients, natural bodybuilders should spread the intake of these substances throughout their day to help guarantee maximum absorption.

Your body can only digest so much protein at any one time. An average bodybuilder looking to assimilate two hundred grams of protein into his body daily should be striving to divide his intake of the nutrient between four and six meals daily. Since you probably can only digest thirty to fifty grams at any one sitting, this is the best way to go. The same applies to carbohydrates, but for a different reason. Consuming too many carbohydrates at any one time may cause the insulin level in your bloodstream to rise to an excess level, causing the body to store the calories from the carbohydrates as fat. Besides, by eating several small meals throughout the day that contain complex carbohydrates and fiber, you will help maintain the glycogen stores in your muscles that are responsible for providing you with the explosive power necessary for your workouts. Another benefit of spreading your daily menu throughout six or more meals is that you will be able to absorb more muscle building calories than if you had tried to stuff yourself in three conventional meals.

Bodybuilders that are new to the sport have a hard time swallowing the concept that they need several small meals a day to build lean muscle without gaining extra body fat. When designing a diet for muscle building purposes, remember that protein assimilation is paramount in realizing success. At the same time, be sure to void your diet of foods high in processed sugars, saturated fat, and empty calories that the fat cells seem to absorb like a sponge. Eating several small meals a day also helps keep your insulin level stable and limits the deposition of fat.

While training with weights provides the resistance needed to stimulate muscle tissue into new growth, the role a properly planned diet has in building and refueling your body after intense training is more important. You could train four hours a day, seven days a week, and your gains would be limited without a well-planned nutritional program. In the previous chapters, we discussed the roles protein, carbohydrates, fats, vitamins, minerals, enzymes, and water play in helping you achieve your goals. Next, we will look at a sample diet to learn how to best consume meals for optimum muscle building gains.

BASIC NUTRITION

Bodybuilding is the scientific application of exercise, nutrition, rest, and a positive mental attitude. For me, nutrition is an easy and the most essential key to the puzzle. The problem with a lot of beginning bodybuilders is that they do not pay enough attention to their diets and eat tons of foods in hopes of gaining muscle; then when excess body fat accumulates in the wrong places they starve themselves to lose the unwanted bodyweight. That is no way to body build! My method is more practical. I eat the same types of foods each and every day. My diet consists of vegetables, fruits, grains, nuts, legumes, poultry, eggs, and spring water. The amount of each food item I consume on any given day depends on how I feel and if I have any set goals in mind, such as losing or gaining bodyweight. By eating the same types of foods every day, at the same times, I find it easy to adjust my bodyweight by slightly modifying my daily nutritional intake. When training to look great at the beach I just lower my fat, carbohydrate, and calorie consumption a bit to bring out the muscular striations. If I want to increase body mass, I move the lever in the opposite direction while maintaining my required protein intake. It is just a numbers game and these slight adjustments are all I need to acquire my desired look. This simple method allows me to maintain my strength and muscular size, while never having to experience hunger pains or any type of physical weakness.

Mastering your diet will not only make you much more in tune with your physique, but more importantly, with your health. Nutrition feeds life and consuming high quality natural foods should be a primary goal for you in building lasting muscle. Learn the nutritional composition of as many foods as possible. Study the amount of calories, fats, carbohydrates, and protein each food contains and design a nutritional program for your own individual needs. Since every one of us leads a different lifestyle, it is impossible for me to prescribe a specific gain or weight loss diet for you in this book without knowing you. What I can do is outline my personal nutritional diet as a reference for you to build off on and then modify to your needs. I'm sure you'll find your base level for the bodyweight you desire.

The following diet helps me maintain a massive bodyweight of 220 pounds at a height of 5'10":

BASIC DIET #1

5 AM	1 Orange
5:30 AM	6 Egg Whites, 1 Egg Yolk Spring Water
7 AM	2 Cups Raw Rolled Oats with Spring Water
9 AM	1 Banana
12 PM	16oz. Skinless Chicken Breast 2 Cups Broccoli Spring Water
3 PM	20 Raw Almonds Spring Water
4 PM	1 Pear (bosc)
4:30 PM	1 Cup Red Grapes
7 PM	16oz. Skinless Chicken Breast 6oz. Lentils, 2 Potatoes (med), 1 Onion Spring Water
8 PM	1 Cup Strawberries
11 PM	1 Cup Raw Rolled Oats with Spring Water

Values: calories 3,095, protein 237g, carbohydrates 431g, fats 45g

Compare this diet to Basic Diet #2 (page 296) to see how slight changes in foods can make a real difference in values consumed.

Please note that all values are approximate. The only liquid consumed is spring water. All foods are eaten raw, boiled, or steamed. Other similar food items may be substituted if desired. For maximum benefit, drink at least one gallon of spring water daily. All of my nutritional needs are fulfilled by the consumption of natural foods. I do not use supplements in any form. No sugar, salt, seasonings, flavorings, spices, sauce, oils, etc. is ever used.

Remember, this is only a sample diet. Each person is unique with different nutritional requirements. Depending in part on your body type, occupation, stress levels, and energy expended during your training, your nutritional requirements will vary from day to day. You may need more calories or protein than stated, or perhaps need to lessen your carbohydrates and fats. Every one is different and it is up to you to find your averages by keeping a record of not only your diet and training, but also of other activities throughout your day. Become a living library of knowledge and monitor your bodybuilding progress each and every day.

One way to make sure you are consuming enough calories and essential nutrients is to keep a daily journal of the foods you eat. Keeping a nutritional log will give you something to refer to when you need to make adjustments in your daily diet. For example, let us say you are trying to gain muscle but the scale does not register a higher bodyweight than your previous measurement. You look into your journal and add up the calories, protein, carbohydrates, and fats that you have been consuming. By studying the averages of these nutrients, you learn how much to increase your consumption of a particular food group in order to help you break through the barrier. Make no mistake about it, nutrition for muscle building is a science and must be mastered if you ever hope to realize your full potential.

PREPARING YOUR MEALS

Eating like a physical culturist does not mean you have to spend hours at the stove to prepare your meals. If anything, it means less time in the kitchen since a great deal of your foods should be eaten in their raw state or slightly cooked. Most of my foods are eaten raw with the exception of eggs, poultry, lentils, and potatoes (boiled) and broccoli (steamed). Everything else is eaten in its pure, natural state. Salads are eaten plain and fresh with no dressing. Fruits are washed and eaten as they come. I only add spring water to grains, and nuts are eaten in their raw natural state. The only thing I drink is the spring water that comes from my underground well in the Catskill Mountains. Even though I enjoy my meals, for me food is more about health than pleasure.

Eating several nutritious meals a day requires some planning and some realism. I understand that most bodybuilders need more of a variety in their diets to keep them from mentally cracking. The important thing when planning your nutritional program is to stay as close to nature as you can and to eat several small meals daily so your body will be fueled to the max and ready for action. The last thing you want to do is miss a meal or two since this can slow your metabolism and decrease your blood sugar levels, which can then cause your muscle tissue to enter a catabolic state from the lack of amino acids.

You have to plan to help guarantee that you will have several well-planned meals throughout your day. To do this, take an inventory of what is in your fridge and on your shelves, then make a list of what you need to buy and stock. When I go shopping, I usually get odd stares from the checkout clerk as she rings up my order of twenty or so large packages of skinless chicken breast. It gets even better when I make my annual purchase of rolled oats. I fill the shopping cart high with eight to ten cases of the nutritious complex carbohydrate and have a ball as I wheel it through the store with my vision blocked by the cases as I struggle to keep the cart from tipping over. Fruits, vegetables, and eggs have to be purchased more frequently since they need to be fresh.

After you have your fridge and shelves stocked, figure how much food you will need for any given day. To make my life simple I usually boil several skinless chicken breasts every three days. I do not have the time to waste every day in the kitchen and preparing six breasts at once frees up my time for other things. When the breasts are finished cooking I wrap them in aluminum foil and put them in the fridge until needed. For dinner, I will usually have one breast mixed in with a fresh salad. If I am going out for an event, I will pack a chicken salad and take it with me. The same goes for all my meals. When it comes to nutrition, I always make sure that I will have my meals at the scheduled time so that I may keep my energy levels and metabolism in check. It is important to be able to eat nourishing meals several times a day and the ability to bring your own meals with you, wherever you go, helps guarantee success in bodybuilding.

When I first started this health regimen in the early 1970s, I use to get strange looks from family and friends when I would show up at a wedding reception or some other gathering with my own prepared meals. While all the guests were enjoying their fancy meals and wine, I was crunching on almonds and gulping spring water. Since I never eat food prepared in a restaurant, I must bring my own food with me and usually get glares of insult from the waiters, who do not understand why their meatballs are not good enough for my taste buds. Eating the way some bodybuilders do can sometimes alienate them from the crowd. Nevertheless, if they wanted to be like the crowd they would not be bodybuilders in the first place...would they?

My advice to beginning bodybuilders is simple. Don't rush! Learn to accept the fact that it takes time to become a true natural champion. It is not an easy path to follow, but once you are on your way, you'll find that it will get a little easier with each step. As your bodybuilding lifestyle progresses, you will see changes in not only your physique, but also in the way you manage the challenges of everyday life.

With each rep you complete the path will become a little wider. With each set it becomes a little smoother, and with each workout a little shorter. Until finally, one day your starship will soar, whistling through the galaxies, as it guides you, the natural bodybuilder, on your *JOURNEY TO THE OLYMPIAN ZONE*!

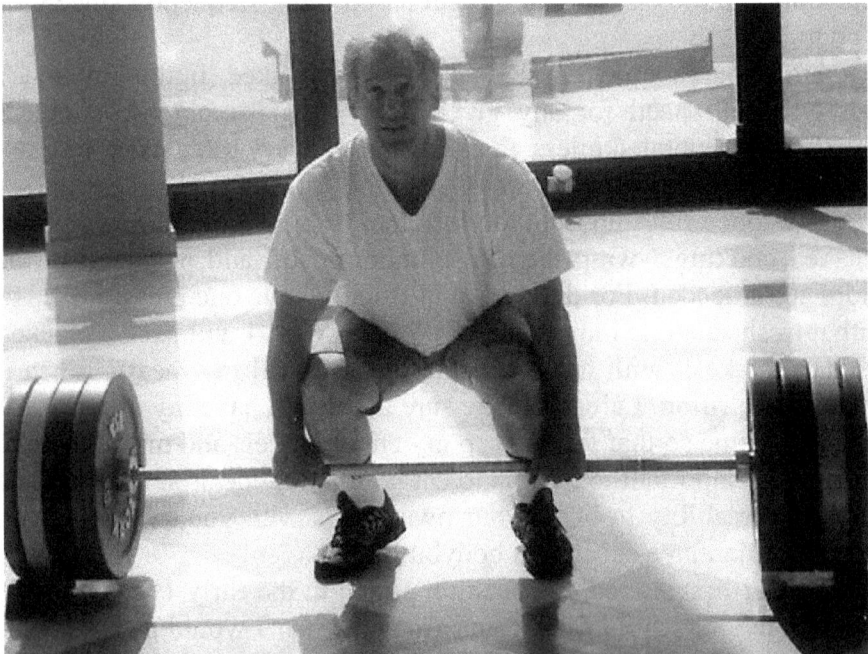

Mario demonstrates the proper technique of performing a heavy pull - 2006

BUILDING MOUNTAINS OF MUSCLE

Bodybuilding is like climbing mountains. To reach your highest summit takes great perseverance and fortitude from deep within yourself. As you climb towards the mountains peak, you are bound to encounter obstacles and dangers that can derail your efforts. By using an intelligent and well-planned exercise program as your compass, you are guaranteed to climb the most awesome mountain imaginable, as your goals become reality.

When you pass the beginning stage of bodybuilding, you should be proud that you made it through the most challenging stage and that you are ready to continue onward to the top of the mountain. As you become an intermediate bodybuilder, your enthusiasm should be burning stronger than ever since you have gained more knowledge on how to achieve your quest in the safest and shortest time possible. By applying this strong desire into your bodybuilding lifestyle, you are sure to succeed.

It is important for the intermediate bodybuilder to plan his training into progressive stages. The last thing you want to do is follow a Mr. America style training program, because you would eventually burn out. You have to build your body's recuperative powers up slowly, increasing the training intensity a little bit at a time. Natural bodybuilders are aware it takes years to become true champions. They also know that once they have achieved their goals, their gains are there to stay for decades.

By applying this bit of sensible advice into your bodybuilding lifestyle, you can be assured of continued gains in the muscle you seek. Realizing that a championship body takes years to develop is a step in the right direction. Too many new trainees think that all they have to do is pop a few Big Ds and presto, instant Mr. Godzilla. It is a shame, because one day they are going to wake up and it is going to be too late. After decades of traveling down the anabolic highway the sport of bodybuilding has finally began to get back on the road towards health and longevity. It is up to you, the natural bodybuilder, to help guide others on this same path by setting an example for the masses to follow. Your presence on the physique stage, at the gym, and in your local community has a positive influence on others…use it and make a difference!

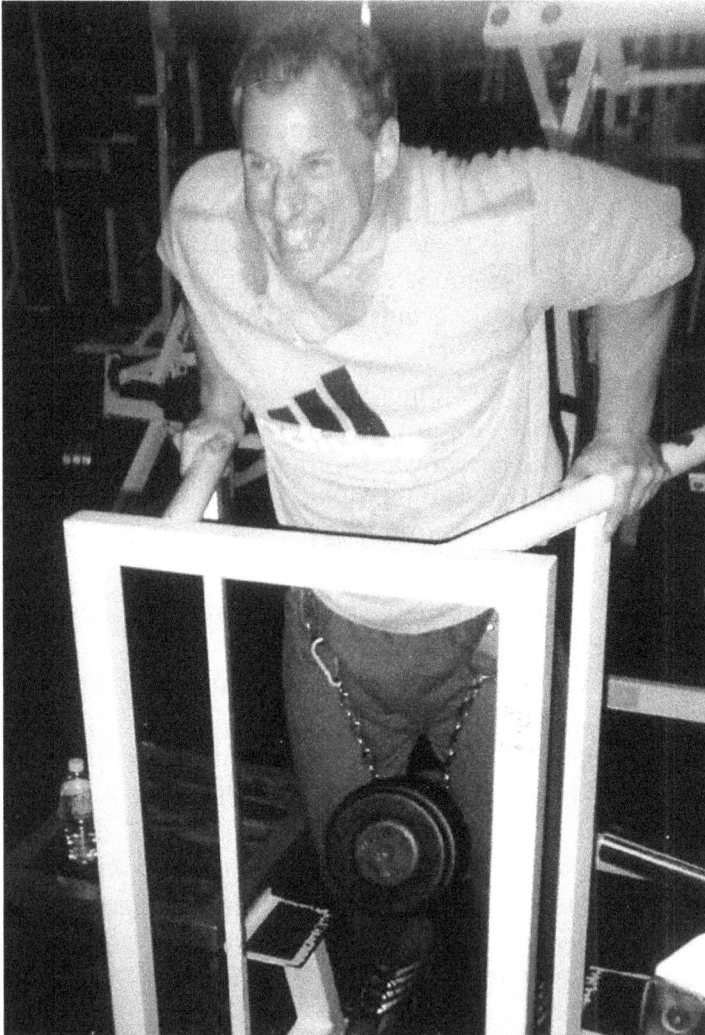

Mario Strong pushing out some heavy reps – 2006

GETTING BIG

I remember when I first reached the level of intermediate bodybuilder. My brother, Johnny, and I would train together three times a week on alternate days. We would follow a schedule of exercises emphasizing the basic movements. Every exercise we performed was a tremendous effort. There was no letting up. We used the heaviest poundage possible on every exercise we performed and made sure to keep the movement strict during the first few reps, adding a slight cheat towards the end of the set. We trained so hard that after every workout we would just collapse and rest for about twenty minutes. Our efforts and dedication paid off. Within six months of intense training, our gains were so miraculous that relatives and friends who had not seen us in a while became astounded when they laid their eyes upon us. We had transformed ourselves into extremely well developed natural athletes. It was hard to believe that only a few months earlier our bodyweights were nearly twenty pounds lighter and now, here we were, with muscles popping out in places that we did not know existed.

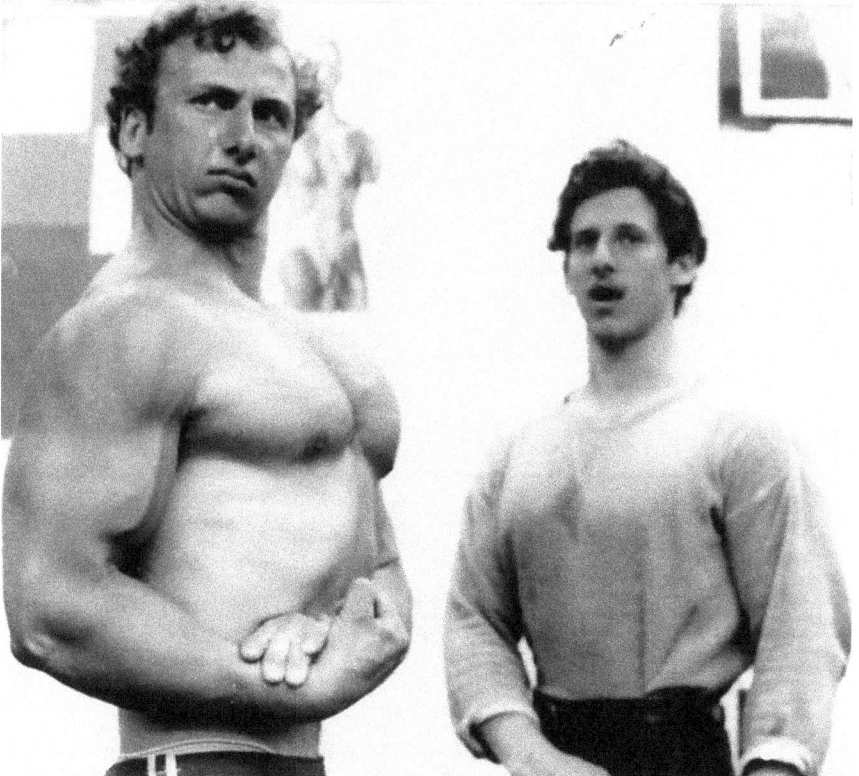

Mario monitors his brother Johnny's progress in a gym mirror - 1979

The following is an exercise routine similar to the one my brother, Johnny, and I used. Many of my students who have trained hard and regularly on this program have enjoyed similar gains. The program should be followed for at least six to nine months:

BASIC WORKOUT #3

EXERCISES	SETS	REPS
Hyperextension	3	15-25
Incline Bent-Knee Sit-Up	3	15-25
Full Squat	3	10-12
Dumbbell Pullover	3	10-12
Stiff Leg Dead-Lift	3	10-12
Standing Calf Raise	3	15-25
Incline Barbell Press	3	10-12
Machine Chest Press	3	10-12
Dumbbell Row	3	10-12
Front Pull-Down	3	10-12
Alternate Dumbbell Press	3	10-12
Triceps Push-Down	3	10-12
Barbell Curl	3	10-12
Reverse Curl	3	10-12
Incline Knee Pull-In	3	15-25

(See ANATOMY OF A BODYBUILDER chapter for technique details)

For best results, follow the guidelines outlined in the beginners section. The only difference is that you should be striving to complete all the prescribed sets and repetitions during every intense workout.

One look at the workout and you will automatically know why we use to collapse after its completion. This program is loaded with growth stimulating exercises; every major muscle group in the body is worked thoroughly and hard. Nothing is left to chance, which is important for the natural bodybuilder looking to develop his physique proportionately. It is an energy demanding routine so be sure to follow a super nutritious diet to help you recover from your workouts. Do not forget about getting plenty of rest and sleep.

Make sure to superset the Full Squat and Dumbbell Pullover together. When combined in superset fashion this dynamic duo is a hard team to beat. Be sure to keep your concentration on the exercises, not allowing your thoughts to drift away. The better you're able to focus, the faster your gains will be realized with these movements. When performing this superset during my teenage years, my ribcage expanded to an unbelievable size. It was tough on my lungs, as they burned while I deeply inhaled and exhaled several times between each repetition of both exercises. Probably the only other superset combo that I have ever performed in the gym that I found more demanding was when I replaced the Full Squat with the Front Barbell Squat. One note worth repeating is to use a full range of motion on all exercises. Especially when performing squats. When I perform squats, I go all the way down until there is nowhere else to go. By performing squats in this fashion, I am guaranteed maximum power and development in my thighs. Too many times I have witnessed trainees at the gym using more weight than they could possibly handle correctly. I doubt if they even completed half the range of motion required. I know squats are very demanding and that they will make you bust your butt. However, the results will be worth it. They will increase your lower body mass, your upper body size, and your power. That is why they are called the king of all exercises.

After following this program for three to six months, you will experience a noticeable increase in muscle mass and overall strength. If you like, you might want to substitute some of the exercises for others. The important thing to remember is to perform the basic type movements through a full range of motion. When trading one exercise for another make sure it will help maintain your physique's balance in the correct proportions.

THE SPLIT ROUTINE

While working out three times a week is a great way to train, chances are that sooner or later you are going to move on to a split system. By applying the split system's principles to your bodybuilding training, you will be able to devote more time and energy to each body part. Just remember not to go overboard by adding twenty different exercises per muscle group. Instead, try keeping it around three with a movement for each part of the muscle group.

For example, the deltoids are composed of three different muscle-heads: frontal, lateral, and posterior sections. Together they make up the entire deltoid region. Now at this stage of the game it would be foolish to concentrate on just one section. Let's say you're training the shoulders. Instead of performing the Behind Neck Shoulder Press, Military Press, and Alternate Dumbbell Press, which concentrate mainly on the frontal deltoid, you'd be better off performing the Behind Neck Shoulder Press, Standing Side Lateral Raise, and Bent Over Lateral, which work all three heads of the deltoid region, giving you a more complete and squared off look. By applying this basic idea to your exercise schedule, you will save yourself a lot of time and energy by not having to balance out your physique's symmetry later on. In addition, you will have a better understanding of your body's proportion, shape, weak, and strong points.

Now, there are many different variations of the split routine. When advancing from training three times a week to the split system, I usually suggest breaking the body parts up into two separate routines, training a total of four times per week. If you have a year or more of steady training, and your goal is to pack on slabs of muscle and gain loads of strength, then four weekly workouts is for you. For example, on Monday and Thursday, you could train your chest, back, and shoulder groups, and on Tuesday and Friday, you could devote your energy to bombing your thighs, calves, arms, and abdominals.

Many of my students do well with this type of training system. The body easily accepts the transition from three workouts per week to four. As a matter of fact, a good deal of my students usually go on to add a fifth training day by performing some light work on their weaker body parts. If you find any exercises or routines prescribed in this book uncomfortable or dangerous to perform because of some sort of physical impairment you may have, please substitute another in its place or do nothing at all.

Here now is such a program followed by many of my students:

MONDAY		
EXERCISES	SETS	REPS
Barbell Bench Press	5	10-8-6-6-6
Incline Dumbbell Press	3	8-10
Parallel Dip	3	6-10
Front Pull-Down	4	8-10
Cable Row	3	8-10
Front Pull-Up	3	6-10
Shoulder Press	4	8-10
Upright Row	3	8-10
Standing Side Lateral Raise	3	12-15
Barbell Shrug	3	12-15

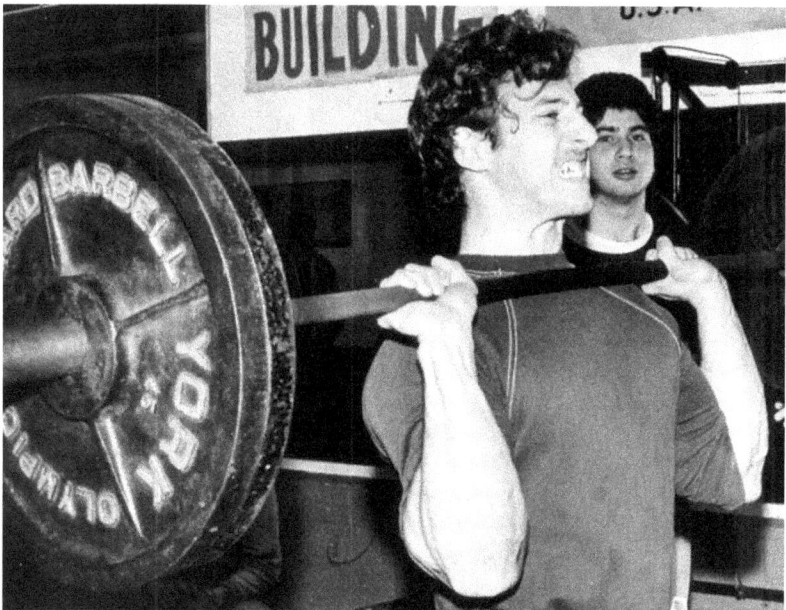

TUESDAY

EXERCISES	SETS	REPS
Triceps Pushdown	4	8-10
Overhead Triceps Extension	3	8-10
Barbell Curl	4	8-10
Incline Dumbbell Curl	3	8-10
Reverse Barbell Curl	4	8-10
Leg Press	5	10-12
Hack Squat	3	8-10
Stiff Leg Dead Lift	3	8-10
Standing Calf Raise	5	15-25
Incline Bent- Knee Sit-up	3	15-25

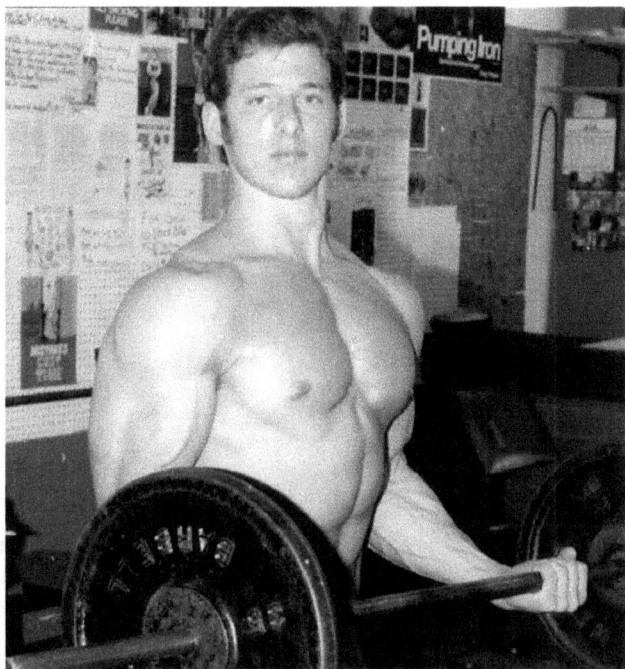

THURSDAY

EXERCISES	SETS	REPS
Incline Barbell Press	5	10-8-6-6-6
Flat Dumbbell Fly	3	8-10
Machine Chest Press	3	8-10
Close Grip Pull-Down	4	8-10
Barbell Row	3	8-10
Front Pull-Down	3	8-10
Alternate Dumbbell Press	4	8-10
Alternate Front Lateral Raise	3	8-10
Bent Over Lateral Raise	3	10-12
Dumbbell Pullover	4	8-10

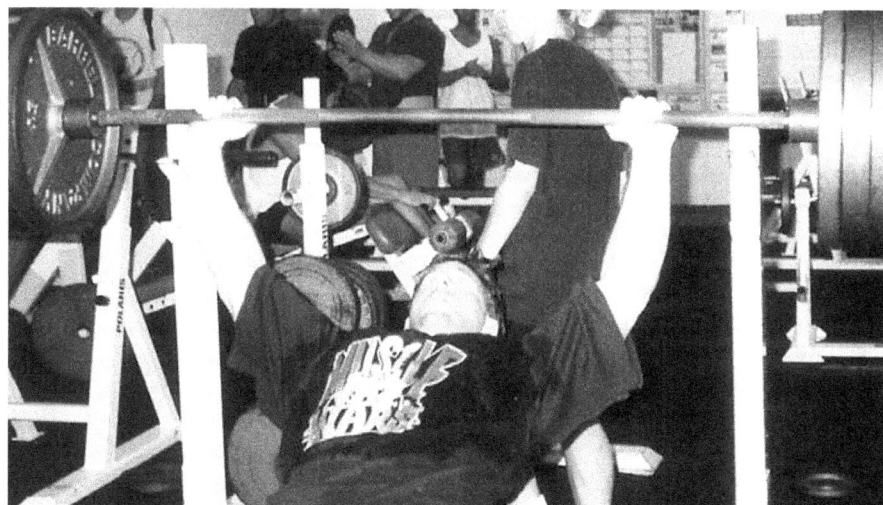

FRIDAY		
EXERCISES	SETS	REPS
Lying Triceps Extension	4	8-10
Dumbbell Triceps Kickback	3	8-10
Barbell Scott Curl	4	8-10
Seated Dumbbell Curl	3	8-10
Barbell Wrist Curl	4	10-12
Full Squat	5	10-10-8-8-6
Leg Extension	3	10-12
Lying Leg Curl	3	10-12
Seated Calf Raise	5	15-25
Leg And Body Raise	3	15-25

(See ANATOMY OF A BODYBUILDER chapter for technique details)

For best results, follow the GUIDELINES as outlined in our beginners section. The only difference is this time you will be training four times a week instead of three and that you should be striving to complete all prescribed sets and repetitions from the first week on.

If you are a more seasoned bodybuilder who likes to workout six days per week, then a further variation of the split routine may be necessary. Weight training six days a week is grueling and taxing on your recuperative powers. On occasion, I use this type of system for several weeks to shock my muscles into new growth before returning to a more sane approach to training. Try the following: On Monday and Thursday train your chest and shoulder region. On Tuesday and Friday train the back, arms, and abdominal areas, and on Wednesday and Saturday bomb your thighs, calves, and abdominals hard. Sunday, try running a fast mile or two to maintain your endurance and stamina. As you can see, each body part is still worked the same amount of times during the week as the four day split routine, with abdominals being the exception by receiving four sessions. The real gem of this system comes from the further splitting up of body parts, resulting in more energy per session with an increased possibility for faster gains.

This system is an old favorite of mine. With each workout being somewhat shorter in duration, I can train harder and with a greater range of intensity while keeping my energy and concentration levels high throughout the entire workout. To me this spells progress. The real secret to making your muscle building goals a reality is to give your training everything you have, each time you enter the gym. Learn to feel the exercises as you perform them.

SUPERSETS

Throughout my decades in the gym, I have occasionally incorporated supersets into my routines with great success. I find that supersets help stimulate my muscles by gorging them with blood, thus giving me a super pump. The difference between a superset and a normal set is that a superset consist of two or more exercises and is performed with little to no rest between sets, whereas you may rest several minutes between individual sets. Personally, I find that supersets are excellent for developing definition but are not effective for building mass or strength. They are not effective because of the reduction in the level of resistance that is used. This reduction in poundage is caused by fatigue due to the lack of recovery time between sets, which results in the decreased level of potential mass to be gained. Supersets save time by reducing the rest interval between two exercises. Shortening the rest period between sets increases the intensity because you are overloading the muscles being trained by performing more work in less time. One of the disadvantages of supersets is that several pieces of equipment are required. This means that a bodybuilder has to prepare his free-weights and machines before he begins his planned movements, and hope that nobody gets in his way during the superset. Having an alert workout partner should keep things in order.

FORCED REPS

Another training principle that I have used on a rare occasion is the Forced Reps Principle. This is one of the most popular and without question the most abused intensity technique. A spotter is needed to provide enough assistance for the trainee to be able to complete the repetition. The purpose of forced reps is to help the trainee realize greater gains in muscle mass and strength by extending the set past the point of failure. With forced reps, a training partner should assist just enough for the trainee to grind out the last rep past the point of failure. The abuse with forced reps comes when the trainee relies on the spotter for assistance during most of the set. In my opinion, forced reps should only be used on the last rep of an exercise to help induce further gains. Properly executed, forced reps are very demanding and can severely tax your recovery systems. Since they can easily tear muscle tissue, use them very sparingly and with great caution.

HIGH OR LOW REPS?

The question of how many repetitions are required to build quality muscle mass has been debated for decades. Some bodybuilders respond well to low reps with heavy poundage, while others enjoy the results that higher repetitions bring to their physiques. Both ranges of repetitions have been demonstrated to work effectively in adding new muscle. In general, the amount of repetitions you should perform on any given set usually depends on your body type and goals.

After training for several decades, I've learned that my body responds best to a low to medium rep scheme, which for me is between three and ten reps. After warming up with a light set or two of high reps, I usually perform my heavy sets in the range of five to six repetitions. On exercises such as the Full Squat, Parallel Dip, and Deadlift, I gradually add weight through the sets until I have reached a peak of one to three heavy repetitions. I like the way the heavy weights feel and enjoy the big gains they bring to both my physique as well as my strength. Remember, when training heavy it is important to warm up by gradually pyramiding the poundage from a light weight to heavier poundage in order to prevent the risk of serious injury.

When teaching beginners how to train, I combine high repetitions (twelve or more) with light weights so the new trainees learn how to perform the exercises prescribed in a proper and complete form. The trainees find that this combination puts little strain on the actual muscles being worked, and helps to ensure that they will continue with their bodybuilding ambitions. Although the higher repetitions provide less resistance than the heavier steel, they do build more endurance than the lower range of repetitions. The higher repetitions also tend to pump more blood into the muscles and help add new growth to the body part being trained. If you have a muscle group that does not respond well to a low/moderate repetition scheme, performing higher repetitions may be what is needed to shock that stubborn area into new levels of growth.

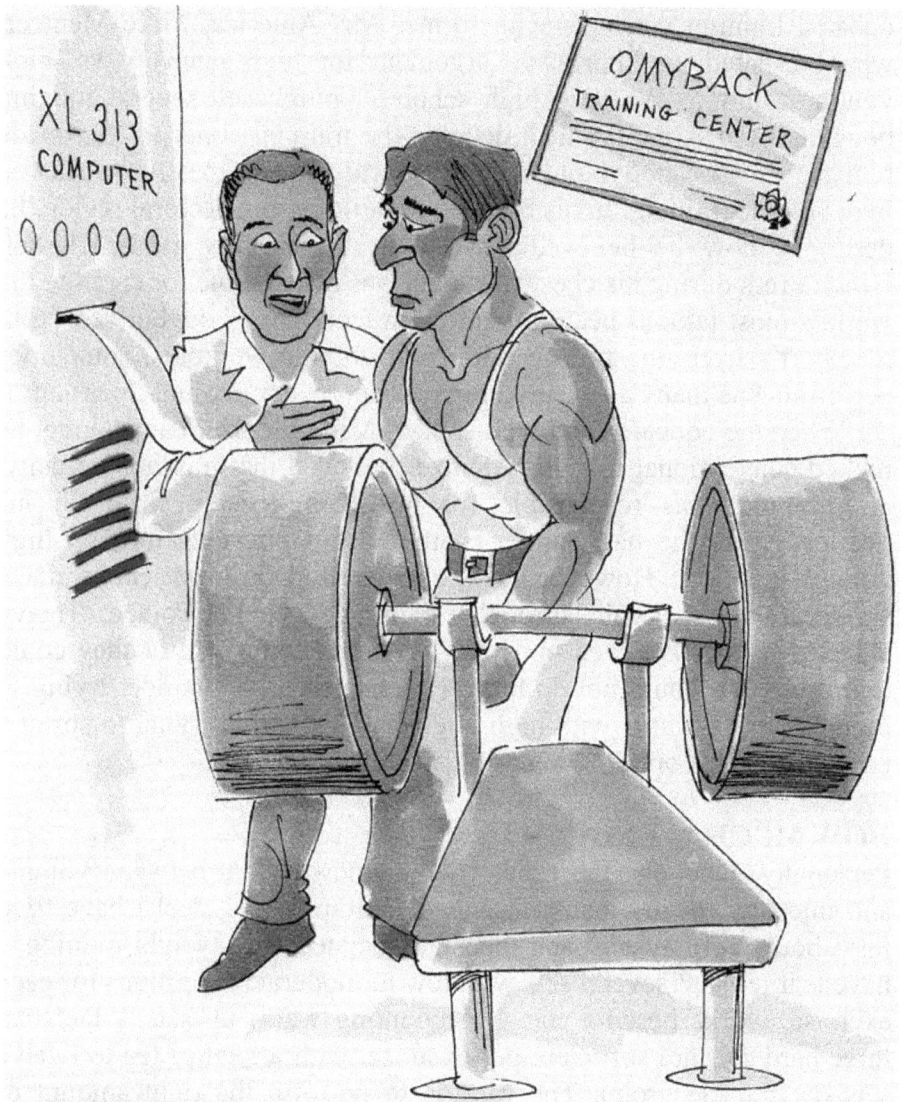

"IT SAYS YOU'D BE NUTS TO TRY IT."

Train for gains not strains. It is a great thing to lift mountains of steel as long as you don't fall and crash along the way. Know your limits! Be patient and give your body time to develop its maximum strength potential. When training with the heavy stuff be sure to have someone strong spotting you as a safety precaution.

HOW MANY SETS?

This has been another hot bed of discussion since the late 1970s, when Arnold Schwarzenegger, who is a proponent of high volume training, debated training concepts with former Mr. America, Mike Mentzer, who presented an impressive argument for high intensity vs. high volume training. When in high school, I purchased several training booklets from Arnold, which detailed the training concepts that made him the greatest bodybuilder in the world at the time. Arnold loved high volume training. In his booklet on building the pectoral region, he described how he believed performing fifteen sets of the Barbell Bench Press during his chest workouts was responsible for creating the world's most famous pectoral region. In fact, many bodybuilders from the sport's Iron Age trained with high volume workouts, sometimes performing as many as twenty, thirty, or more sets per muscle group.

When the educated and well-spoken Mike Mentzer came along, he rocked conventional thought. Mentzer believed that training intensity, not volume, was responsible for his championship form. In his younger years, he had built a championship physique through high volume training. However, he believed bodybuilders could make similar if not better gains through a training concept he coined, "Heavy Duty." Mentzer believed bodybuilders could train hard or they could train long, but could not do both. He equated a bodybuilder trying to perform high volume with high intensity to a runner trying to sprint a marathon. In his opinion, it was impossible to do both.

HOW MUCH IS ENOUGH?

Personally, I believe the answer lies somewhere in between volume and intensity. In my many decades of pumping the steel I have tried just about every system and theory associated with weight training. I have learned that several sets with low to moderate repetitions for each exercise, works best for me. Not counting warm up sets, I feel that three hard sets are sufficient per exercise, with a total of ten to twelve sets per muscle group. The trick is to perform the right amount of muscle stimulation without overtraining and wasting the workout.

Too many exercises, sets, and reps will only hamper your ability to recover from your grueling workouts. Through many decades of training at various gyms, the one mistake that I have repeatedly witnessed by bodybuilders is that they continuously overwork the muscles that they are trying to grow. Unfortunately, this only leads to fatigue, decreased strength, loss of muscle mass, and an increased heart rate, with little desire to return to the gym. When searching for your training threshold, gradually increase your workload to meet your body's recuperative powers. Be patient. It will take some trial and error to find your training limit, but once you do, you will be better able to navigate your training towards greater gains without having to worry about the negative effects caused by overtraining.

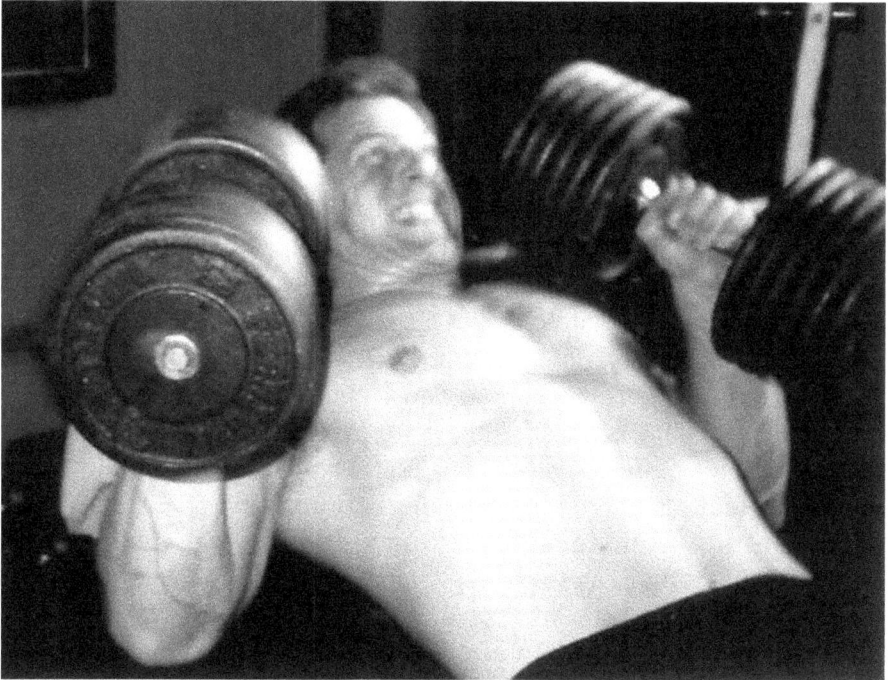

Mario Strong crashing through the pain barrier - 1995

DANGERS AT THE GYM

Bodybuilding is an endless pursuit! It takes years of commitment, desire, effort, and guts to pump muscle with steel so that we may realize our goals in this world of muscle and strength. Unfortunately, the journey to Muscledom is filled with roadblocks that can sometimes derail a bodybuilder and put him on the disabled list. This sport of ours requires pushing, pulling, and straining against heavy metal. It demands our constant attention and focus in the gym, and punishes us when our thoughts wane or our technique becomes sloppy. Over the decades, I have witnessed as well as personally experienced many different types of physical injuries. To make lasting gains in the gym I like to train heavy and with great intensity. While I find this type of training is best to stimulate growth it also brings me into the danger zone as I continually flirt with the chance of experiencing a serious injury. Workout after workout, bodybuilders push their physiques to the max, and unfortunately, they sometimes suffer from some sort of injury as a result. Whether it is a tear in their flesh or a bone snapping from the stress placed on it, bodybuilders are often reminded of their human limits. Injuries are a common problem in all forms of athletic endeavor but are even more prevalent in the bodybuilding community. Gyms, by themselves, are inherently dangerous places to be without adding the careless factor into it. To last in this iron game you need to have common sense in the gym and learn how to avoid injuries before they happen. Having the thick head that I do, I learned the hard way a long time ago. After experiencing several serious injuries, something registered in my old cerebrum and advised me to smarten up before I became permanently disabled. Today, I listen to my body's feedback and make the appropriate changes in my training when warranted, so that I may avoid any potential injury. In the gym, I have witnessed plenty of torn biceps, muscle spasms, and ruptured disks caused to bodybuilders. This is mostly due to the physical and psychological stress muscle builders place on their bodies through the heavy resistance they use. Whether you are new to the iron game or have decades of intense training under your lifting belt, you need to pay particular attention to any warning signs your body may be giving you. If you ignore a warning, you will undoubtedly pay for your carelessness with pain and forced time away from the gym.

Here are a few of the types of injuries bodybuilders experience when pushing past their limit or just being careless:

Types of Injuries
A. Avulsion: A body part is forcibly torn away by trauma or surgery. This usually occurs along the convergence between the muscle and its tendon.
B. Tendonitis: Inflammation of the tendon connecting muscle to bone.
C. Fracture: A complete break or partial impairment of a bone.
D. Strain: Injury or impairment caused by overuse or overexertion.
E. Sprain: Painful wrenching or laceration of the ligaments of a joint.
F. Bursitis: Bursitis is the painful inflammation of the bursa, a pad-like sac found in areas subject to friction.
G. Contusion: An injury in which the skin is not broken; a bruise.

Common Injuries In The Gym

A. Pectoral Avulsion: A tearing of the tendon connecting the Pectorals Major to the Humerus Bone. This painful injury that may result in a balling of the muscle towards the sternum. A significant amount of bruising and swelling can be expected.

B. Neck Strain: Caused by stress placed on the tendons or muscles of the neck.

C. Knee Strain/Sprain: Indicated by pain along the joint-line of the knee, behind the knee joint, or just below the kneecap along the patellar tendon. Various injuries include meniscal tears, patellar tendonitis, ACL tears, and bursitis.

D. Back Strain/Sprain: Resulting from lifting poundage incorrectly. Pain may be centered in the lower back, gluteus area, or muscles that surround spine.

E. Delayed Onset Muscle Soreness: Soreness in a muscle that has been worked. Usually occurs within a 24-48 hour period after training and diminishes within 72 hours. Resulting from a build-up of cortisol, lactic acid, or micro-tears in muscle tissue.

F. Elbow Tendonitis:
   1. Lateral Epicondylitis: Indicated by pain along the outer-bone on the upper portion of the forearm. Results from strain placed along the origin of the extensor muscles of the forearm and may result in tearing of these muscles.
   2. Medial Epicondylitis: Inflammation of the tendons that attach the forearm flexor (wrist) muscles onto the medial epicondyles of the humerus, on the inside of the elbow.
   3. Triceps Tendonitis: Inflammation or swelling of the triceps tendon where the triceps muscle connects to the elbow.

PREVENTING INJURIES

Bodybuilders experience injuries because of poor exercise technique and lack of focus. Incorrect exercise form can pull, rip, spasm, and tear muscle and delicate connective tissue. Our bodies and limbs have very specific biomechanical pathways and muscle builders need to be precise when it comes to performing each exercise with the proper technique. To prevent serious debilitating injuries it is imperative for bodybuilders not to deviate, twist, or misalign their bodies while lifting heavy weights. I always find it amazing at how many trainees cause injury to themselves because they fail to use caution during their workouts. To avoid injuries in the gym I handle weights that I know I can handle in a safe, correct form, and through a full range of motion. To me, it is just common sense. Here are a few of the things to avoid while climbing the mountain.

Probably, the biggest reason for injuries in the gym is when trainees try to lift more weight than they could possibly handle correctly. When it comes to using too much weight, I can write volumes on this. We are all guilty of pushing beyond our normal limits and I am no exception. I have crashed to the floor plenty of times when squatting heavy and have had more mishaps than I care to remember. However, if there is one exercise that trainees love to push more weight than they can handle, it is the Bench Press. Don't ask me why, but the Bench Press has become the standard in the gym by which we measure our strength. In the old days, when someone asked how much you could lift, he or she was referring to the Military Press. This lift has been replaced by the Bench Press, which in my mind is an inferior upper body movement when compared to the Parallel Dip. Using too much iron in any exercise is a sure way to experience a serious injury. If you cannot control the poundage you are lifting within its biomechanical boundaries and if you have to jerk the weight in order to lift it, then that is a good indication that you are using more weight than you could handle.

Personally, I rarely use spotters. Nevertheless, if you have been training for a year or so you might want the benefit a spotter can bring to your workouts. Spotters are of particular benefit when maxing out on power-lifts such as the Bench Press and Squat. Many bodybuilders have seriously been injured while performing these movements and having a spotter by your side is one way to avoid injury. Make sure the person spotting you is strong and focused on what you are doing. The last thing you want is for him to be checking out some fitness babe while you are attempting a new, personal record.

The Cheating Principle allows muscle builders to train beyond their normal capacity and therefore should only be used by advanced lifters. This principle takes the muscle beyond its point of failure and can literally force it to grow. I like to use cheating movements to further my gains. Being a bodybuilder that likes to train heavy, I incorporate the cheating principle quite a bit into my training, but as I perform an exercise, I am sure to feel the resistance constantly in the muscle desired as I move the weight in the line of the exercise. When applying this principle to your training, make sure not to overdo it as so many trainees do. You must feel the weight in the muscle being worked. For example, when performing the Cheating Curl movement you should feel the biceps receiving stimulation throughout the entire exercise. If your back starts to spasm, it's probably a good indication that you're handling an excessive amount of steel.

Overtraining drains the bodybuilder's energy and retards his progress in the gym. It is virtually impossible for the bodybuilder to make gains when in an over-trained state. Overtraining interferes with both the muscle and the nervous system's ability to recuperate because it severely depletes our body's glycogen stores and puts our metabolism in an unsettled state. We have all over-trained at one time or another. When I'm at the gym and have some extra time, I like to keep lifting the steel until the gym closes for the night. Sometimes this can be up to four hours of heavy bombing, which definitely falls into the category of overtraining. Have your basic workout planned before you enter the gym and when you are finished, put the barbell back on the rack and leave. Use your time wisely.

Another neglected factor in the gym is priming the muscle area to be trained. I remember Bill Pearl's words in an article he wrote about warming up. Simply put, Mr. Pearl stated that if you did not have the time to warm up, then you did not have the time to train. Makes sense to me. Think of it as getting in your car on a cold winter morning. You wouldn't just start the car and speed off…would you? If you had any kind of sense you would let the engine run a while as it primed its pistons for the road ahead. The same rule applies to weight training. If we neglect to prime our muscles before we lift the heavy stuff we are definitely going to breakdown our motors and crash before we get on the highway. A warm up is usually a high rep, low intensity, quick-paced exercise, or two, used to increase blood flow to the muscles. Performing a few light movements raises the temperature of the involved muscle, while decreasing blood viscosity and promoting flexibility and mobility. This is because a muscle with blood coursing through it is more elastic and pliable than a cold, stiff muscle. When I begin my workouts I start slowly, using very light weights, and increase the poundage with each set I perform. I am especially sure to warm up on every power movement I perform. For example, I usually perform the Barbell Squat in the middle of my thigh routine. Now, even though my thighs are burning by the time I get to the squats, I am still sure to start the exercise with a very light weight and get my form in a correct line before I increase the poundage. Warming up is necessary for a safe journey.

In addition to warming up with light weights, I also perform several stretching movements before and during my workout to prevent injuries. I not only stretch the muscle group to be trained, but the entire body as well. When stretching, I bring a joint to the end of its range of motion and hold it there for a period. As I feel my muscles relax and elongate I am careful not to bounce them, since this could result in an injury. You should perform your stretching exercises in not only the gym but also whenever you have a few spare moments. Stretching can be done anywhere and at anytime. Incorporated with your weight training, stretching helps loosen the muscles and make them more neurologically alert, thus helping them to become more pliable and injury resistant. Stretching between sets also helps to build muscle by promoting muscular circulation and increasing the elasticity of the fascia. An important point to remember is that flexibility is joint specific. Some joints can be more or less flexible than average. Flexibility in a joint depends upon the joint surface, the length and elasticity of ligaments, and the elasticity of muscles. Flexibility can be improved upon by anyone and at any age. If you stretch regularly and correctly, it can be tremendously beneficial. Stretching allows for maximum muscle repair and decreases soreness resulting from exertion. Most importantly, stretching regularly can help you prevent injuries. Good forms of stretching are tai chi, yoga, pilates, and some callisthenic exercises.

Negative Reps is another training principle that can cause muscle builders painful injury. I find that negative reps are one of the most difficult and dangerous of all weight-training principles. This is because the amount of resistance used is overloading the muscle that is being trained. When bodybuilders train, they normally use weights that they are capable of moving in a positive motion. When negative (eccentric) movements are incorporated into the workout, heavier resistance is needed. To train in this manner you need an experienced spotter or a machine designed to move the poundage from you in a concentric motion.

Keeping your mind focused on what you are doing in the gym can prevent disaster. The easiest way to hurt yourself, or someone else, is not to pay attention to what you are doing. Years ago, while getting some 45lb weight plates off the plate-rack, I accidentally dropped one on my foot and instantly felt an intense pain that sent me soaring. Now, I did not drop the weight because it was too heavy, I dropped it because my mind was elsewhere and not focused on the task. The same applies to your training. When in the gym, watch the advanced bodybuilders and see how focused they are in their training. It is this kind of intense focus that helps prevent them from experiencing injuries. Their minds are in tune with their muscles. Once you acquire this same ability to focus, you too will enjoy years of injury-free training. One ounce of prevention is worth more than a pound of cure!

When it comes to training accessories I have never had the need for knee-wraps or a lifting belt, but I have used training gloves and do use wrist-wraps on rare occasion to aid in my grip when pulling very heavy steel. Using knee-wraps during heavy squats may help to protect your knee joints. They do this by helping to increase external pressure and by distributing the strain across a larger area. Similarly, a lifting belt acts like a layer of muscle across your lower back as it distributes the strain of the weight away from your lower lumber area and into the belt itself. Bodybuilders find wrist-wraps useful during heavy lifts such as the Deadlift, Shrug, and Row. Wrist-wraps not only help prevent the lifters from dropping the heavy steel, but also allow them to lift heavier because they are attached to the bar and don't have to worry as much about their grip. Earlier in my bodybuilding career, I experienced a tremendous amount of callus buildup on my hands. I was training several times a day and the calluses were very thick and covered my entire palm as well as my five fingers. I bought a set of weight training gloves and they seemed to help a bit with the callus problem. However, because of my intense lifting, the gloves kept tearing apart. Finally, after a dozen or so pairs I decided to call it a day and just train bare handed.

IF YOU EXPERIENCE AN INJURY
A. For serious injuries seek medical attention immediately. Postponing the inevitable will only delay recovery time.
B. If the injury is to a bone or joint, protect the area by supporting it with a brace or splint.
C. Give the injury plenty of time to heal. Minor injuries should resolve themselves within several days. Serious injuries may take weeks.
D. Treat the injury with ice or cold packs to help limit inflammation, swelling, and internal blood loss.
E. Use a wrap or towel as a compression on the injured area to limit swelling.
F. Elevate the injured area above the level of your heart to reduce blood flow to the area and to help decrease blood loss and swelling.

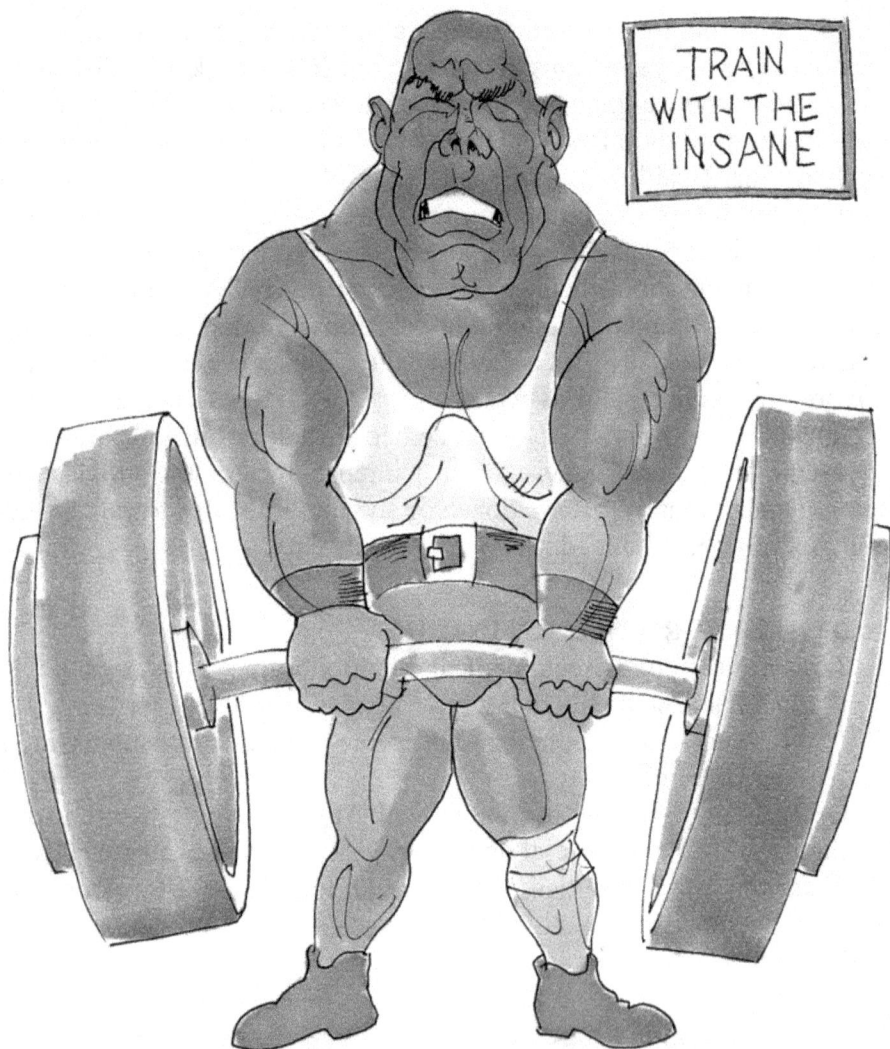

Be sensible when planning your training routines

COMMON SENSE BODYBUILDING

If performing an exercise causes injury or exasperates a condition, stop immediately! Give your body time to rest so the injury can properly heal. I have been knocked down plenty of times during my many decades in the gym. The one thing that I have learned, is that when you experience an injury in the gym, stop training. Missing an exercise, workout, or even a week or two from the gym, is better than turning a minor problem into a major one.

Train for gains not strains. It is a great thing to lift mountains of steel as long as you do not fall and crash along the way. Know your limits! Be patient and give your body time to develop its maximum strength potential. When training with heavy steel be sure to have someone spotting you as a safety precaution. A good way to help guarantee steady gains with your training is to have a workout partner who is motivated and willing to push to the limit. Having someone there when you need to force out an extra rep or two is a great and safe way towards continued progress. Train with a partner who's at the same stage of development and strength as you and who will be there to motivate you on days when you are down in the dumps.

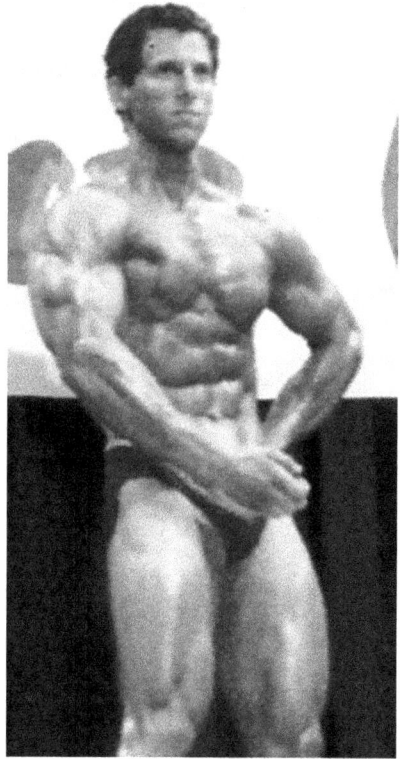

Have you ever noticed that guys with he-man size physiques tend to get some extra respect wherever they go? Make no mistake about it, size matters, and the bigger you are the more you're going to standout. Once you reach he-man proportions, you may be surprised to notice that people who were a bit unkind to you in the past have now become downright friendly. Now on the other hand, nothing turns a woman off more than an egomaniac who is full of himself. Learn to act in a low-key fashion while in the public view, and take an interest in what others have to say. The bigger and stronger you become the more essential it will be to develop a friendly personality. It's just not all about you, and the sooner that sinks into your muscle-man brain the better off we'll all be. While being dedicated to your bodybuilding is great, don't forget to enjoy the simple pleasures in life. Every once in a while take some time out from your training and experience the world around you. When on vacation forget about the steel and take a hike, swim, or just relax and take it all in. Advanced bodybuilders are like living works of art. Wherever they go, they bring their creation with them. Some guys like to display their masterpieces every chance they get. Men with muscle cars don't race them at every corner they turn; the same principle applies to you, save it for the competition.

Bodybuilding is an extremely scientific sport. By attaining as much knowledge as you can on the subject, you will not only realize your goals sooner, but also understand how you got there. Make it a habit to buy and read as much literature on the subject of physical culture as possible. Evaluate what you learn and apply what works best for you and your natural bodybuilding lifestyle. With this newfound knowledge, your visions and dreams of the future will transform into the realities of the present, as you, the natural bodybuilder, thrust into warp drive, on your *JOURNEY TO THE OLYMPIAN ZONE*!

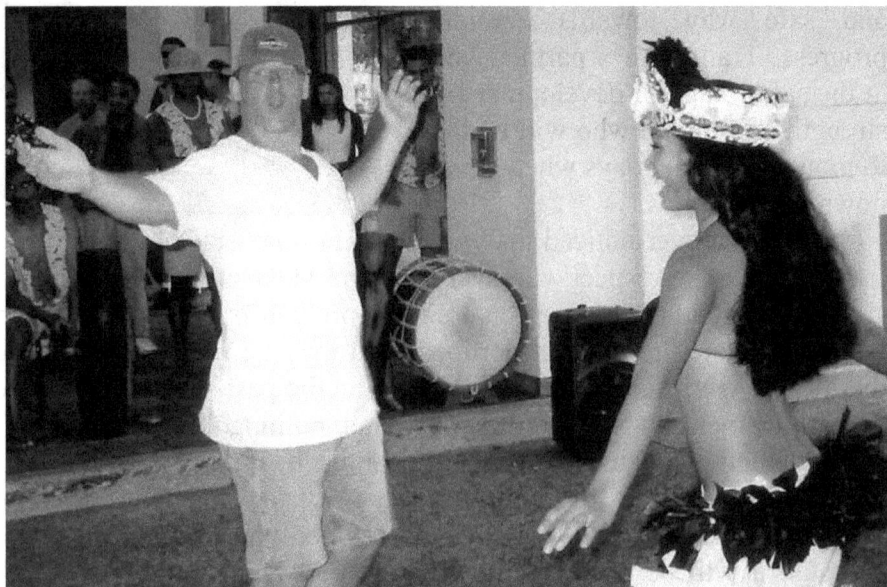

Mario Strong performing with a Hawaiian hula girl in Waikiki - 2002

GETTING READY FOR THE BEACH

EATING TO LOSE UNWANTED BODY FAT

Occasionally you may feel the need to shed some excess body fat. Perhaps you just want to look good at the beach or maybe just trim up a bit for your health. Following a well-designed exercise and nutritional program is necessary for maximum results. When following a weight loss program, the goal is to retain muscle mass while losing unwanted body fat. After training hard for several years and successfully building a he-man physique, the last thing a bodybuilder wants to do is lose the muscular gains he worked so hard to achieve. Following a diet that severely reduces calories is difficult for most bodybuilders. The best way to lose weight and retain muscle mass is to do it slowly over an extended period. When bodybuilders lose weight too quickly some of their weight loss may be in the form of muscle and not fat. This is because the human body has a survival mechanism designed to hold on to its fat stores in order to prevent starvation.

The more overweight a person is the faster he or she will lose bodyweight. This is because the heavier person creates a greater calorie deficit. As an example, Person A is 50 pounds overweight and consumes between 1,800 and 2,200 calories daily. Person B is only 10 pounds overweight and consumes the same 1,800 and 2,200 calories. The heavier person will lose more because it takes more calories to sustain a heavier bodyweight. If you are extremely overweight, you can expect to lose an average of 1.5 to 2 pounds of fat a week. If you are between ten and fifteen pounds overweight, your weight loss will average 0.5 to 1.5 pounds of fat a week. For most bodybuilders, two pounds is the maximum amount of body fat they should strive to lose in any given week. Any additional weight loss is probably only a loss of muscle tissue and not fat.

Be sure to drink adequate amounts of water daily to help curb your appetite and maintain your health. Forget the fallacy about gaining weight from drinking lots of water since this is probably a result of poor mineral balance in your diet or some underlying medical condition. This alone should be reason enough for you to follow a well-balanced nutritional program and seek medical advice when needed.

When on a fat loss program it is important to understand the scientific principles involved in the process. To lose one pound of fat (3,500 calories), your consumption of food must be 3,500 calories less than your calorie expenditure. Although this process is slow, there are other factors to consider.

Breaking the "base level" is an important factor to understand when trying to lose unwanted body fat. The base level is a particular bodyweight the body maintains when calories are not restricted. Your body has its own level of fat that it wants to store, regardless of slight variations in everyday caloric intake and expenditure. One way to manipulate your base level to a lower point is to perform cardio exercises each and every day.

Natural bodybuilders should strive to lose no more than two pounds per week. More than that may result in the loss of muscle tissue. To regulate your weight loss you need to know exactly how many calories you are eating every day and to adjust them until you begin to lose body fat. It may take some experimentation on your part, but knowing how many calories you are consuming before starting a diet gives you a good point of reference.

Remember, it is calories that are of prime importance when losing body fat. Many bodybuilders make the mistake of severely reducing their carbohydrate consumption or eating lots of protein with the belief that this is the best method in becoming more muscular. While these nutrients are important, the first consideration should always be the calories consumed. A good starting point to losing body fat is to learn how many calories are needed to maintain your current bodyweight and then gradually decrease your caloric intake by 300-500 calories a day. It is also important to monitor your condition and determine if you are losing body fat or muscle tissue.

When following a fat loss diet, consuming a sufficient amount of protein is of prime importance. Protein is responsible for repairing and rebuilding muscle tissue, and since retaining muscle mass is a primary goal of natural bodybuilders, they should be sure to consume enough high quality amino acids daily in order to maintain a positive nitrogen balance. To accomplish this, muscle builders that train intensely should consume between 1.0 and 1.25 grams of protein per pound of bodyweight daily. That means that a two hundred pound bodybuilder needs to consume between 200 to 250 grams of protein a day. To properly digest and assimilate this much protein, bodybuilders should eat several small meals per day, spread out over every two to three hours. This practice will help keep the body in a positive nitrogen state by constantly feeding the muscles with protein and other nutrients. Spreading your daily nutritional requirement through several small meals also helps with absorption and prevents indigestion.

Carbohydrates are a primary source of energy. When on a fat-loss diet, they must be adjusted to meet the goals of the bodybuilder. The trick is not to lower the carbohydrates to the point where the body has to rely on muscle tissue for energy. In order to retain muscle mass and strength it is imperative to include some carbohydrates in your diet. Some bodybuilders make the mistake of drastically cutting their carbohydrate intake while increasing their fat consumption, believing that fat is a better source of energy. Fat contains twice as many calories than protein or carbohydrates, and since it is more difficult for the body to breakdown its fatty acids, this does not seem like a reasonable practice. The bottom line is to keep your fat intake to thirty or less grams per day. All animal products have fat, so be careful in the type and amount of foods you consume.

At the beginning stages of a reduced calorie diet, most of the initial weight loss may be in the form of water. As your body burns it's most accessible fuel, which is the glycogen stored in your muscles, it releases three to four grams of water for each gram of glycogen. During the first week of your fat-loss program, you may lose several pounds of unwanted bodyweight. This reduction in poundage is dramatic and should motivate you to stay on your program. As you continue on your reduced calorie diet, your body will start burning fat more readily. Because fat contains many more calories per pound than glycogen, it takes longer to lose. Patience is the key!

METABOLISM ADAPTATIONS

A common mistake bodybuilders make is to limit their consumption of calories, fats, and carbohydrates severely in an attempt to lose pounds in a short period. This type of diet lacks food variety and the essential vitamins and minerals the body needs to function properly. Luckily, your body has a survival mechanism (base level) that holds fat stores if your nutritional consumption is limited for a period. Severely restricting your intake of nutrients turns on your body's survival mechanism and causes your body to respond by slowing down its metabolism to save energy. While this survival mechanism helps us stay alive in times of need, it can nevertheless stop you from losing the unwanted bodyweight you desire. This means that even though you are eating very little you will not be able to lose bodyweight because your body has drastically slowed down its metabolic rate. It all comes down to a balanced exercise and nutritional program when trying to lose excess body fat.

One important thing to remember when first undergoing a fat-loss program is patience. If you do not see your bodyweight dropping after adopting such a program, do not worry. Your weight training might be creating new muscle and causing you to weigh the same or more. Just stay with your nutrition and exercise program. After the muscle growth stabilizes, you will eventually start losing unwanted bodyweight as your body begins to tighten and firm up.

DAILY MEAL PLAN

If you are currently on a high calorie/fat diet, do not immediately jump into a low calorie/fat regimen. Let your body and mind adjust to your new nutritional plan gradually. Never let yourself become weak from hunger. Remember, while you are burning away the fat, you are also building a fortress of long lasting health and vitality.

Since natural bodybuilding is the scientific application of exercise, nutrition, rest, and positive mental attitudes, it's important to apply each of them to your life in a reasonable fashion. Many bodybuilders do not pay enough attention to their diets and eat tons of food to gain weight, and then starve themselves while trying to rid their bodies of excess fat accumulations. That is no way to body build! My method is more practical. I eat the same types of foods each and every day. My diet consists of vegetables, fruits, grains, nuts, legumes, chicken, eggs, and spring water. The amount of each food item I consume on any given day depends on how I feel and if I have any set goals in mind, such as losing or gaining bodyweight. By eating the same types of foods every day at the same times, I find it easy to adjust my bodyweight with some slight modifications to my daily nutritional intake. When I desire to look great at the beach, I just lower my fat, carbohydrate, and calorie consumption a bit to bring out the striations. If I want to increase my body's mass I move the lever in the opposite direction while maintaining my required protein intake. It is just a numbers game and these slight adjustments are all I need to acquire my desired look. This simple method allows me to maintain my strength and muscular size, while never having to experience hunger pains or any type of physical weakness.

Mastering your diet will put you in tune with your physique and your health. Nutrition feeds life and consuming high quality natural, organic foods should be a primary goal for you in building lasting muscle. Learn the nutritional composition of as many foods as possible. Study the amount of calories, fats, carbohydrates, and protein each food contains and design a nutritional program for your own individual needs. A nutritional adviser can help you do that. What I can do is outline my personal fat-loss diet as a reference and you can adjust it as needed. Most importantly, be patient. It takes time to accomplish your goals, but rest assured that they will be realized by you if you consistently follow the advice given in this chapter.

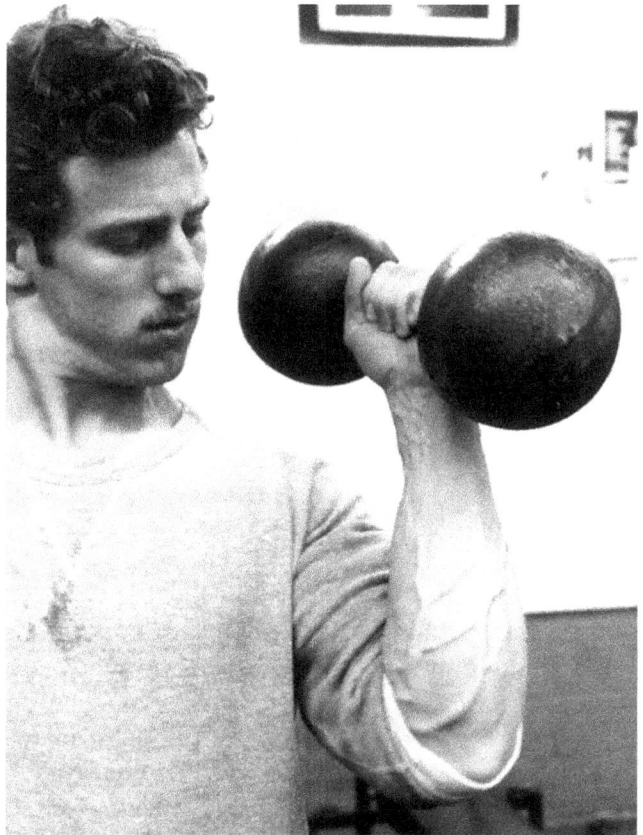

The following diet helps me maintain a lean muscular bodyweight of 200 pounds at a height of 5'10":

BASIC DIET #2	
5 AM	1 Orange
5:30 AM	6 Egg Whites, 1 Egg Yolk Spring Water
7 AM	1 Cup Raw Rolled Oats with Spring Water
9 AM	1 Banana
12 PM	16oz. Skinless Chicken Breast 2 Cups Spinach Spring Water
3 PM	10 Raw Almonds Spring Water
4 PM	1 Apple
4:30 PM	1 Cup Pineapple
7 PM	16oz. Skinless Chicken Breast 2 Cups Broccoli Spring Water
8 PM	1 Banana
11 PM	1 Cup Raw Rolled Oats with Spring Water

Values: calories 2,401, protein 204g, carbohydrates 325g, fats 28g

Compare this diet to Basic Diet #1 (page 265) to see how slight modifications in foods can make a real difference in 'values' consumed.

Diet notes: All values are approximate. The only liquid consumed is spring water. All foods are eaten raw, boiled, or steamed. Other similar food items may be substituted for the above. For maximum benefit, drink at least one gallon of spring water daily. All of my nutritional needs are fulfilled by the consumption of natural foods. I do not use supplements in any form. No sugar, salt, seasonings, flavorings, spices, oils, sauces, etc. is ever used.

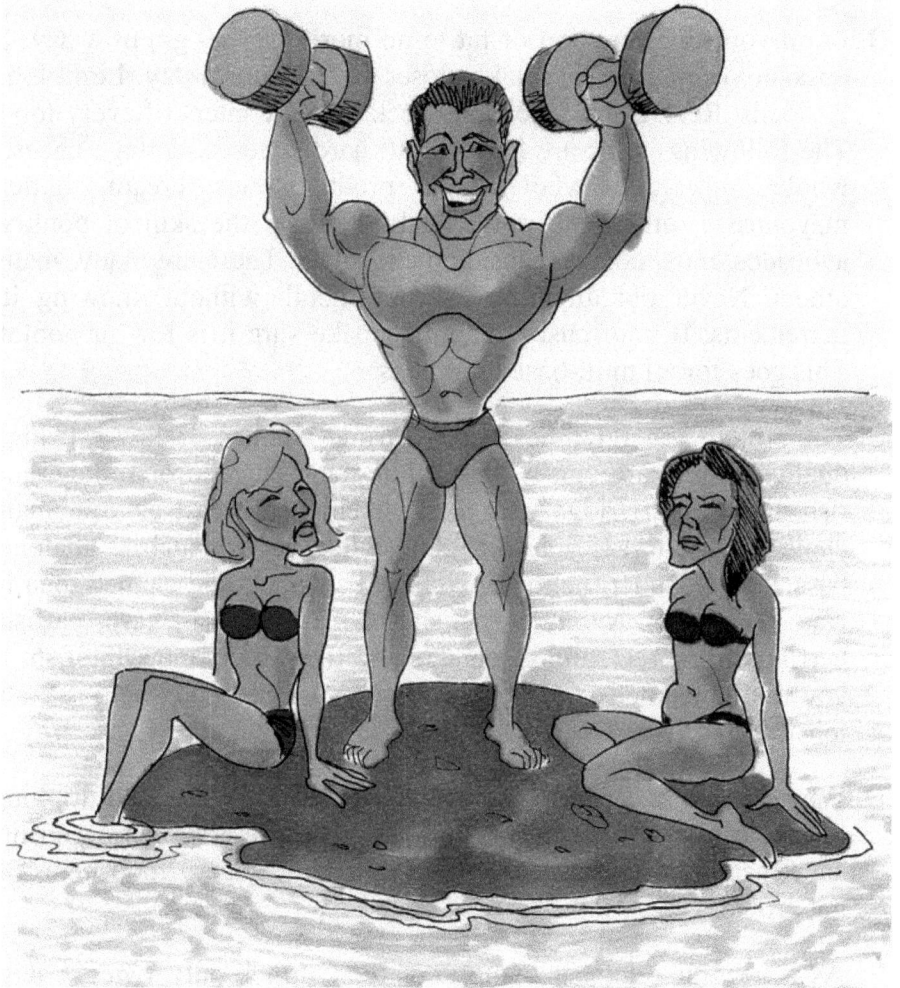

While being a dedicated bodybuilder is great, don't forget to enjoy the many simple pleasures in life. Every once in a while take some timeout from your training and experience the world around you. When on vacation, forget about the steel and take a hike along a mountainside or a tan on a tropical beach. Relax and take it all in!

NUTRITIONAL TIPS FOR WEIGHT LOSS

A. Reduce your calorie intake by 300 to 500 calories per day. A calorie deficit will help you lose the visceral fat, which is the fat that wraps around the abdominal organs. Give your body time to adjust to your new nutritional program. Reduce or eliminate those foods that are high in fat. Remember that a gram of fat has more than twice as many calories than a gram of carbohydrate or protein does.

B. Limit your consumption of fat to no more than 30 grams a day. If possible, keep your fat intake closer to 25 grams a day. Limit high fat foods. Read every label and check the fat content of every food. The following items are high in fat: hard cheeses, cottage cheese, whole milk and whole milk products, ice cream, butter, mayonnaise, oils, beef, pork, lamb, sausage, the skin of poultry, avocados, nuts, potato chips, and chocolate. There are many, many others. Never put anything in your mouth without knowing its ingredients. If you must have milk, make sure it is low or nonfat. This goes for all milk-based products.

C. Eat protein several times a day. Prime sources of low fat, high quality protein are egg whites, white-meat chicken or turkey, and fish. Stock your fridge with skinless chicken breast as your main choice of poultry. If you like, choose low fat fish such as abalone, bass, cod, flounder, halibut, perch, red snapper, and canned tuna in water (no salt). Avoid fatty fish such as bluefish, carp, catfish, herring, mackerel, salmon, shad, swordfish, trout, and whitefish. If you are concerned about cholesterol, avoid seafood such as crab, lobster, and shrimp.

D. When possible, eat fruits in their natural form rather than drinking their juices. The fiber in the fruit slows calorie assimilation. Fruits have macronutrients and fiber that manmade sugary food items do not provide.

E. As a general rule, eat complex carbohydrates only twice a day. Complex carbohydrates tend to satisfy hunger. They also have a calming effect and slow the metabolism slightly. Limit the complex carbohydrates to the scheduled planned meals. Eat plain cereals (hot or cold) such as rolled oats. If you eat bread, use grain or whole wheat instead of white.

F. Avoid eating foods that are fried or cooked with butter, oils, commercial dressings, or any other fatty substance. When you cook, boil, steam, broil, or poach your foods. When possible, steam vegetables rather than boil them. Boiling removes many valuable micronutrients. Do not add table sugar to your foods or drinks. Do not use butter, sour cream, jams, peanut butter, or margarine. If you must, use spices, herbs, lemon, or lime juice as seasoning. Sodium encourages water retention. Do not add table salt to your foods.

G. Drink several eight-ounce glasses of spring water daily. Drink water with your meals and throughout your day. Also, be sure to drink water before, during, and after your workout to avoid dehydration. Never drink coffee, caffeinated tea, soda, or diet drinks, and never consume beer or other alcoholic beverages.

H. Eat high-fiber foods. Fiber is great for the digestive system. It has a low caloric value and helps prevent some calories from entering the bloodstream. Fiber also contains cholesterol-reducing properties that can keep blood levels in a healthy range.

TRAIN HEAVY OR GO HOME

One of the biggest sins I see bodybuilders commit when on a fat loss regimen is to train with light weights. Training in this fashion while losing body fat will only cause you to lose the hard-earned muscle you built through the lifting of heavy steel. If you diet correctly, you should experience no drastic changes in your strength while losing body fat. Remember, to retain their mass and strength, muscles need to be stimulated often. When training for a competition, or just to look good at the beach, I always lift heavy, right through the entire sculpting process. It is what I know and what has worked best for my students and me. Training with light weights in order to get cut for the beach scene will most likely cause you to lose quality muscle size. If you find yourself to weak to use the same heavy steel that you were previously using before your fat loss program, then chances are you are probably not consuming enough calories and are losing bodyweight too fast. It takes time to build mountains of muscle and it takes time to lose excess body fat and reveal your rock-hard ridges.

Another mistake natural bodybuilders make when trying to lose body fat is to increase the volume of their training by adding sets, exercises, and even workouts in the assumption that the more time they spend in the gym, the more calories they will burn, and in turn the more buffed they will look. Unlike the anabolic androids, natural bodybuilders have to depend on their bodies' own recuperative powers, so the last thing you want to do is over train while dieting and cause your body to halt its progress. Forget about the marathon workouts you read about in the muscle magazines. Many of the so-called champions are on the *juice* and have little credibility in my book. If they were so knowledgeable about muscle building, they would not be relying on chemical enhancements to create their Herculean forms. The bottom line – do not train to increase your endurance, that is not your goal. Train in accordance to your recuperative powers while following a sensible calorie and fat restricted diet such as the one outlined in this chapter.

For these reasons, natural bodybuilders on restricted diets should not train every day of the week. At most, seasoned muscle builders should train each body part once every four to seven days, while intermediate bodybuilders should target each area twice weekly, since their training intensity is not yet at peak levels. It is also important not to weight train more than two days in a row so your muscles will have a chance to recuperate and rebuild. Body parts should also be broken down into groups so as not to directly work any muscle group on two consecutive days. Retaining muscle tissue while simultaneously increasing the separation and hardness of the individual muscle should be of prime importance when training to lose body fat.

A favorite advanced split-system of mine for losing body fat is to weight train each body part once every four days, with a rest day in between each workout. I group the body parts into two sections: one is the torso group (chest, back, and shoulders) and the other group is the limbs (arms and legs). For example, based on the following workout charts, on the first week you would perform Workout 1 on Monday, Workout 2 on Wednesday, Workout 3 on Friday, and Workout 4 on Sunday. On the second week, you would perform Workout 1 on Tuesday, Workout 2 on Thursday, Workout 3 on Saturday, and Workout 4 that following Monday. It is a continuous pattern that produces big results.

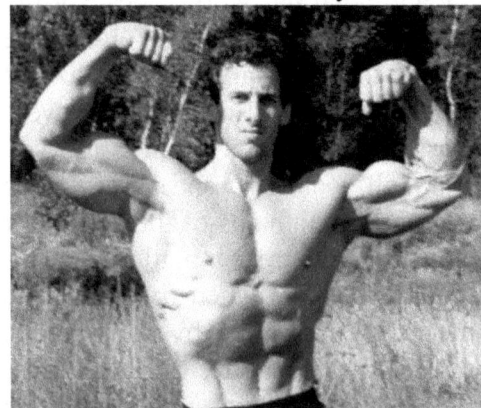

This system has always produced solid results for me when training for that he-man look at the beach. It looks something like this:

WORKOUT #1		
EXERCISES	SETS	REPS
Bench Press	5	10-8-6-6-6
Incline Dumbbell Press	3	6-8
Machine Chest Press	3	6-8
Front Pull-Up	3	8-10
Dumbbell Row	4	8-10
Close Grip Pull-Down	3	8-10
Shoulder Press	4	8-10
Alternate Front Dumbbell Raise	3	8-10
Barbell Shrug	4	8-10
Abdominal Crunch	3	15-25
Incline Knee Pull-In	3	15-25

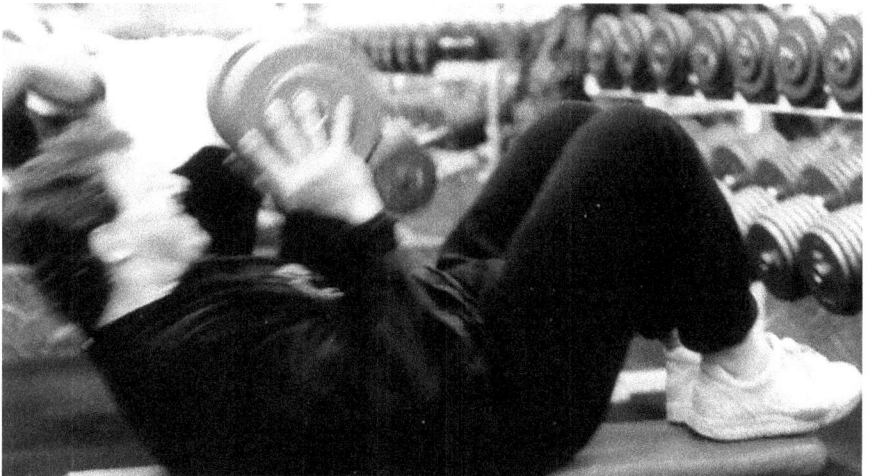

WORKOUT #2

EXERCISES	SETS	REPS
Dumbbell Triceps Kickback	4	8-10
Overhead Triceps Extension	3	8-10
Barbell Scott Curl	4	6-8
Seated Dumbbell Curl	3	6-8
Wrist Curl	4	10-12
Leg Press	5	8-10
Hack Squat	3	8-10
Stiff Leg Dead Lift	3	8-10
Standing Calf Raise	5	15-25
Hanging Knee Pull-Up	3	15-25
Leg and Body Raise	3	15-25

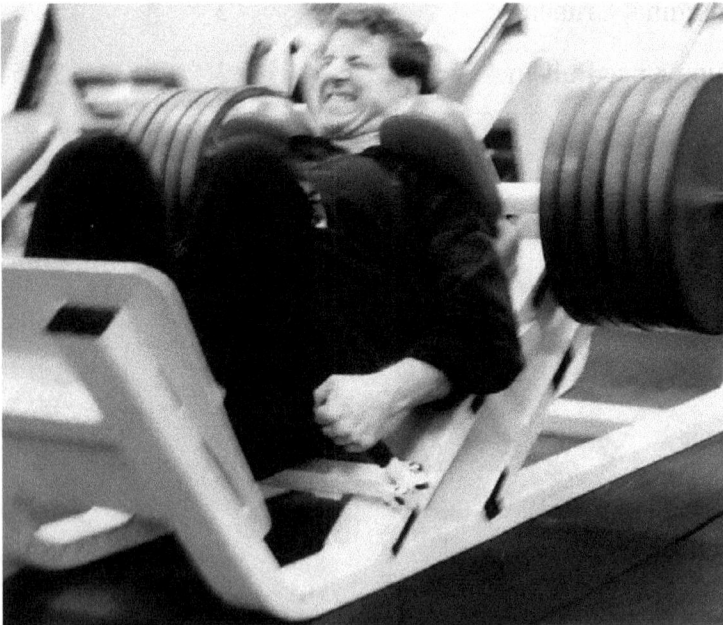

WORKOUT #3

EXERCISES	SETS	REPS
Incline Press	5	10-8-6-6-6
Parallel Dip	3	8-10
Flat Dumbbell Fly	3	8-10
Front Pull-Down	4	8-10
Cable Row	3	8-10
Barbell Row	3	8-10
Alternate Dumbbell Press	4	8-10
Upright Row	3	8-10
Standing Side Lateral	3	8-10
Abdominal Crunch	3	15-25
Dumbbell Side Bend	3	15-25

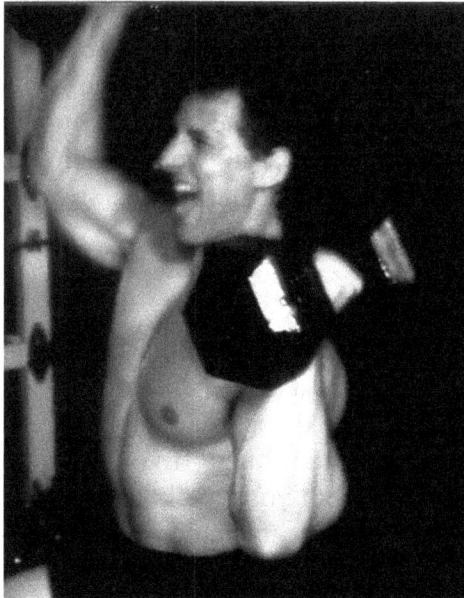

WORKOUT #4

EXERCISES	SETS	REPS
Triceps Pushdown	4	8-10
Lying Triceps Extension	3	6-8
Barbell Curl	4	6-8
Incline Dumbbell Curl	3	6-8
Reverse Barbell Curl	4	8-10
Leg Extension	3	10-12
Full Squat	5	10-8-6-6-6
Lying Leg Curl	4	8-10
Seated Calf Raise	5	15-25
Incline Knee Pull-In	3	15-25
Incline Bent Knee Sit-up	3	15-25

(See ANATOMY OF A BODYBUILDER chapter for technique details)

This daily training sequence should be followed throughout the weeks. Some weeks you will train four times while other weeks you will perform just three weight-training sessions. On your off days, it would be wise to include some light cardio work to help raise your metabolic rate. This way you can continue burning calories while your muscles are rebuilding.

WORK THAT BODY
It is vital that you weight train when on a fat-loss program. If you do not pump the iron while on a reduced calorie diet your muscle mass will diminish. Lifting steel keeps your muscular gains intact as your body begins to become more refined. If you go off your diet for a few days be sure to continue with your workouts so that you will continue to burn calories and not gain unwanted bodyweight. If you do gain while not exercising, the pounds will be fat, not muscle. Stay active!

Similar to your mass-building workouts, the majority of exercises performed while on a weight loss program should include the same basic movements that got you to the level where you could even consider trimming up for the beach. As explained earlier, it is imperative to include the heavy mass-building movements in your workouts and not replace them with inferior light isolation exercises. The basic exercises help you retain muscle mass while you diet. If you stop doing them, you run the risk of not only losing muscle mass but strength as well. The basics include the: Full Squat, Leg Press, Bench Press, Deadlift, Row, Upright Row, Shoulder Press, Power Clean, Parallel Dip, Front Pull-Up, etc. These types of movements work several muscle groups across several joints, which means you can use heavy weights and retain more muscle mass.

While the basic exercises should constitute the majority of your weight training movements, occasionally performing a few isolation exercises is a great way to help striate, define, and separate the individual muscles. These exercises will add polish and refinement to your physique. Make sure to use proper form when performing them and use a weight heavy enough to give the muscles some real stimulation. Some examples of isolation exercises include the Side Lateral, Leg Extension, Incline Fly, and Concentration Curl.

CARDIO TRAINING

Because a slow metabolism burns fat slowly, it is important to increase the metabolic rate while retaining as much muscle mass as possible. The faster your metabolism, the quicker you will burn fat. To accomplish this you need to raise your metabolic rate up to the point where you can practically see and feel the fat melting off your body. One tool in your fat loss program is cardio exercise. Cardio exercises not only promote fat loss, but also help strengthen the heart and lungs as well. The heart is a muscle, and just like the skeletal muscles, it needs to be exercised vigorously to become strong and healthy. Although it will take a bit of time before you realize the benefits of cardio work, you will almost immediately benefit from the oxygen delivered to your heart.

Many bodybuilders overdo aerobic training when trying to lose body fat and unfortunately lose muscle tissue as well. You have to find the right balance between weight training, cardio, and a nutritional plan to help guarantee maximum fat loss while retaining muscle mass. To help keep excess pounds from accumulating on your body, perform cardio work several times a week (on non-weight training days). By performing cardio exercises for 30-45 minutes on your off days, you'll have more stamina for the steel and prevent overtraining, because the exercise load is spread evenly throughout the week. This will help retain your muscle mass while shedding away-unwanted body fat. The well-being of your heart and lungs will also improve dramatically. For you to realize the benefits of aerobic training, try getting your pulse rate up to 70-80 percent of its maximum capacity and keep it there for at least twenty minutes (to determine your maximum pulse rate, just subtract your age from 220). You can accomplish this with any number of activities, such as cycling, jogging, running, elliptical, step-master, swimming, etc. Whatever activity you prefer is fine, as long as you sustain the elevated pulse rate for at least twenty minutes, several times a week. Be patient when first beginning a cardio program and gradually increase the workload on the heart and lungs to prevent possible medical problems.

Remember, while on a fat loss program you should be training hard and heavy while simultaneously following a fat/calorie reduced diet. If you perform an excess amount of cardio work, you run the risk of losing muscle tissue and that is the last thing you want. As a natural bodybuilder, your primary goals are to retain as much muscle and strength as possible, while losing body fat and improving the function of your heart and lungs as well.

Personally, my favorite form of cardio training is running. Since my body fat is already in check, all I need is a good one to two-mile run once a week to keep off any excess fat that might accumulate on my physique. I also include several 100-yard sprints after my run to help bring out the definition in my thighs and keep them agile and mobile. Find out what works best for you and apply it to your fat-loss program.

Exercises to Stimulate the Aerobic System

For Weight Reduction
Walking, Long Distance Swimming, Slow Paced Stationary Cycling

For Cardiovascular Conditioning
Running, Treadmill Running, Jogging, Jumping Rope
Elliptical Trainer, Rowing, Fast Paced Stepper, Fast Pace Bike Riding,
Fast Paced Stationary Riding, Basketball, etc.

CALORIE EXPENDITURE LIST	
ACTIVITY	PER HOUR (APPROX)
Archery	270
Basketball	560
Bowling	215
Calisthenics	200
Cycling	300
Dancing	450
Golf	340
Gymnastics	257
Jogging	750
Racquetball	870
Running	950
Sitting	90
Sleeping	70
Swimming	500
Watching TV	90
Volleyball	250
Walking	180
Weight Training	550
Wrestling	790

Look at the chart above to see how various activities expend energy. Intense aerobic movements use the most calories, while less active movements expend less energy.

FLEX THOSE MUSCLES!

Another way to bring out the separation and detail in your physique is to practice flexing each muscle group during and after the workout. When bodybuilders flex their muscles, their physiques become refined and take on a polished look. Although your goal may not be to compete on the physique stage, it is nevertheless strongly recommended that you add some muscle flexing to your fat loss program. The isometric tension involved in flexing and squeezing the muscles striates and refines your muscular structure.

Performed correctly, flexing can be extraordinarily hard work, especially for beginners who find themselves shaking wildly as they tense their muscles with every ounce of energy they have. As you continue to practice flexing your muscles several times a week, you will notice that not only will your physique begin to look more complete but that you'll also have better control over the individual muscle groups being flexed. Onstage, professional bodybuilders look relaxed when posing for the judges and audience, yet they are tensing extremely hard to bring out the clarity of the muscle being displayed. It takes time to become a great poser, but the rewards of mastering this art will add greatly to the quality of your physique. Try it!

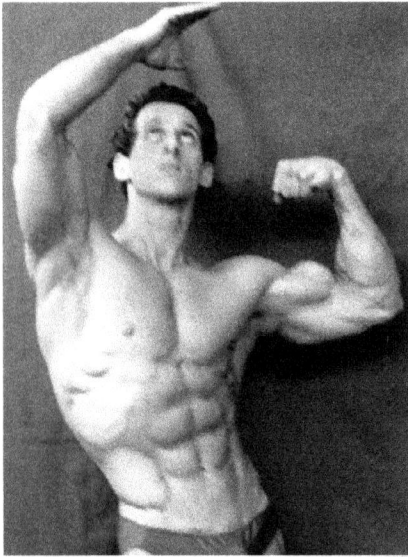

MONITOR YOUR PROGRESS

While on a fat loss program be sure to monitor your progress on a steady basis. This will help you find weak points and correct them as you continue with your training. The mirror is one tool to evaluate your progress and help determine where extra work might be needed. Be sure the mirror is full length so that your legs are not overlooked. While it is great to build huge pectorals and biceps, many bodybuilders often neglect the foundation of their physique, which are their thighs and calves. A full-length mirror will remind you of this. A mirror will also let you know if you are carrying too much fat around the middle.

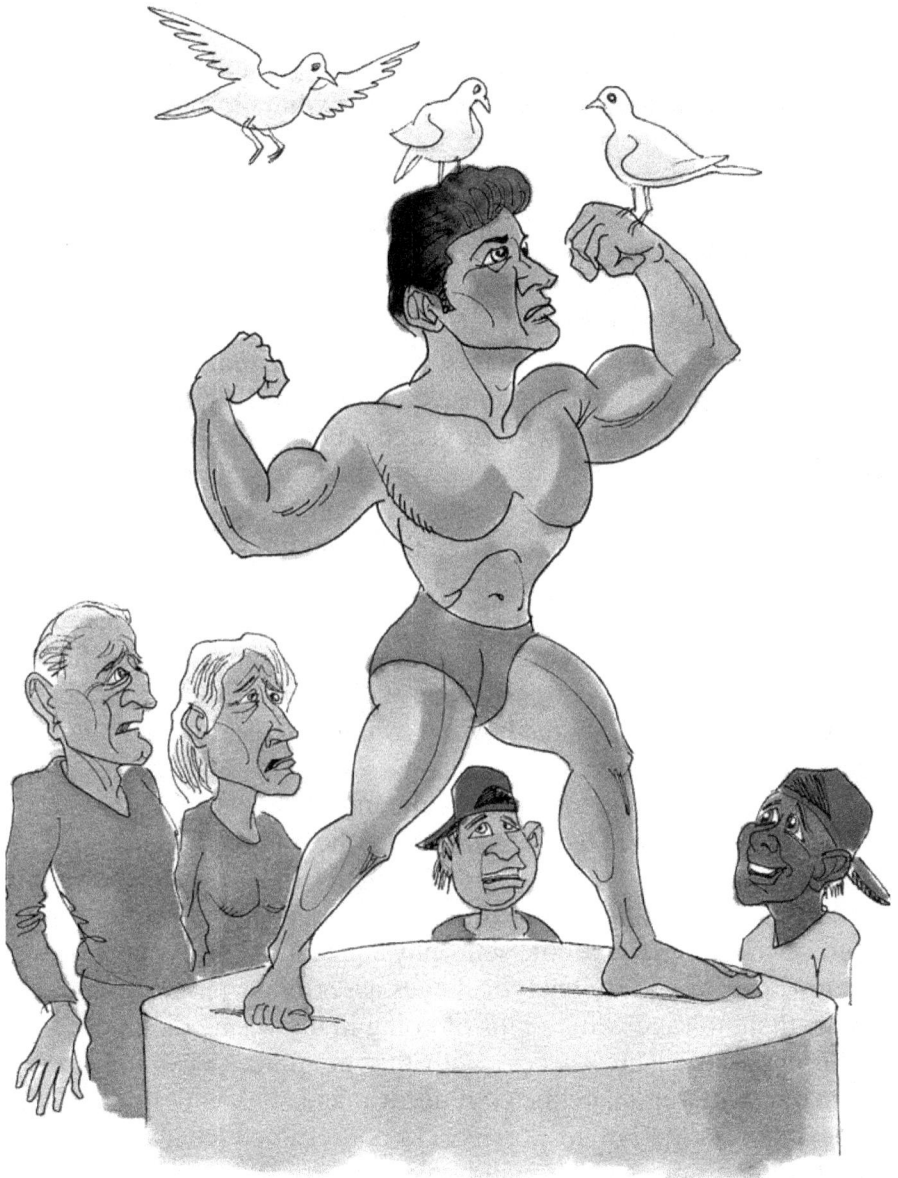

Advanced bodybuilders are like living works of art. Wherever they go, they bring their creation with them. Some guys like to display their masterpieces at every chance they get. Men with muscle cars don't race them at every corner they turn. The same principle applies to you; save it for the competition.

Seeing a jellyroll covering your abs should motivate you to perform some cardio work and pay special attention to your diet. Be sure to study your physique from the front, back, and both sides.

Another way to monitor your progress is through photographs. Once a month have photos taken of your physique from all angles and place them in an album for future reference. Study the photos for comparisons and look for any weaknesses your physique may have. Take the photos under the same lighting (indoors) so variations in contrast can be avoided. Also, wear the same posing trunks or swimsuit and record the date, bodyweight, and measurements when the photos were taken.

Two additional ways to monitor your progress are the tape measure and the old reliable scale. If the scale reads twenty pounds less than the previous month this could be an indication that your weight loss is not only fat, but muscle tissue as well. This is something you must avoid. Another way to gauge whether you are gaining the wrong type of bodyweight is when your body measurements increase drastically in a relatively short period. The probability here is that you added unwanted body fat as opposed to the quality muscle you seek.

Another method of measuring body fat is with calipers. Calipers measure the thickness of your skin by measuring the subcutaneous fat located between the muscle and skin. The less subcutaneous fat you have the more defined your physique will become. Most calipers can be purchased with a chart showing where to measure and how to record your subcutaneous levels. Be sure to also record your bodyweight at the same time using calipers.

Having someone that understands the sport of bodybuilding evaluate your physique can be a big assistance in achieving your goals. Try to find someone that has judged physique competitions and is not afraid to be too critical of your physique and hurt your feelings. Having a pair of honest, analytical eyes assess your physique could be just the thing to save you months of going in the wrong direction.

In order to ensure success with this program, you must make a commitment. If you make the commitment and stick with it, results are as inevitable as the law of gravity. Do not let impatience prevent you from having a muscular he-man body and a more positive outlook on life. Believe that you can, and you will!

By ridding your starship of excess poundage, you, the natural bodybuilder, will travel at warp speed, as you *JOURNEY TO THE OLYMPIAN ZONE*!

RUNNING IS A BODY BUILDER

The following event actually happened to me in the summer of 1980. It was mid-August in the Catskill Mountains of New York. What began as a beautifully clear summer day suddenly became cloudy, with cooler ranging temperatures. I was about two miles from my home and the weather was threatening. After a minute or two of hustling down the road, I was surprised by a powerful gust of wind that slapped me swiftly across my face. I realized a cold front was quickly moving into the area and that a storm was about to break loose. As I looked towards an open valley, I felt the wind's gale grow in intensity. The sky quickly changed dark in color with grayish and blackish hues dominant. Suddenly, a bolt of lightning struck nearby, as a loud booming thunder rattled the ground I stood on. Another lightning bolt exploded its blinding light close to me; it could not have been more than a few feet away. More thunder, more lightning, increasing until it sounded like tons of dynamite bombing the very countryside where I stood. What had been a calm summer day became Hell on earth as the storm's gale force winds stung my body with cold rain and chunks of sharp hail.

Boom! Crack! Snap! I jumped into the air, not knowing which way to go. I looked back to where I had just been standing and stared in disbelief. The storm's axe had just sliced a large granddaddy oak in half, leaving its giant trunk across the road. Immediately, a voice in my head screamed out: Run! Run! Run! I ran for my life!

I ran with everything I had as I pumped my thighs like a hotrod's pistons. I pulled my knees up high and stretched my legs as far as I could with each stride I took. As I ran, I felt like a plane racing down the runway moments before take-off. As I jumped over fallen branches and dodged flying debris, I prayed that nature's axe would miss on her next swing. Within a few minutes, I was back at my home, huffing and puffing, wishing I had a stopwatch. Who knows, the world record might have just been broken. I knew for sure that I'd broken my own record!

You never know when you'll need to fly with the wind. Having a good pair of running legs is a sure way to help guarantee that you will be able to respond to the call when summoned. To prepare for those times, read this chapter.

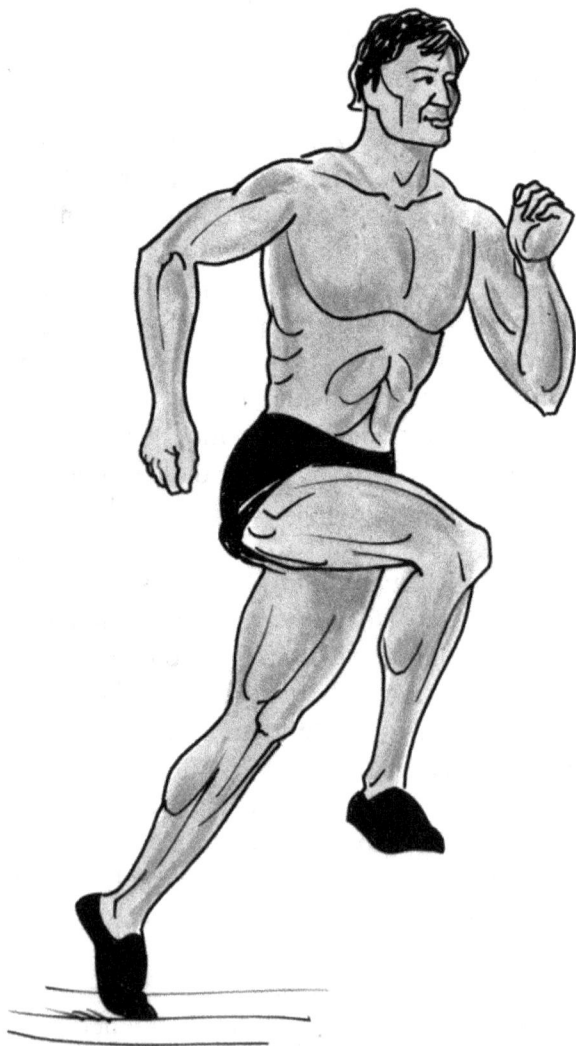

RUNNING AND THE BODYBUILDER

Being a natural for life bodybuilder I know the importance running has on my health, muscular development, and training. Because of my running program, I am able to weight train with greater intensity and confidence, knowing that my endurance and stamina are tough enough to withstand any Herculean workout. My body actually pumps up faster with a more fulfilling feeling of self-satisfaction. The same thing happens when I run as blood starts to rush and gorge itself into all of my muscles. After I run a short distance my physique starts to transform; my size increases, my cuts become more pronounced, and my body begins to experience a super pump.

Running also has many other benefits. It helps to remove unwanted fat from your body by placing demands on your energy system, which in turn breaks down fatty tissues to release energy into your bloodstream. By following a consistent running program, your abdomen and leg muscles will begin to reveal their true shape and proportions, helping you to realize their full potential. Running is also an excellent way to relieve unwanted stress, anxiety, and worries. Next time you feel uptight, go for a fast, brisk run, and see how relieved and full of life you feel afterwards.

Two extremely important factors of running are the heart and lungs. Our hearts have been pumping steadily, since before birth, and as with many people have undergone periods of dangerous abuse. Poor nutrition, smoking, lack of exercise, pollution, drugs, and other factors have made this a heart attack-prone society. You really have to give this muscle a lot of credit and should treat it as a pot of gold, for it controls the keys to your health. Participating in a running program will help you build a strong, healthy, and lasting heart.

INCREASE CARDIOVASCULAR FITNESS

As with other muscles in the body, the heart gets stronger with regular exercise. Performing aerobic type exercises increases cardiovascular fitness by improving blood circulation throughout the body. The more a bodybuilder becomes cardiovascular efficient, the more vigorous and longer he will be able to train while experiencing less tiring. When we improve our cardiovascular condition, we also improve the efficiency of our heart, lungs, and other organs. A fit cardiovascular system also helps us meet the every day physical and emotional demands of life more readily.

The better fit our cardiovascular system is the less chance of heart disease. In addition, the better conditioned your heart is the less effort it will have to expend to circulate blood through your body because it can pump more efficiently with each beat. Many factors produce a strong and lasting heart. Because of this, our cardiovascular system has an important role in the quality of our health and lives. Be sure to pace yourself when beginning a cardio program so as not to tire too quickly. Pacing yourself is especially important if you have been relatively inactive.

Your target heart rate is an effective tool in measuring your initial fitness level and in monitoring your progress after you begin a fitness program. This approach requires measuring your pulse periodically as you exercise, so be sure to stay within 50 to 75 percent of your maximum heart rate. This range is called your target heart rate.

The following table provides estimated target heart rates for different age categories. Look for the age category closest to yours and read across the page to find your target heart rate:

Age	Target Heart Rate Zone	Heart Rate Max
20 years	100-150 beats per minute	200
25 years	98-146 beats per minute	195
30 years	95-142 beats per minute	190
35 years	93-138 beats per minute	185
40 years	90-135 beats per minute	180
45 years	88-131 beats per minute	175
50 years	85-127 beats per minute	170
55 years	83-123 beats per minute	165
60 years	80-120 beats per minute	160
65 years	78-116 beats per minute	155
70 years	75-113 beats per minute	150

Your maximum heart rate is approximately 220 minus your age. The figures above are averages and should be used as general guidelines.

Our lungs are also vital. In our busy and mobile society, the lungs are exposed to thousands of different pollutant particles daily. The main function of the lungs is to intake energizing gases through its respiratory channels and expel toxic gaseous end products of energy production. Our trachea, bronchi, alveoli, and other segments of this system may become clogged and irritated through the inhalation of pollution. This impairment of the exchange of gases, which take place in our lungs, can lead to serious illness and possibly even death. Running, especially sprinting, will help promote heavy breathing, which in turn might help breakdown and release some of these unwanted pollutant particles from our respiratory system.

PACE YOURSELF
During the first few weeks of your running program stay at the lowest part of your target zone (50%). As the weeks and months go on, gradually increase to the higher part of your target zone (75%). After six months or more of consistent running, you might be able to run comfortably at up to 85% of your maximum heart rate. Although this is fine, you do not have to train at a maximum level to get or stay in good cardiovascular condition. Perform at a pace safe for you.

PRIMING THE PISTONS
Prior to running, it is important to warm up. Lacking the time to warm up means you do not have the time to run. Back, front, and side leg raise movements should be performed, also rotate your ankles in all mobile plain directions. Perform a few free-hand squats, toe touches, jumping jacks, and knee pull-ups to help activate the lower extremity major muscle mass areas. Make sure your body, especially your legs, is primed before you begin to run.

TECHNIQUES OF RUNNING
There are many different techniques, styles, and reasons for running. Ours is going to be geared for bodybuilders. I have found that the more I lower my hips while I run, the more quadriceps and hamstring stimulation I receive. It might look funny to on-lookers but believe me the pump you will receive will be worth it. There are many other important factors to note when running. Styles in foot placement, body arch, and arm movement all have their part and kinetic effect.

At the beginning of the run, I drop my heels and roll off them. As my foot rolls forward, I move the pressure towards its outside edge.

Nearing completion of the roll, I reverse the process, bringing the pressure back inwards so that I am kicking up with all my toes. This technique acts as a shock absorber for the feet. It also works my calves thoroughly and improves my coordination.

A vital element in smooth and efficient running style is the position of the body carriage. Try running erect by keeping your upper body's posture upright. To do this, pull back the shoulders, lift the chest high, and keep the back straight. Next, balance the trunk over the legs and the head over the trunk. Run on the legs.

The arms are a source of speed and power because they have important balancing and driving functions. Keep your fists loose, wrists fixed, elbows unlocked, and shoulders leveled when you run. Remember, hands and arms influence the movement of the legs and body carriage tremendously. Getting your techniques down correctly will make you a precision runner.

RUNNING BAREFOOT

During my teens and early twenties, I seldom wore sneakers when I ran. I just enjoyed the feeling of the rough pavement pounding against my feet and ran barefoot at every chance I got. It did not matter what season it was or what location I was at. If I was going to run, it was going to be barefoot. There were plenty of times during the deep cold of winter when the road was frozen from the sub-freezing temperatures that I would run barefoot for miles. There were also many times when upstate at my Catskill Mountain home, when I would run on the dirt path that encircled my properties lake, which was loaded with pebbles and rocks. The conditions never stopped me from running barefoot, and after awhile, I developed extremely thick calluses on the bottom of my feet that acted as cushions and prevented me from damaging or feeling pain in my soles. These days, I have gotten into the habit of wearing sneakers when I run and I like the variety of footwear available today to meet the biomechanical needs of my feet. Running has become a science and today technology offers us the best products to help us excel at it. Although I will probably take up running barefoot again sometime down the road, for now I'll just stick to my Nikes and watch for any stones in my path.

COMMON SENSE RUNNING

Now that we understand the proper techniques of running, let's move on to the next steps. At first, I recommend that you run on a track so your timing and rhythm can be achieved. After a while, you may want to run on roads, beaches, or even across mountains. Wherever you decide to run, make sure that the air quality is the best you can get. Running along fume-spewing highways, factories, and chemical plants is not just stupid, but downright deadly. Use common sense.

When bodybuilders workout, they usually perform a set or two of light weight warm up exercises. The same principle applies to running. After I finish my stretching exercises, I start to run a slow quarter mile. This primes and prepares my body for the real thing. After the brief run, I stop and rest for about one minute. This lets blood pump through my body and helps me to build inner confidence.

RUNNING HARD NOW

So, are you're ready to run? Here's what I do. I start out slow with short strides and knees low. As I continue to run, I pick up the pace a little at a time, keeping my feet, arms, and body working in rhythm. I am planning to do just one mile, for experience has taught me that this is all I need for a thorough heart, lung, and thigh workout. I divide my mile into four parts, increasing the intensity with each lap until I am in an all-out sprint for the last quarter mile. This is where most of my gains are realized! As I come around the turn on that last lap, I am really flying. I am pulling my knees almost up to my chest and stretching my thighs with each stride until they are nearly ripping apart. You need a lot of mental discipline and willpower during this explosive part of the run. It's either you make it or you don't.

After this intense run, you will experience feelings of exhaustion, accomplishment, and self-satisfaction. Now, one mile may be less than some of you have been doing, but it is the quality and not the quantity of work output that serves our purpose. After completing the run, I perform a series of one hundred yard sprints. This shocks my thighs and heart muscle, making them work overtime. It also gives the lungs a real boost, cleansing them through forced breathing.

An important note: Right after completing such an intense run, it is very important to cool down by jogging or walking a quarter to one half mile in distance. When you drive a car and hit the brakes, it sometimes stalls out. The last thing we want is heart failure by not giving this vital organ a chance to slow down to a normal rhythm.

I run just once a week and feel this is all I need to make continued gains with my size, endurance, and recuperative power. I actually become stronger and bigger with these weekly runs. However, when a contest or guest appearance comes around I change my running instinctively to fulfill my immediate goals. When on vacation I usually do a lot of distance running which adds variety to my program. Find out what works best for you.

Enjoy running! It's healthy, fun, invigorating, satisfying, and best of all, running will explode your gains throughout the universe, as you, the natural bodybuilder, travel on your *JOURNEY TO THE OLYMPIAN ZONE*!

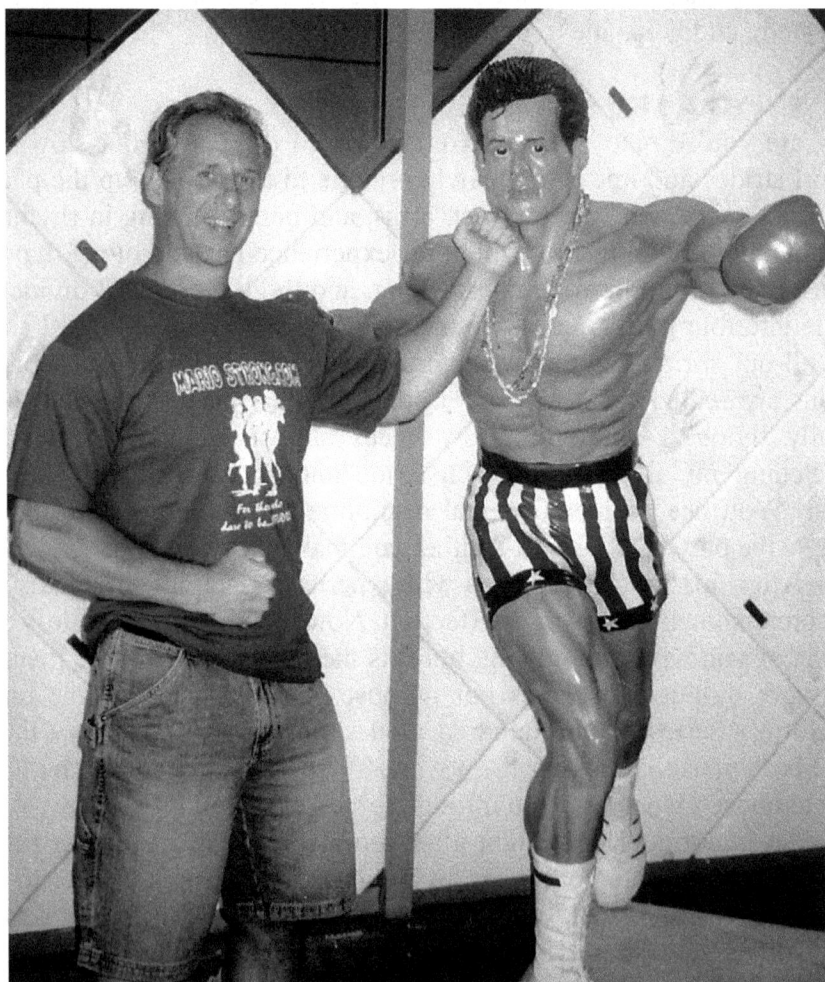

Mario Strong greets Rocky Balboa at Planet Hollywood in Waikiki - 2007

PRINCIPLES OF LONGEVITY

Natural bodybuilding is a path towards health, radiance, and longevity. That being said, it should be clearly noted, that the keys to living a long, healthy life are more than just lifting steel and eating chicken breasts. There are many facets that come together to help insure one's continuance on this planet. Sure, big biceps are nice but what's even greater is to be able to flex those mighty guns throughout the decades to come. To be lucky enough to reach such a plateau takes a lifestyle that leaves little to chance. The following is a set of rules to help guarantee your success in bodybuilding and more importantly, in life.

THINK POSITIVE   There is no power greater than that of a positive thought in action. Be optimistic with your life. Believe that you can and you shall. In 1969, I witnessed the amazing Mets win the World Series against all the odds. The slogan, *You Gotta Believe*, was amplified that year as spectators proudly held banners and signs to cheer on their team to victory over the Baltimore Orioles. Bodybuilding requires a great deal of positive thinking. When you are training, you've got to believe in your workout. When eating, you've got to believe in your diet. When planning, you've got to believe in your course of action. Most important of all, you've got to believe in yourself. If you do not, you are bound to failure. You need to apply a positive plan of action to your muscle building lifestyle and believe that you can succeed in the sport of bodybuilding. *You Gotta Believe*!

EAT TO LIVE Learn as much as you can about nutrition and apply this knowledge to your daily diet. Avoid junk food and eating at fast foods restaurants. Try to consume only that which is pure and natural. Do not consume any cakes, candies, sodas, pastries, fried foods, fatty animal products, etc. Stick to one-ingredient natural foods and cook only when necessary. Learn how to combine your foods for maximum health. When attending dinner functions or on a cruise I stand out from the other folks when I eat my prepared meals and everyone else is feasting on delicacies and wine. It is a sacrifice to be different but sometimes that is what's needed to succeed. Remember, you are what you eat, so be wise as to what you put in your mouth.

WORK THAT BODY Train as if your life depended on it. Give it everything you have and then some. You have to lift the heavy steel with every once of energy you can muster. Set goals for yourself often and conquer them one at a time. Make the gym your battleground and fight until you are victorious. When I enter the gym, I leave the problems of the world outside. I am there for some serious business and my training requires maximum mental focus and physical effort. Nothing else would be acceptable. Find your performance zone and *Go For It*!

REST THAT BODY Try to maintain a regular bedtime and rising schedule. Take a power nap (about 20-30 minutes) during the day to help you recuperate and re-energize for your grueling workouts. You can do all the training in the world but without sufficient rest, your gains will be minimized. Without enough rest, I find it nearly impossible to train at the same intensity, as I am use to. Getting enough sleep and rest are key ingredients to being successful in bodybuilding. After putting so much of your hard-earned time in the gym, you deserve to take a snooze on a comfortable mattress. Besides, that is when you will make most of your new gains. Personally, after a heavy bombing session, I find there is nothing better than to relax for a while, as my body rebuilds the muscle I just tore down and my strength grows to a new, higher capacity. Make the time to rest!

BE PATIENT Patience is a great virtue when striving towards any worthy goal. It takes time to become what your dreams are made of, and it is important to take each new day as it comes. Wanting everything to happen overnight will only result in despair and anguish. Let the flame of desire burn strong, but watch closely or it may burn out of control, stopping you in your tracks, long before you realize the results you seek. Be grateful for your blessings and give each new day a little bit extra. Before you know it, you'll be on top of the mountain. Remember, time has no limits and neither should you.

TREASURE YOUR HEALTH Your body is the temple of your greatest wealth. Never neglect or abuse that which can easily be lost forever. When you abuse your body through drugs, cigarettes, alcohol, etc., you are traveling on a dead end street. Put the brakes on your bad habits and get on the highway of health. Maybe I am a little boring but I have never been high from drugs, alcohol, or anything in my life. Throughout my teenage years, I never had the desire for such ill practices, or for that matter, could ever understand what the big attraction was to being a space cadet. In high school, I had several friends who use to get high from sniffing glue, popping pills, and smoking weed. To me this was insanity and I continually fought with them to stop their bad habits before it was too late. They just laughed at my well-intended efforts and today they are just shadows of what they could have been. I followed a different path than most of my generation, and today I am still going strong and trying to help those who will listen to my warnings about the dangers of drugs.

RESPECT NATURE Spend as much time as you can where the air and water are fresh and clean. Never pollute or abuse the land in which you live or visit. Every week, I visit my home in the Catskill Mountains and smile at the beauty of nature. There is always something to do up in the hills. Whether it is axing firewood, cutting acres of grass, or carrying boulders down from the mountain top, I have always enjoyed the challenges of the great outdoors as it removes me from the raft of society and puts me more in touch with the nature I desire. When possible, take a trip to some place secluded and enjoy the gifts that nature provides. Remember, this is the only world you will ever get to live on, so enjoy its endless wonders while you can.

329

REDUCE STRESS   In this high-paced society of ours, it is sometimes easy to get lost in all the confusion. Find harmony within yourself and stay focused on the big picture. Through the years, I have learned how to block negativity from my thoughts so as not to be distracted in my training. One day in 1979, while driving to my gym for an early morning workout I accidentally left my gym bag (containing my wallet and house keys) on a busy sidewalk as I drove off. Soon after arriving at my gym, I discovered what I had done. Immediately, I blocked the mental stress of my mistake from derailing my workout and put the problem on the back burner to be dealt with after the workout (luckily, an honest person found my bag and returned it later that day). On another morning, I opened my club and found that a back window of my gym had been smashed during a failed burglary attempt. I simply swept up the glass and proceeded to train, again putting off the problem for later when I could think more clearly. It's important to figure out when something is really an emergency and when it could wait for a bit. I have plenty of such examples to share but I believe you get the idea. You have to be focused on your goals, and not let negativity sidetrack you on your path to success.

DO NOT LIVE RECKLESSLY   Your most precious gift is your life. Do not risk losing it to an error in judgment. Drag racing on the local highway is a sure way to a dead end. Be careful with each step you take in life and never let complacency derail you. As a teenager, I suffered the loss of a cousin who was killed while joy riding on a mini-bike without a helmet. Years later, I lost a workout partner because he was killed while racing his motorcycle at an excessive speed. It is this kind of irresponsible behavior that all too often leads to pain and sorrow. Think before you act!

BE PREPARED   In our crazy world, it is important to always be aware of your surroundings. Whether crossing a street, shopping, or just home watching your favorite sports program, you must always be prepared for the unexpected. There are many in this world that would uncaringly steal your property, and there is always that potential accident just around the corner. To survive in life you must be physically and mentally prepared for any event that arises. Expect the unexpected and you'll be able to handle whatever comes your way!

LIVE LONG AND BE STRONG Hopefully, with a little luck and decades of discipline towards your health, you will be able to enjoy a long, vibrant, and rewarding life. There are no guarantees in life, so it is imperative that you learn as much about fitness as you can. The application of proper nutrition, exercise, rest, and positive thinking are necessary for a vibrant life. There is nothing more precious than the gift of life and the best time to start a healthy lifestyle is now. Make each day count by living life to its fullest through healthy living and enjoying the fruits of your labor.

GET SMART Your greatest tool to gaining that which you desire is knowledge. Learn as much as you can and apply it to your life. In today's world, it is virtually impossible to land a good paying career without a good education. You have to get your head into the books to be able to meet the challenges of your changing world. Be informed. As you read these words, the world is changing around you. In order to meet the demands of your future you must be prepared with knowledge to meet the challenges that await you. Knowledge is strength!

ENJOY YOUR LIFE You only get one shot at this party so make it a good one. Learn to be happy with yourself and the world in which you live. When possible, take in the mountains, oceans, or the wind flowing through the trees. It is all there for you to see and enjoy. Remember, there is more to life than pumping iron and big biceps. Visit your family and friends. Spend time with those you care about. Learn to find peace, joy, and love within your heart and share these feelings with others.

ASK QUESTIONS The only foolish question is the one you don't ask. Save yourself worry and get the answers to your problems. How many times have you gotten lost and found yourself going in circles? Asking simple questions can save you loads of frustration and time. Like most men, I am a little stubborn about asking directions when I'm lost or driving in an unfamiliar area. This usually results in lost time that can be put to better use at the gym or event I'm going to in the first place. A simple question is all it takes to set us on the right path, so why not ask it? Getting the answers to what, why, where, when, and how, can make your life run a whole lot smoother.

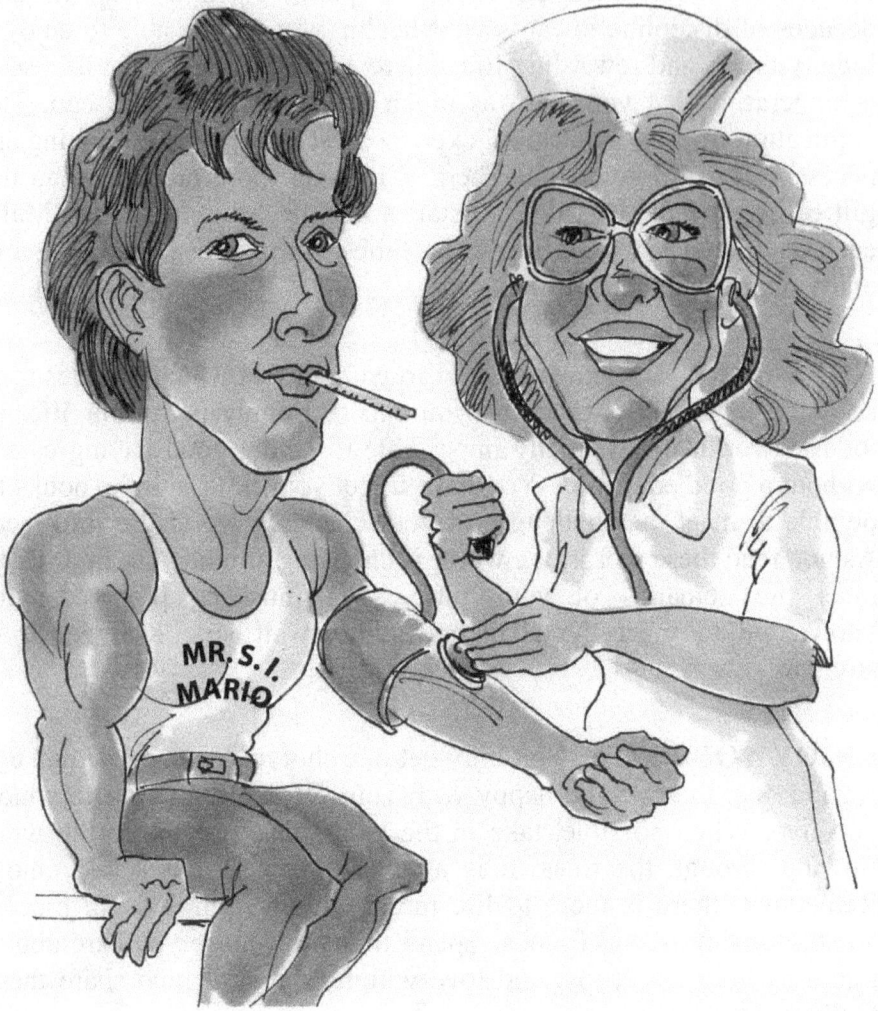

GET REGULAR MEDICAL CHECKUPS Routinely visit with your health care provider. Build up a working knowledge of your health and maintain it. Over the years, we all get knocked down with some form of illness. Seek medical attention when needed and keep a record of what medical therapy helped you in your time of need. Thanks to the benefits of living a healthy lifestyle through natural bodybuilding, I rarely need to seek medical advice for a problem. It has been decades since I have contracted the common cold or caught the flu, but on occasion, I do catch poison ivy and treat it before it spreads like wildfire, saving myself some grief and agony. In this country, we have some of the best medical professionals. When you need help, seek their advice!

SAVE FOR TOMORROW By working hard now and saving some of your earnings for the future, you will have more time to enjoy the fruits of your labor later on. It is easier to put in long hours at the job when you are young and ambitious, than when you are over the hill. It is also more enjoyable to be able to sit back and watch the waves hit the shore while you are older. Take the time today to invest in tomorrow. Live within your means and not larger than life! Forget about the Joneses next door. The time to save is now! A dollar saved is a dollar earned! Invest in your savings with the same enthusiasm you have for your training and tomorrow you will be able to reap the benefits of both disciplines.

BE VIRTUOUS Have strength, courage, and honor in your bones; tranquility and honesty in your blood; and compassion, hope, and love in your heart. Doing the right thing should be as natural as the sun that rises. We are all accountable for our actions in life and being true to others and ourselves will help make this a better world for you and me. You do not have to be a superman to do the right thing!

FREEDOM In our land of the free, we all have the right to choose our own path in life. Never take for granted what millions of others are denied throughout this world. If necessary, defend the liberty of your nation with every ounce of strength and determination your will can muster. Do not become complacent and believe that our way of life cannot be changed for the worse. As we sadly saw on 9/11, there are those who want to destroy what we as a nation have created and it is up to us to defend what our forefathers envisioned for us.

FAMILY One of the biggest challenges in life is to bring another being into this world. It is a very demanding, self-sacrificing, time-consuming, and endless effort to raise a son or daughter. Yet, it is the most rewarding of nature's gifts when they become responsible adults because of your efforts. Before beginning a family, be sure you are prepared both physically, mentally, and financially for the long haul.

There can be great joy in raising a family and great tragedy as well. Do your best to enjoy the moments you share together, for you never know what tomorrow will bring.

TIME   The clock ticks 24/7 and stops for no one. As the world spins, love, friends, battles, laws, fortunes, hopes, and dreams are being made and lost. Decide what is important to you and manage your time to fulfill your goals. Now that I am in my fifties, I see friends and family I have known for decades, age with every tick of the clock's secondhand, while I chronologically age at a much lower pace. Natural bodybuilding is a great way to preserve your health and radiance through the decades. Even though we cannot turn the clock back to the days when we were younger, we can slow its pace by living a healthy lifestyle. It is all up to you.

DEATH   The cycle of life on our planet is never ending. In with the new and out with the old. The process can be somewhat overbearing, even for the strongest among us. Although there are no guarantees, practicing a healthy lifestyle is almost certainly a sure way to keep the Grim Reaper away from your door for a long, long time. Make the most of your time here by living a full, healthy, and happy life, and help others by striving to make their lives just as rewarding as yours.

By carefully guiding your starship through the perilous obstacles of the galaxies, you, the natural bodybuilder, are on your *JOURNEY TO THE OLYMPIAN ZONE*!

THE NATURAL OLYMPIAN

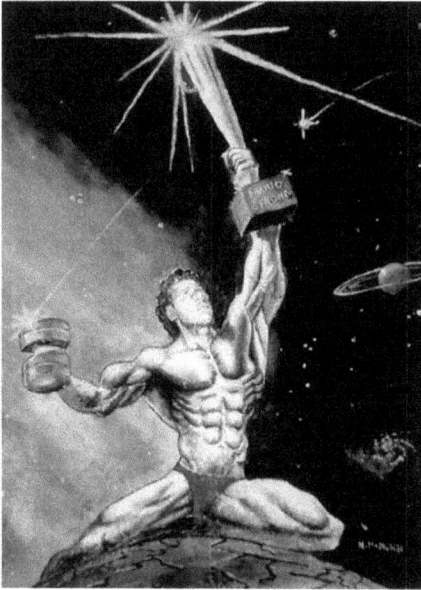

Natural bodybuilding is the scientific application of nutrition, exercise, rest, and positive thinking. The natural bodybuilder combines these factors into developing his body and athletic capabilities further than the average person does. In the advanced stage of natural bodybuilding, the bodybuilder masters these and other factors to create a healthy and radiant form of physical culture. Therefore, it should be clearly understood, that the advanced natural bodybuilder has achieved a state of being that relatively few people ever enjoy. He is a rare breed of human, having a close relationship with nature and a strong desire to live. Through trial and error, the advanced natural bodybuilder has found the way. Thanks to his focus and dedicated efforts, he has cleared a path to master the scientific principles needed to reach the Olympian Zone.

Look at yourself, chances are you would not be reading this book if you were not interested in improving your physique. As a natural bodybuilder, you are trying to learn, absorb, and apply as much knowledge about the art of physical culture to your life as possible.

When bodybuilders find something new, they try it to see if this newly discovered "secret" works for them. If it does not, they store it in their minds to be retested later. However, if it works, they immediately apply it to their bodybuilding lifestyle for further gains.

The more you learn about building your physique naturally, the faster your progress is going to paramount. Over time, natural bodybuilders gather volumes of muscle building knowledge to help them travel from the mere mortal cloud of existence into the realms of the Olympian Zone.

FEEL THE PUMP

If the advanced bodybuilder has one advantage over the others, it is his ability to feel each exercise. He knows how to perform every moment in a complete and absolute style. It is because of his many years of weight training that he has developed a sixth sense for the weights he uses. For example, when the advanced bodybuilder performs the Bench Press or Barbell Curl, he becomes one with the exercise. From start to finish, whether he uses a strict or cheating style, he receives maximum stimulation from the movement. He gets those muscles into the exercise, contracting them right from the start. Every muscular section receives its fair share of the work. No fibrous tissues are excused. As he reps the weights, he constricts and expands his Herculean physique into new and seemingly endless boundaries. He is doing what comes naturally to him, reaching out, and holding onto his number one friend, the pump.

When training, I use the pump as a guideline to ensure that each muscle receives its proper level of stimulating intensity. For example, when I work my quadriceps, I am careful not to let any one section get more than its share of work. The feeling the pump gives me in my thighs helps guide me in the way I distribute the resistance throughout my quadriceps. Through the pump, I am able to feel my way right into new levels of growth. Depending on what I am after, I can either gorge the muscle with loads of blood or strive for a deep pure burn. It's instinctive and the ability to realize this is one of the advanced bodybuilder's greatest weapons. Through time, the advanced bodybuilder has learned to depend more and more on his instincts. The more instinctive he becomes the less he is able to follow a set course. His muscles have become so accustomed to lifting that he has to literally feel his way through his workouts. It is a constant effort to get those seasoned muscles to respond to the resistance placed upon them, and it is the advanced bodybuilder's awakened instincts that give him the ability to do so properly.

If you follow the same workout schedule for too long your muscles will become stubborn. It is not for lack of desire or training, but simply because your muscles know which way they are going to be stimulated. By changing or adding a new exercise to your routine you will be able to attack their fibrous tissues where they least expect it. Advanced bodybuilders know this and through their acquired knowledge are able to select and apply different exercises and principles into their workouts, bringing them further into the zone.

Before every workout, I declare war on my muscles. I bomb and attack them with new combinations of exercises whenever their defense becomes aware of my previous plans. When I train, it is an all out effort! I grind every bit of human intensity (and then some) into my sets and feel the muscular tissues pleading for mercy as they constrict and stretch with each repetition I demand them to perform.

I am a natural for life bodybuilder that likes to train heavy. Sometimes the poundage becomes so monstrous that my muscles feel like they are exploding off my body and are being replaced by plates of hardened steel. When I am finished with my workouts, I feel like a Greek statue, freshly poured from the mold of perfection. It is because of my super heavy, high intensity training rituals that I am able to enter this realm of the Olympian Zone.

Once you learn how to incorporate the pump into your training, the level of intensity your body is capable of exerting will increase tremendously. Through time and experience, your muscle building instincts will make working out seem as natural as breathing the air. When the bodybuilder's lifestyle becomes one with nature, he leaves the everyday existence of the average mortal to become a super healthy and radiant being.

LIVE LONG AND BE STRONG

Bodybuilding is much more than a sport. It is a way of life! Too many guys lose touch with this concept. Sure, it is nice to enter and win a physique contest. I think bodybuilding is the greatest sport in the world, believe me. However, there is more to it than that.

Radiant health is what natural bodybuilding is all about and that is what you should be striving to achieve. It is the most rewarding accomplishment imaginable and yet the most difficult possession to maintain. Without it, you are nothing more than a mere mortal!

The bodybuilder who is able to realize true health in his lifetime is the Natural Olympian. Through hard work and endless dedication, he has reached his pinnacle of success. His life shines like a burning star, beaming its glowing force so that others may also find the way.

As important as exercise equipment is to the gym, so too is proper nutrition to the natural bodybuilder. Taking sufficient amounts of proteins, fats, carbohydrates, minerals, and vitamins (not to mention spring water) is only part of the game. The natural bodybuilder must learn what amounts and combinations of these substances work best for him. Every muscle builder is different. As stated previously, advanced bodybuilders have reached their level of development through years of endless trial and error to learn what worked best for them.

When striving to incorporate the best foods possible into your diet, select those with the least amount of artificial ingredients. In today's modern world it seems as if everything consumed causes cancer or some other type of serious illness. My advice to you is to learn as much as you can about nutrition and apply this knowledge to your muscle building lifestyle. In the end, it is not whether you win or lose that counts the most, but rather the fact that you tried and gave it everything you had. That is what is truly important!

When you get the chance stop by your local health food store and ask the manager which books he recommends on nutrition. Buy one or two and read their contents. Begin to learn and experience the different theories in the field of nutrition. Build a library of knowledge, not only on your bookshelf, but also within yourself. The more you understand what the word natural means, the better you will be able to select and apply foods to your diet that work best for you.

Nature is the mother of the Natural Olympian. She houses and provides him with all the essentials of life. In turn, the Natural Olympian uses these provisions as the tools in which he builds his fortress of health, thus creating his Herculean physique. The combination of nature and the bodybuilder create the highest force imaginable. This dynamic duo is a team that climbs far into the limitless boundaries of the Olympian Zone.

The mind is the most complex database known to man. For the advanced natural bodybuilder it is his means for storing, solving, and updating his mountain of knowledge. The enormous positive attitude that is generated from this intricate computer is in itself a chief factor for the advanced natural bodybuilder's success.

BELIEVE

Like all bodybuilders, the Natural Olympian was an average person when he first began to expand his physical horizons. Through time, his positive attitude and strong belief in himself ignited with a burning desire to achieve. With this fire raging deep inside of him, he trained relentlessly through many decades of high intensity workouts. In his heart, he knew that one day his goals would be achieved and with this burning belief, he marched on until his dreams became a reality. The sky is the limit and the advanced bodybuilder knows this. All physique champions have had a dream of what they wanted to accomplish in bodybuilding. They projected a belief in themselves that one day they would succeed and with this positive attitude, they continued on their journey, until success was realized. By visualizing what kind of physique you are after, you too, can accomplish your goals in bodybuilding. Knowing which path to follow early in your bodybuilding career will save you lots of time and energy. The mind is a wonderful thing. When your levels of concentration become focused and in tune with the body, nothing will be able to penetrate its dense force. Learning how to develop these powers will prove to be a great asset towards your future success, not only in bodybuilding but also in every endeavor of your life.

CONCLUSION

When the Natural Olympian trains, it's like a sixth sense to him as he masterfully conducts his workouts like a symphony orchestra. Each exercise, set, and repetition he performs is united together to create a living work of art. His naturally balanced foods are the musicians he directs. If his proteins are playing too low, he will raise his mighty wand as a signal for them to increase their performance. If his carbohydrates are sounding a bit weak, he will pick up his hand just enough to balance out their tone. If his fats begin to overpower the others, he will sweep both his hands down swiftly, silencing their shouting at once. To help his worn muscles recuperate from his intense performances he calls upon his chorus to sing him a relaxing lullaby, so that he can reenergize, to play harder and louder another day. The Natural Olympian formulates his workouts, nutrition, and recuperation into a song of harmony. A melody so harmonic and positive in nature that it creates an entity of strength, honor, and self-belief. It is with this song of life that the Natural Olympian marches on, through the many suns that will rise and shine as he journeys to the realms of his destiny.

The Natural Olympian is the maestro, harmonizing his bodybuilding lifestyle to form the perfect masterpiece. He unites the instincts he has for bodybuilding with those he has for life in an attempt to form the ultimate entity. An entity, so advanced and in tune with nature that no mortal man could dare imagine. An entity, so healthy and glowing in radiance that the Herculean Gods cry out in envy. An entity, whose presence here is but a stepping-stone towards his *JOURNEY TO THE OLYMPIAN ZONE*!

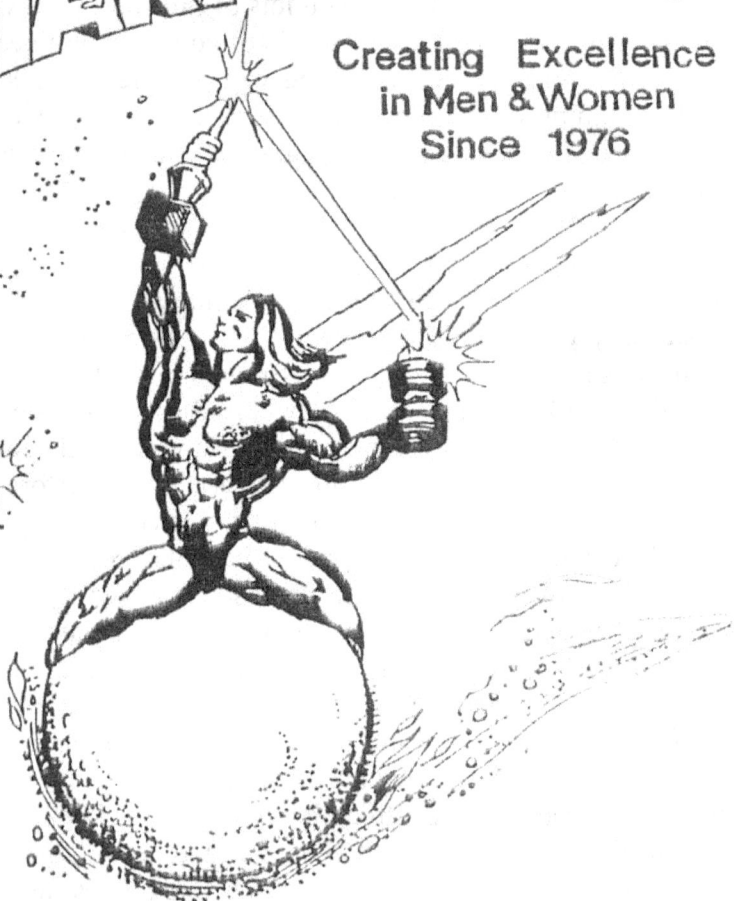

MARIO-STRONG

Creating Excellence
in Men & Women
Since 1976

ANATOMY OF A BODYBUILDER

Natural bodybuilding is the scientific application of exercise, nutrition, rest, and positive thinking. While wanting bigger biceps and six-pack abs are worthy goals, it is important to know which tools to use to help you achieve them. One of the tools natural bodybuilders use is resistance training, primarily with the use of free-weights and related machines. Since the early 1970s, the evolution of exercise equipment has been nothing short of phenomenal. As much as it has evolved, one simple fact remains; the basic bodybuilding tools provide the best results for the effort. The good old barbell, bench, and squat rack may have some competition for attention in the gym, but they will never be topped in their ability to bring lasting results.

Because of the hundreds of exercises to choose from, many beginners are confused about which exercises to include in their weight training routines. Through trial and error, bodybuilders have come to recognize several key exercises that best stimulate the individual muscles and their groups. This chapter will discuss those key exercises, which have lasted through the test of time, and are still heavily relied upon today for greater mass and strength. Knowing what exercises to perform is one thing, knowing what body part they effect and how to perform them correctly is another. It is important that you learn the proper technique while performing each exercise. In the following pages, I have detailed what I believe the best manner for doing so. Remember, it is up to you to learn which exercises and techniques works best for you. Everyone is different, and only through time and sweat will you learn what exercise systems and tools brought you gains and which ones didn't register with your muscle's receptors.

MR. MUSCLES

Biceps

Neck Rotators

Triceps

Pectoralis Major

External Obliques

Hip Adductors

Rectus Femoris

Vastus Lateralis

Gastrocnemius

Tibialis Anterior

Anterior Deltoid

Forearm Flexors

Serratus Anterior

Rectus Abdominus

Hip Abductors

Quadriceps

Vastus Medialis

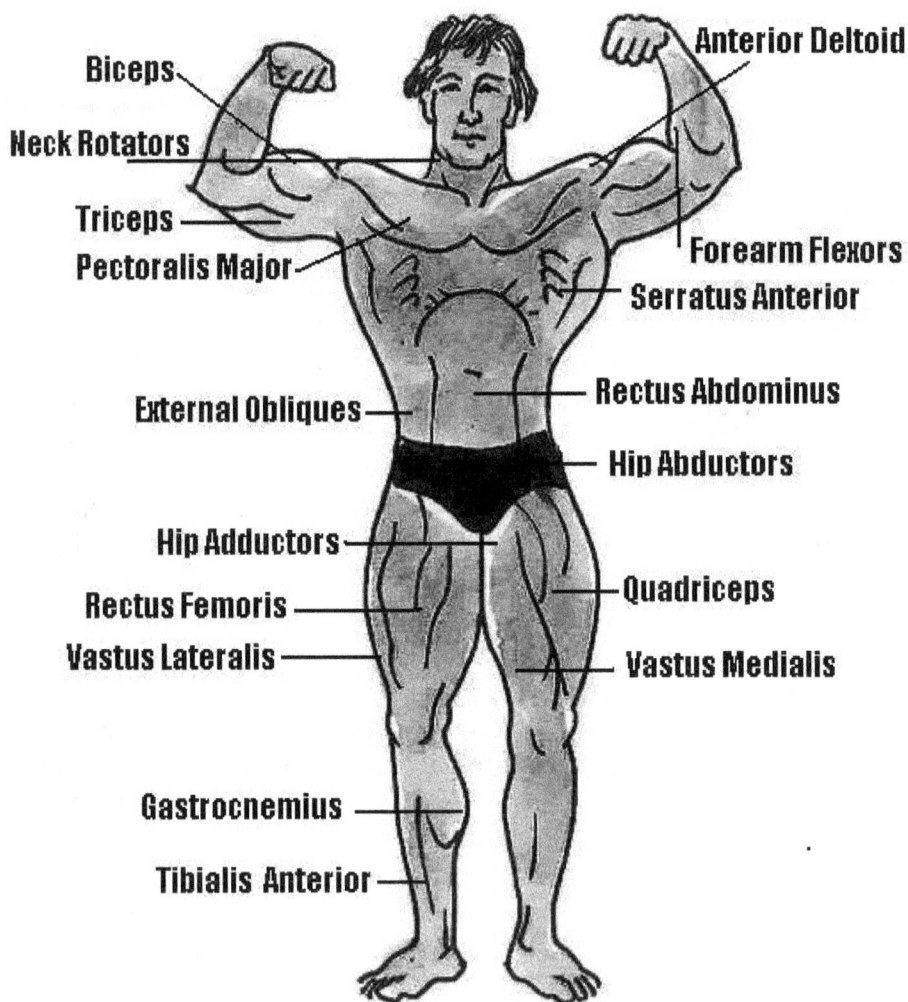

All drawings in this chapter with permission of Bernie Shuman

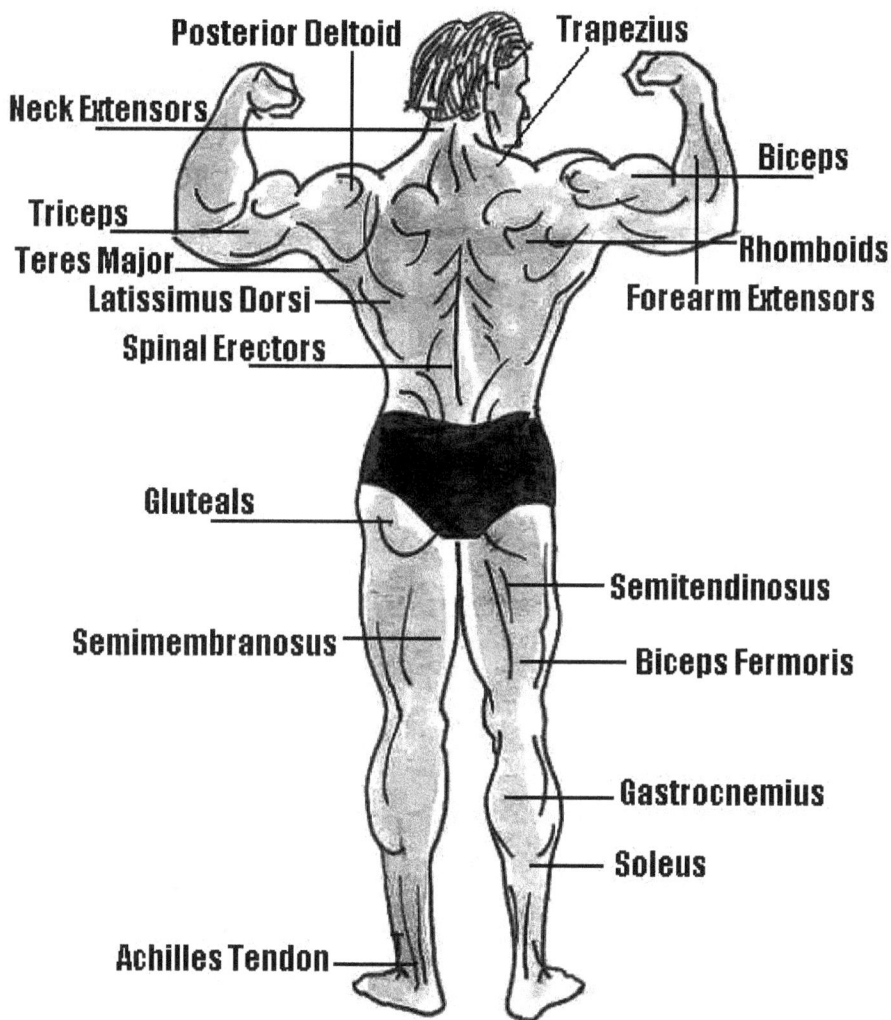

Posterior Deltoid

Trapezius

Neck Extensors

Biceps

Triceps

Teres Major

Latissimus Dorsi

Spinal Erectors

Rhomboids

Forearm Extensors

Gluteals

Semitendinosus

Semimembranosus

Biceps Fermoris

Gastrocnemius

Soleus

Achilles Tendon

THE INDIVIDUAL BODY PARTS

THIGHS

The thighs are among the largest muscle group in the body. They are designed to withstand a lot of work and are capable of lifting extremely heavy poundage. Any muscle builder planning on competing on a physique stage or just looking good at the beach should be focused on training his thighs from the first day he picks up a barbell. The thighs are an important body part and the last thing a bodybuilder wants to do is neglect this area and play catch up.

This major muscle group consists of two main sections, the quadriceps and hamstrings. The quadriceps is a group of four large muscles that can be viewed on the front of the thigh. These muscles are the vastus mediali, vastus intermedius, vastus lateralis, and the rectus femoris. The front part of the quad is the rectus femoris. Directly beneath, it is the vastus intermedius. On either side of the rectus femoris and vastus intermedius you will find muscles that run parallel. These muscles are the vastus medialis, which is located on the inside of the thigh, and the vastus lateralis, which is located on the outside. These four muscles begin at the top of the femur and travel down to the tibia, forming the quadriceps. The one exception to this is the rectus femoris, which originates on the pelvis and crosses the hip joint. Its function is to extend the knee, and act as a hip flexor. The main function of the quadriceps is to straighten the leg by extending the knee.

The hamstrings are located on the back of the thighs and consist of three separate muscles. These muscles are the biceps femoris, semitendinosus, and semimembranosus. All three muscles originate on the pelvic bone and attach down on the tibia of the lower thigh. The lateral hamstrings are the short and long head of the biceps femoris.

The medial hamstrings are the semitendinosus, which joins the sartorius muscle and gracilis muscle at the pes anserinus on the tibia, and the semimembranosus, which is the largest hamstring muscle. The tendons for these muscles begin at the ischial tuberosity and attach on the outer edges of the shinbone, just below the back of your knees to help stabilize them. Your hamstrings also have many soft connective tissues and are innervated by your sciatic nerve. The hamstrings are primarily fast-twitch white fiber muscles and respond best to low reps and powerful movements. Their main functions are knee flexion and hip extension. An example of knee flexion would be the Leg Curl movement, where the heels are brought towards the glutes. An example of hip extension would be the Stiff-Leg Deadlift, where the thighs are moved towards the rear. The hamstrings are also involved with eccentric movements that increase the length of the muscle while it is under tension. An example of this is when the muscle acts as a brake to stop an action. You can feel this when walking or running downhill, landing from jumps, or performing squats, and when trying to stop quickly after sprinting.

It is important to note that to maintain balance in the thigh, bodybuilders should train their hamstring group just as hard as their quadriceps. Personally, I like to train my hamstrings after my quads. This is because my hamstrings receive a lot of indirect stimulation from the mass-building exercises that I perform with my quads and therefore are thoroughly warmed-up for the intense work that I demand of them.

The adductors are a group of muscles that include the adductor magnus, longus, brevis, gracilis, and the pectineus. The adductors originate on the pelvic bone and attach at intervals along the length of the femur. This interval attachment provides the most power and stability for the hip joint and the femur. The primary function of the adductors is to move the leg in towards the centerline of the body. The adductors also serve to stabilize the hip joint.

The gluteus maximus (glutes) is one of the largest and strongest muscles in the body. It is mentioned here because it receives a great deal of direct stimulation through exercises such as squats and lunges. The glutes originates along the pelvic bone crests and attaches to the rear of the femur. Their primary function is hip extension, which is moving the thigh to the rear.

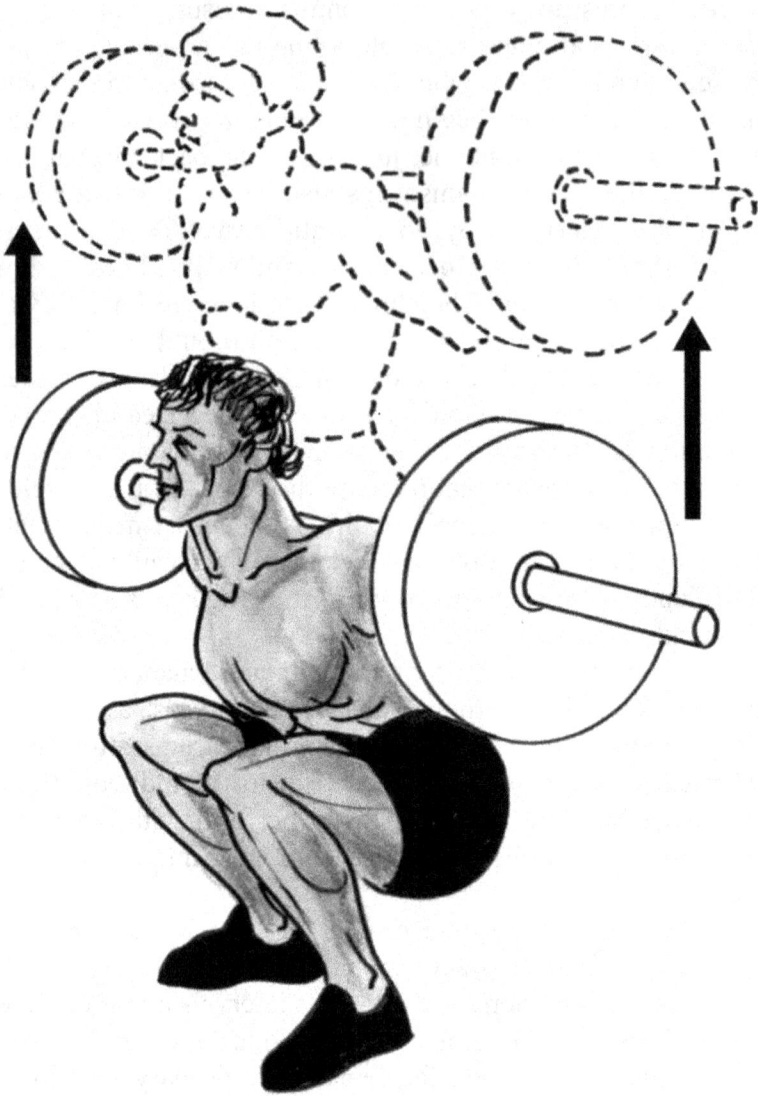

FULL SQUAT – Quadriceps, Hamstrings, Gluteus Maximus

- Place barbell on upper back.
- Use comfortable handgrip.
- Head up, back straight, feet firmly on the floor about 16" apart.
- Squat, until upper thighs are at least parallel to floor.
- Keep head up, back straight, knees positioned slightly outward.
- Return to starting position.
- Inhale down, exhale up.

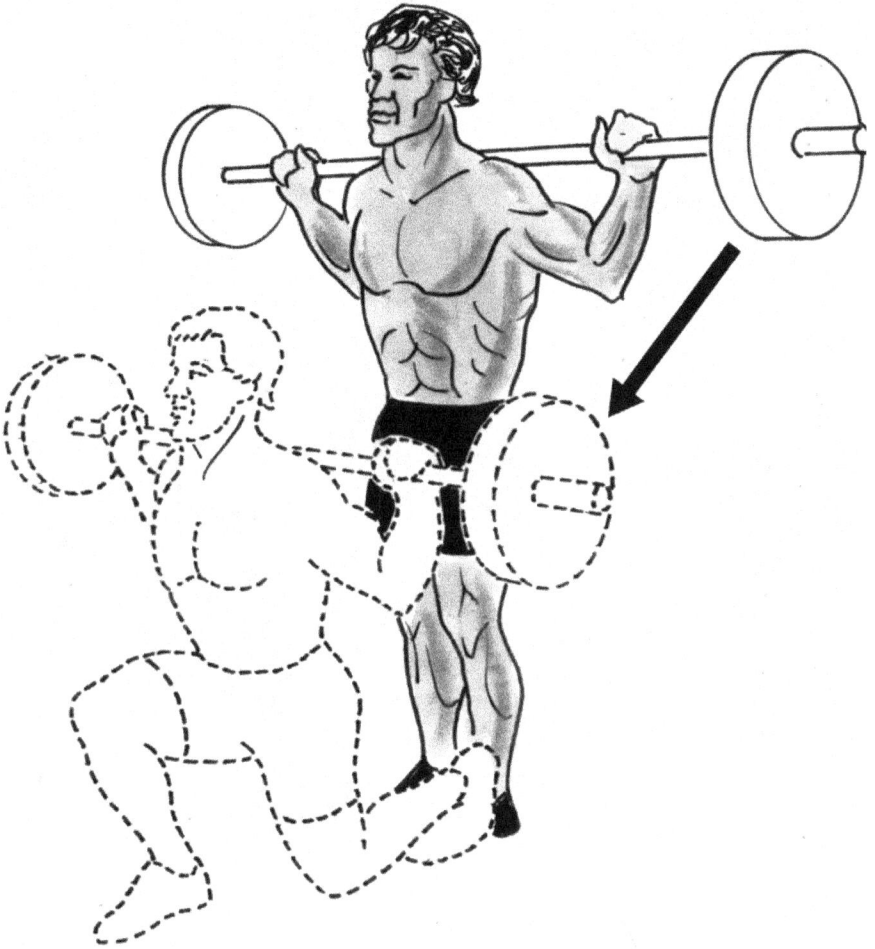

BARBELL LUNGE – Quadriceps, Hamstrings, Glutes

- Place barbell on upper back.
- Head up, back straight, feet about 6" apart.
- Kneel forward as far as possible with left leg until upper left thigh is almost parallel to floor and then straighten it.
- Keep right leg as straight as possible throughout movement.
- Repeat with opposite leg.
- Inhale down, exhale up.

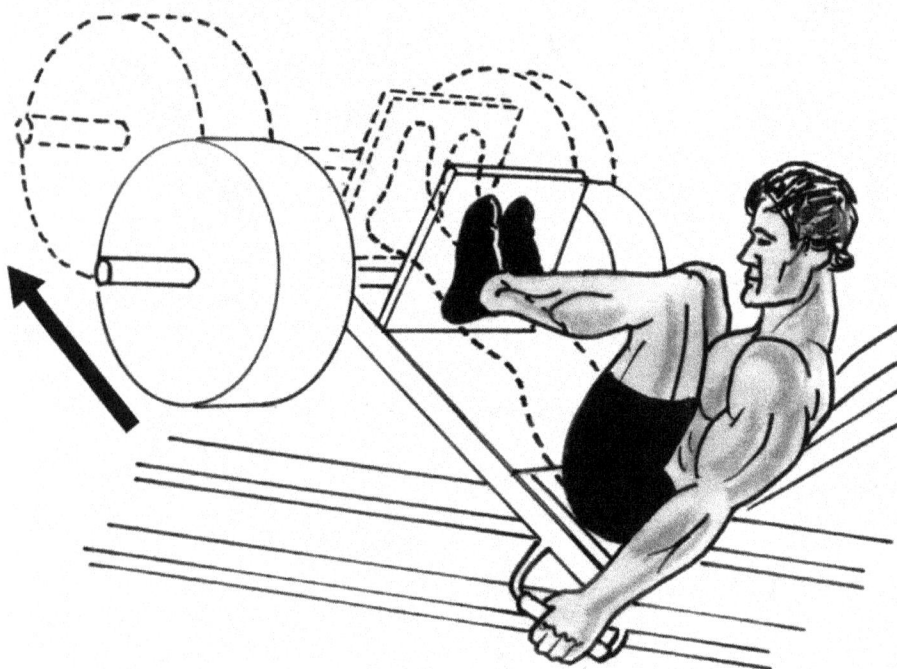

LEG PRESS – Quadriceps, Hamstrings, Gluteus Maximus

- Position yourself on machine with your back firmly against the support pad and your feet firmly on the footboard about 16-18" apart. Knees should be positioned slightly outward.
- Press the resistance out to full extension, release the support pins and then lower the weight carriage until your upper thighs are near the sides of your torso.
- Do not let your upper thighs bounce off your chest.
- Return to the starting position.
- Inhale down, exhale up.

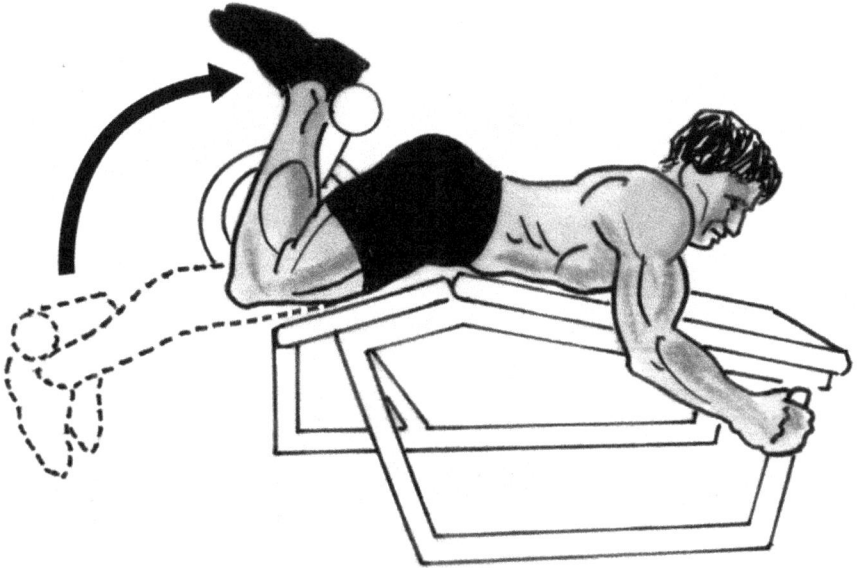

LYING LEG CURL – Hamstrings

- Lie face down on machine.
- Place heels under foot pad.
- Hold front of machine for support.
- Curl legs up until calves touch thigh biceps.
- Return to starting position.
- Inhale up, exhale down.

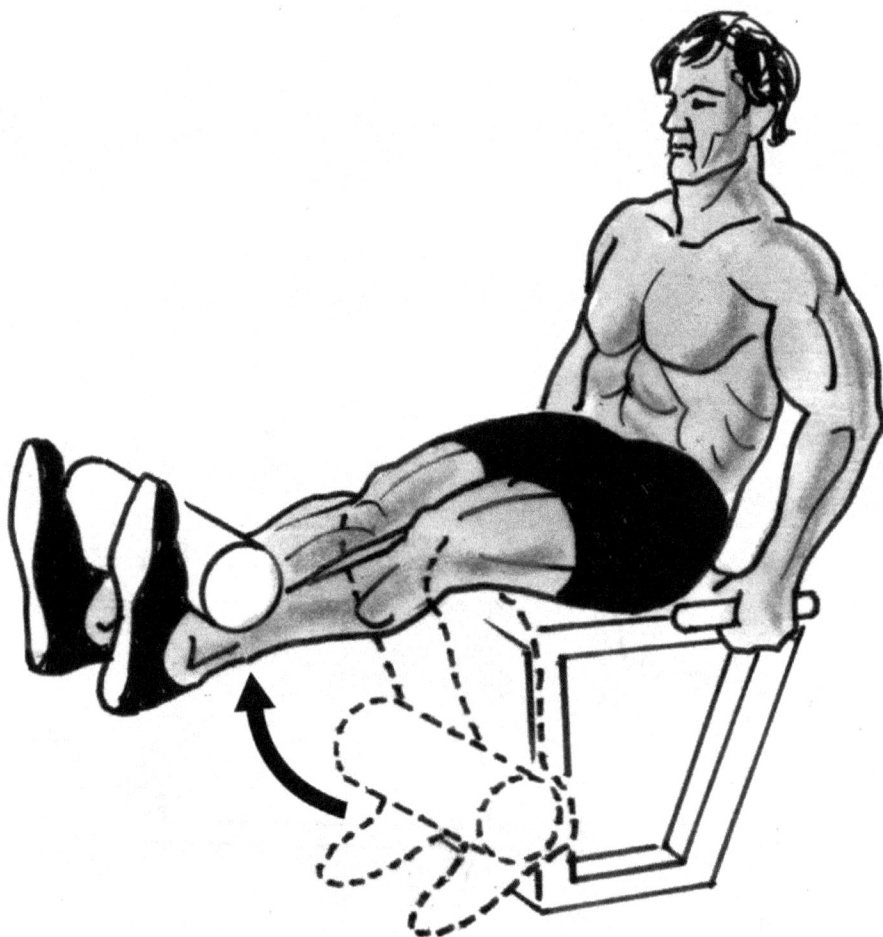

LEG EXTENSION – Quadriceps

- Sit on machine with ankles behind footpad.
- Place back of knees against seat.
- Grip handles for support.
- Point toes slightly down.
- Raise resistance up until legs are at least parallel to floor.
- Return to starting position.
- Inhale down, exhale up.

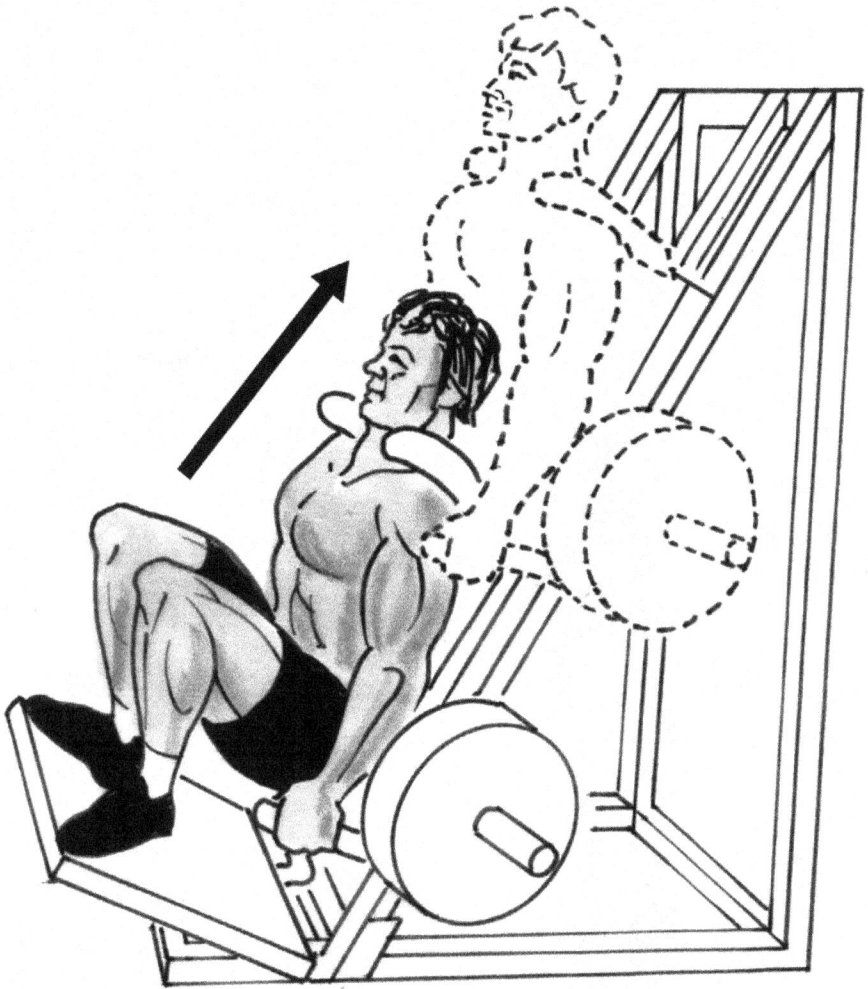

HACK SQUATS – Quadriceps,   Hamstrings,   Gluteus Maximus

- Position yourself in machine.
- Place shoulders under pads.
- Plant feet firmly on angled footboard.
- Stand erect, head up, back straight. Knees positioned outwards.
- Release weight support pins.
- Squat, until upper thighs are at least parallel to machine.
- Keep head up and back straight.
- Return to starting position.
- Inhale down, exhale up.

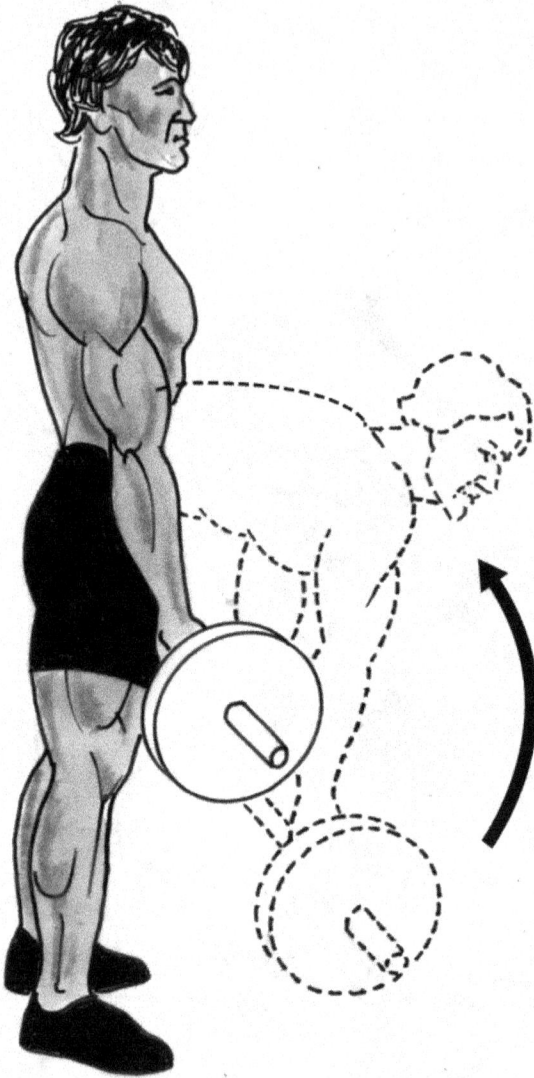

STIFF-LEG DEADLIFT – Hamstrings, Gluteus Maximus

- Place barbell on rack above floor.
- Stand on platform.
- With feet 16" apart, bend and grasp bar using a shoulder width grip.
- Keep knees locked, back straight, head up.
- Using only your back muscles, stand erect with arms locked.
- Lower resistance to platform, then return to erect position.
- Inhale up, exhale down.

CALVES

The calves are one of three vital areas, along with abdominals and deltoids, which add greatly to the symmetry of a bodybuilder. Diamond-shaped calves add an illusion of mass to the legs, even if the thighs are not well built. However, as important as calf development is, it is one of the least favorite body parts for bodybuilders to train, mostly because of their stubbornness to grow. The calves consist of two separate muscles and each has a specific function.

The diamond shaped muscle that makes up the largest portion of the calf is the gastrocnemius. The gastrocnemius crosses two joints by originating behind the knee on the femur and attaching itself to the heel with the Achilles tendon. This main calf muscle consists of the medial and lateral heads, and when fully developed takes the shape of a diamond. The medial head originates on the posterior tibia and the lateral head on the posterior fibula. Both heads come together and insert into the calcaneal tendon. The soleus portion of the calf is located on the rear of the lower leg and is not visible because it lies beneath the gastrocnemius. The function of the soleus is the same as the gastrocnemius, which is to raise the heel. The only difference is that the soleus is best worked when performing calf exercises where the knee is bent, such as in the Seated Calf Raise. The plantaris is a small muscle located at the bottom of the calf, which passes between the gastrocnemius and soleus, and inserts itself into the calcaneus. It originates at the lateral epicondyle of the femur, just above the origin of the lateral head of the gastrocnemius.

Over the decades, I have tortured my calves with every conceivable exercise and training routine possible. I have trained them with heavy steel in the gym, performed both high and low rep schemes, used supersets and giant sets, hit them twice a day for weeks at a time, sprinted up hills and even run on sand (while carrying an extra 50 pounds). My calves are stubborn and the one thing that I have learned which brings me the best results is to train them consistently and with some new routine each workout. Training the calf muscles can be like a war and its imperative for guys like me to attack this dense fibrous muscle group continually in ways it least expects it. Be creative and bomb them like there is no tomorrow!

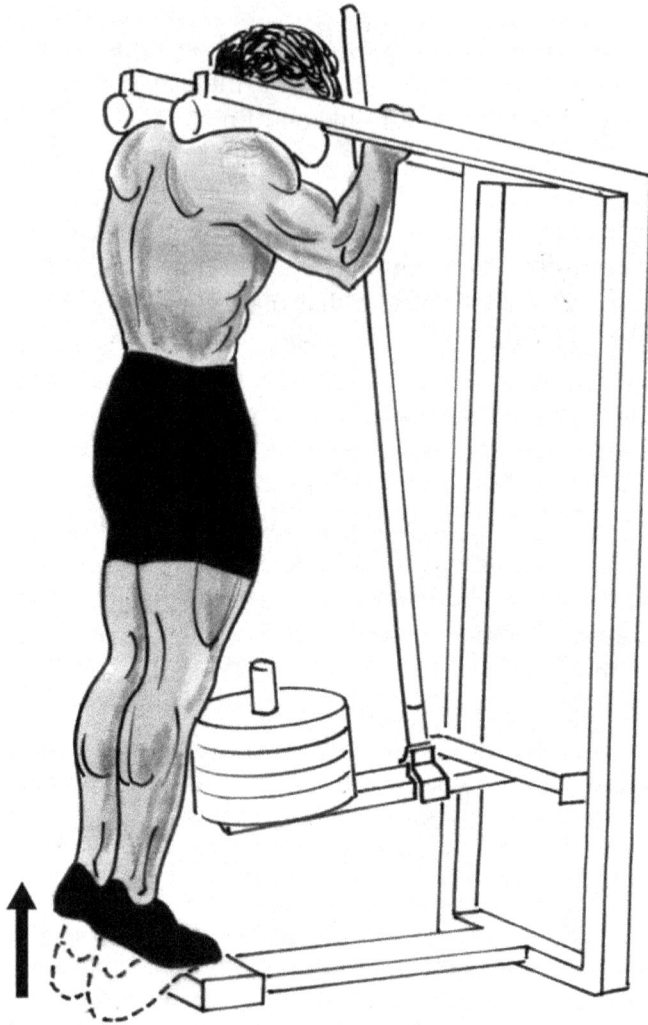

STANDING CALF RAISE – Gastrocnemius

- Position shoulders under pads of machine.
- Stand erect with balls of feet on footboard.
- Keep back straight, head up, legs locked.
- Do not let hips move backward or forward.
- Rise up on toes as high as possible.
- Hold position shortly and then lower heels to lowest comfortable position.
- Feel stretch, then rise back to top.
- Inhale up, exhale down.

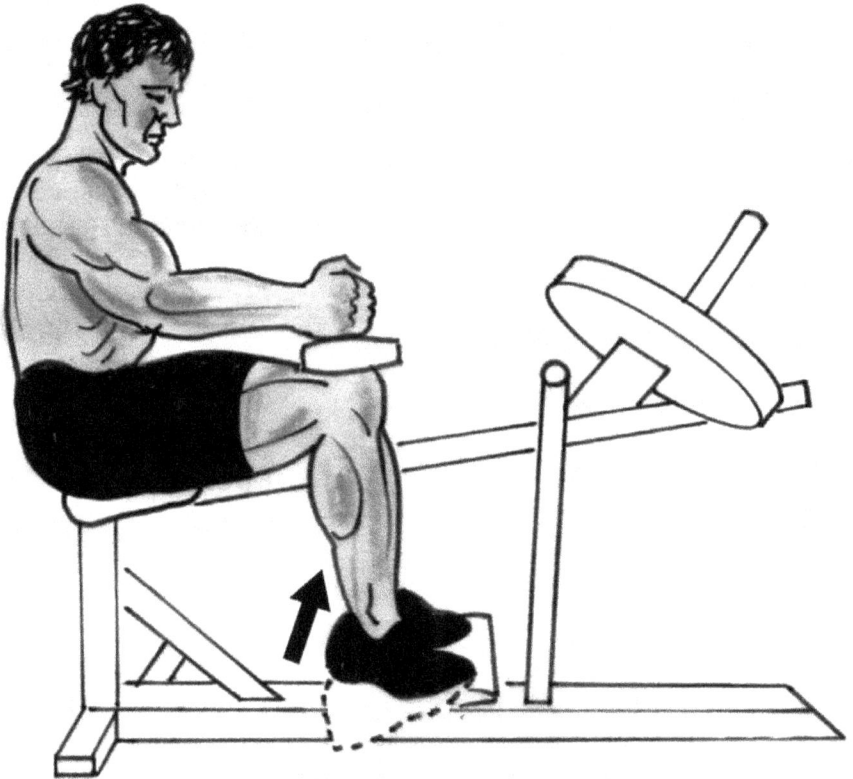

SEATED CALF RAISE – Soleus

- Sit on seat of machine. Place balls of feet on footboard.
- Place upper thighs under leg pad just above knees.
- Rise up on toes and release safety stop.
- Lower heels to a comfortable position.
- Rise up on toes as high as possible.
- Hold shortly and then return to starting position.
- Inhale up, exhale down.

BACK

The back is one of the largest muscle groups to develop. On the physique stage, it is a body part that can be seen from most angles while posing. A well-proportioned muscular back says volumes about the bodybuilder who posses it and such development has been a constant factor in determining many bodybuilding championships. Bodybuilders often neglect this vital body part because of the hard work it takes to develop it. Personally, I find that the heavier and more intensely I train this area, the more powerful and massive my entire physique becomes, resulting in gains that have lasted a lifetime.

The back is a complex and multi-layered body part. Its muscle group consists of the latissimus dorsi, trapezius, posterior deltoid, teres major and minor, rhomboids, erector spinae, and the external abdominal oblique. The latissimus dorsi muscles (lats) are the largest and most visual muscles of the back. They start at the upper end of the humerus and travel down to the pelvic girdle. The function of the lats is to pull the arm down towards the pelvis. An example of this would be the Front Pull-Down movement.

The trapezius (traps) is an extremely powerful and complex muscle section of the back. Its long trapezoid-shaped muscle originates at the base of the skull and attaches down in the middle to lower back. The angles of the traps provide pull in three different directions: up, down, and in towards the centerline of the body. The traps have several functions including bringing the shoulder blades together, pulling the shoulder blades down, and shrugging. The back also consists of several other smaller muscles, namely the teres major and the rhomboids, which assist in various movements. The teres major is located at the outside edge of the shoulder blade and attaches itself to the humerus. Its main function is to bring the arm towards the back. The rhomboids are located on the spinal column and attach themselves to the middle of the shoulder blade. Their main function is to bring the shoulder blades together. There are also many smaller muscles in the back that travel along the spine. Located in the erector spinae, they include the longissimus, spinalis, and the iliocostalis. The functions of the erector spinae are to support the spine as well as extend it. The muscles of the erector spinae are attached to the vertebrae, pelvis, and to the ribs.

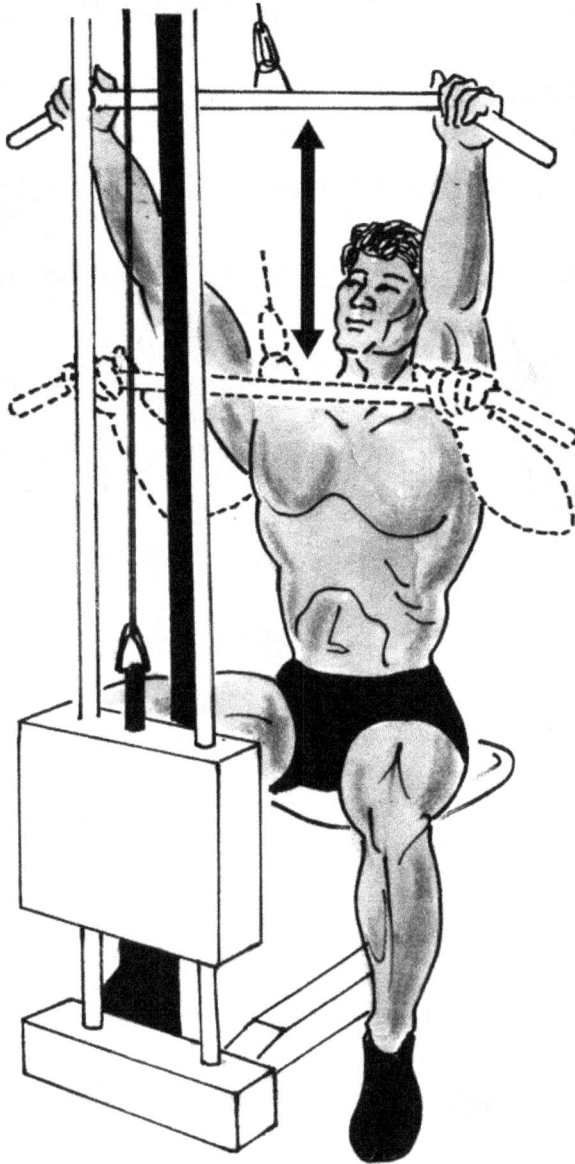

FRONT PULL-DOWN – Latissimus Dorsi

- Hold lat-bar with hands about 36" apart.
- Sit down on seat and support resistance with arms fully extended overhead.
- Pull bar straight down until it reaches upper chest.
- Return to starting position.
- Inhale down, exhale up.

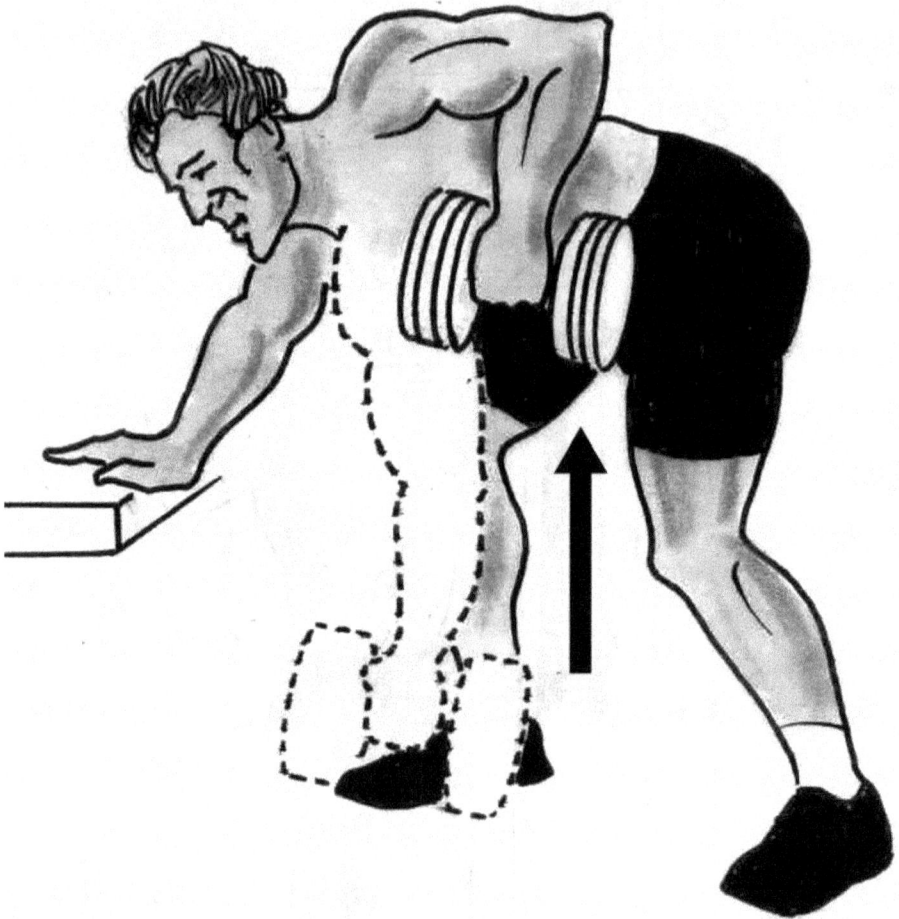

DUMBBELL ROW – Rhomboids, Latissimus Dorsi

- Place a dumbbell on the floor in front of a flat bench.
- Put left leg back, knee locked.
- Bend right knee slightly. Place right hand on bench, elbow locked.
- Keep back straight, eyes forward.
- Bend over and hold dumbbell with left hand, palm in, about 6" off floor.
- Pull dumbbell straight up to side of torso, keeping arm close to side.
- Return to starting position using same path.
- Inhale up, exhale down.
- Reverse position and repeat movement on opposite side.

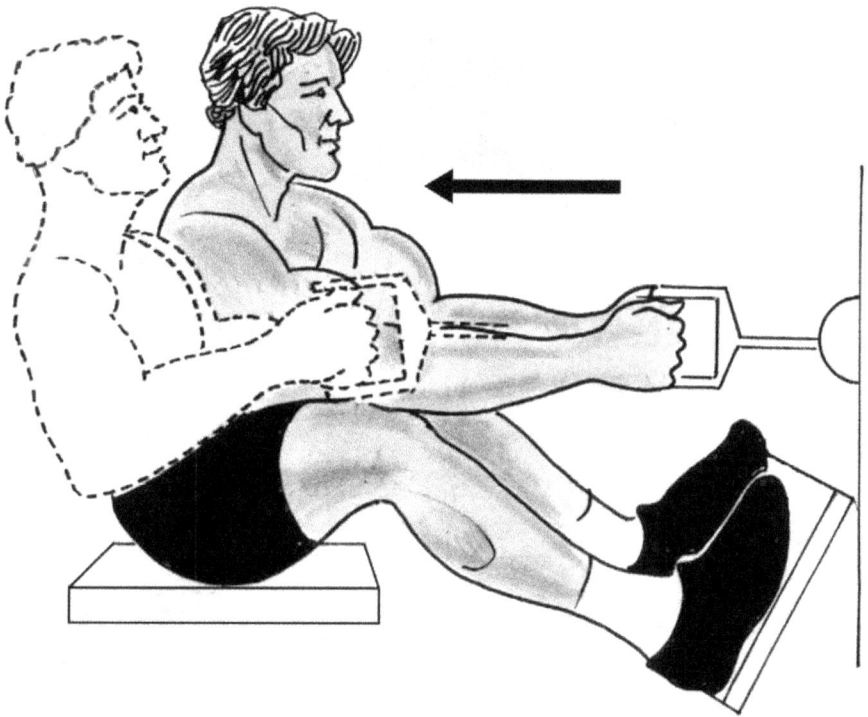

CABLE ROW – Rhomboids, Latissimus Dorsi

- Sit on bench in front of low pulley.
- Place feet on footboard.
- Grip pulley handles.
- Bend slightly forward at beginning of movement; straighten torso as resistance is pulled inwards.
- Pull handles just below pectorals.
- Return weight stack to starting position.
- Inhale in, exhale out.

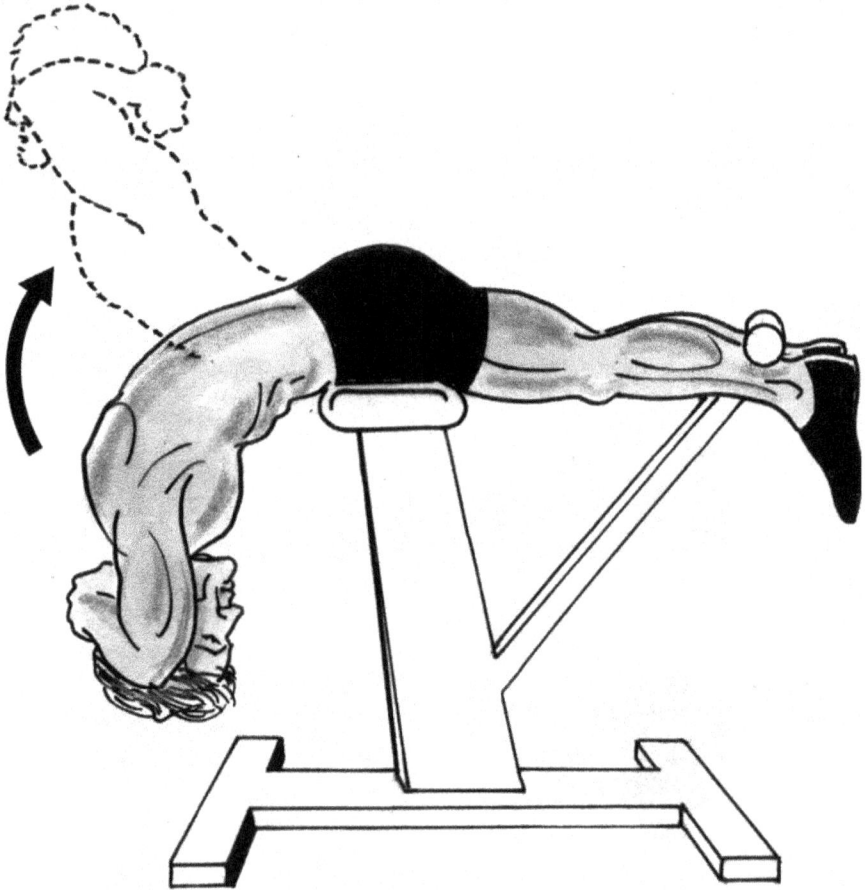

HYPEREXTENSION – Lumbar, Spinal Erectors

- Extend upper body over end of hyperextension bench.
- Lock legs under support.
- End of bench should be at hips.
- Bend down at waist so upper body is vertical to floor.
- Place hands behind head.
- Raise torso straight up until slightly past parallel.
- Return to starting position.
- Inhale up, exhale down.
- Can also be done with added resistance.

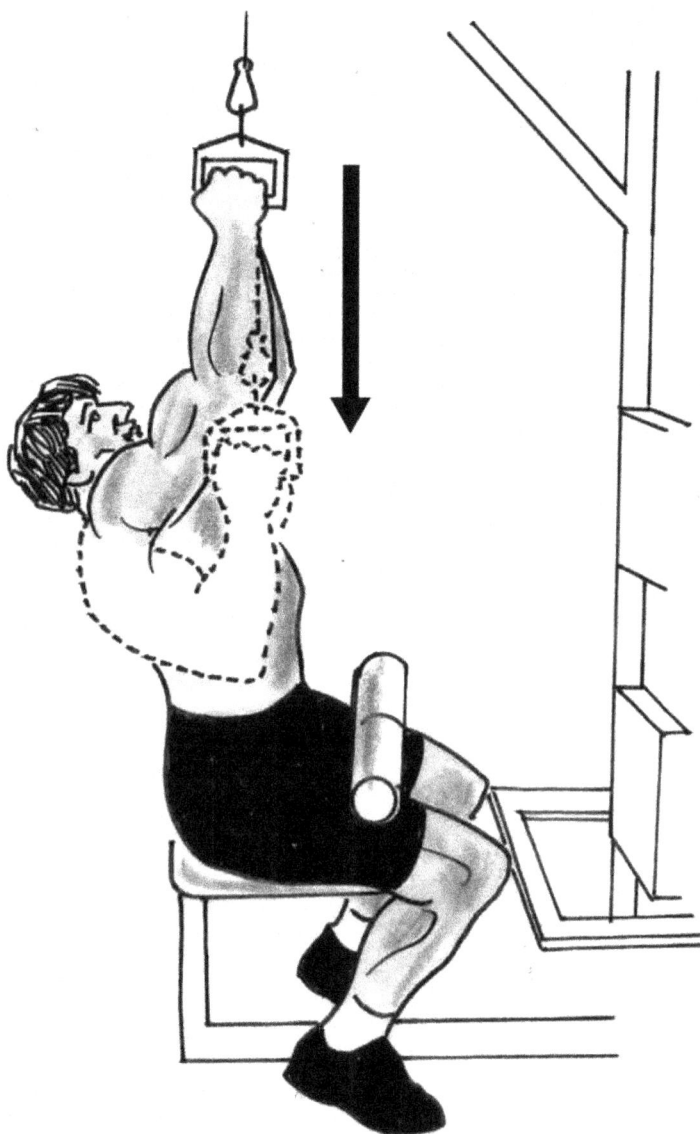

CLOSE GRIP PULL-DOWN – Rhomboids, Latissimus Dorsi

- Grip handles with palms facing in, about 6-8" apart.
- Sit down far enough to support resistance with arms extended overhead.
- Pull handles straight down until it reaches center chest.
- Return to starting position.
- Inhale down, exhale up.

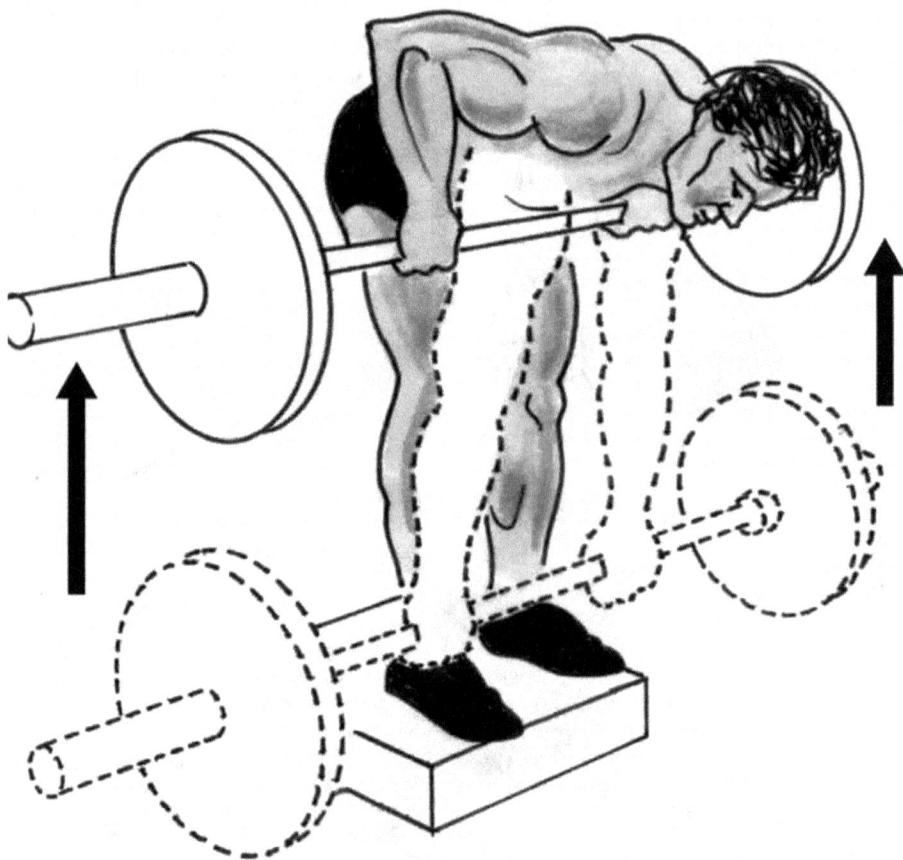

BENT OVER BARBELL ROW – Latissimus Dorsi, Rhomboids

- Place a barbell on the floor in front of you.
- With your feet about 18" apart, bend forward and hold a barbell using a shoulder width grip.
- Keep the legs bent and the back parallel to the floor as you inhale and pull the barbell directly up to the lower part of the chest.
- Inhale up, exhale down.
- Do not let the barbell touch the floor once you have begun the exercise. A foot block may be used for added stretch.
- Keep your head up and the back straight.

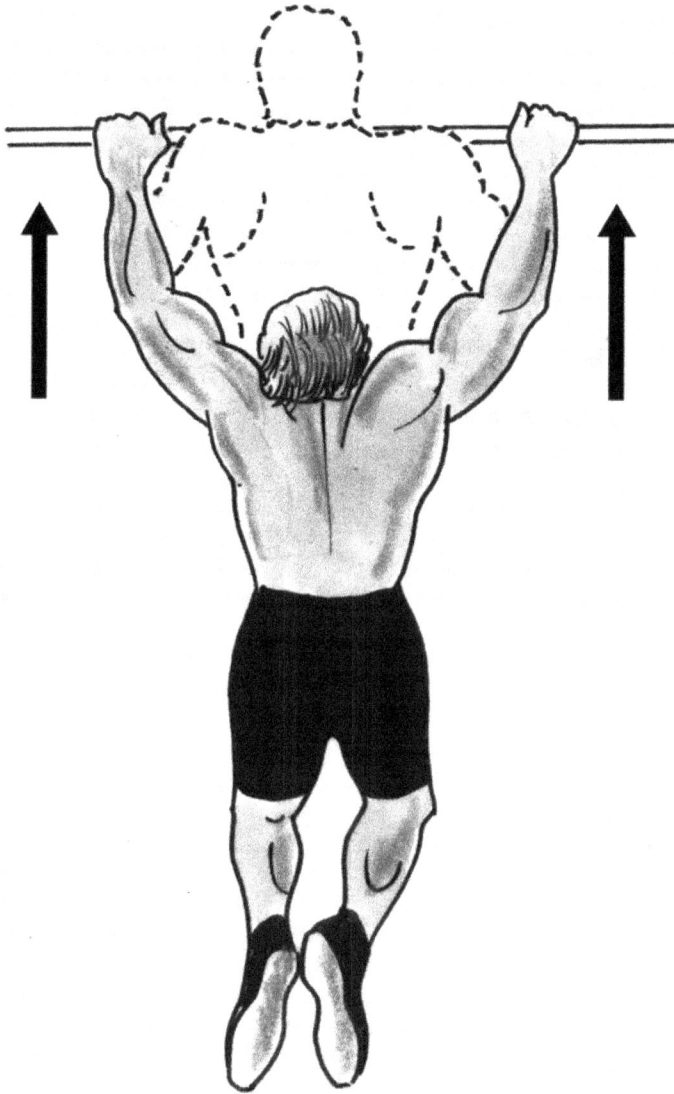

FRONT PULL-UP – Latissimus Dorsi, Rhomboids, Teres Major

- Hang from chinning bar with arms extended overhead.
- Hold bar with hands approximately 18-20" apart.
- Pull up, raise chin above bar.
- Return to starting position.
- Try to keep back slightly hyper-extended.
- Do not swing back and forth.
- Inhale down, exhale up.

CHEST

Next to the biceps, the chest area is the muscle builder's favorite body part to train and display. A well-developed chest represents masculinity and strength. It also helps to protect your most vital organ (your heart) from trauma. Remember the 99-pound weakling in the old Charles Atlas advertisements? His sunken-in chest was a sure sign of a frail, weak body. Understanding the anatomy of the chest area will help you develop that steel plated pectoral he-man look.

This important muscle group consists of the pectorals major and the pectorals minor. The pectoralis major originates on the breastbone, which is located at the center of the chest and is attached to the ribcage, and to the humerus near the shoulder joint. The function of the pectoralis major is to bring the humerus across the chest. Its muscle is shaped like fan-blades, which allow the humerus to move in a variety of planes across the body. An example of this is the Dumbbell Fly movement. The pectorals minor is located beneath the pectoralis major. It originates on the ribs and is attached to the scapula at the coracoid process. The function of the pectoralis minor is to move the shoulder area forward. An example of this would be when the shoulders are shrugged forward. The pectoralis major brings the humerus across the body while the pectoralis minor moves the shoulders forward. Thus, this muscle group serves to adduct, horizontally adduct, and internally rotate the arm.

The chest is one muscle group that I like to train with heavy steel. While performing the main pressing movements (including the Parallel Dip) I gradually pyramid the poundage until I am maxing out with one or two reps. As a result of this, the power I feel throughout my body gives me an impenetrable sense that stays with me throughout the entire workout and afterwards. I also feel that by using the heavy poundage that I do, it not only builds muscle and strength but also lasting health and vitality as well.

One very important note: Repeatedly, I have seen bodybuilders cause injury onto themselves while training the chest area because they had egos that were bigger than their pectoral region and used poundage that far exceeded their normal limits. In the iron game, you are only as good as your weakest link. One sure way to find that link is by using more steel than you can handle. Be smart, train according to your body's abilities and not beyond.

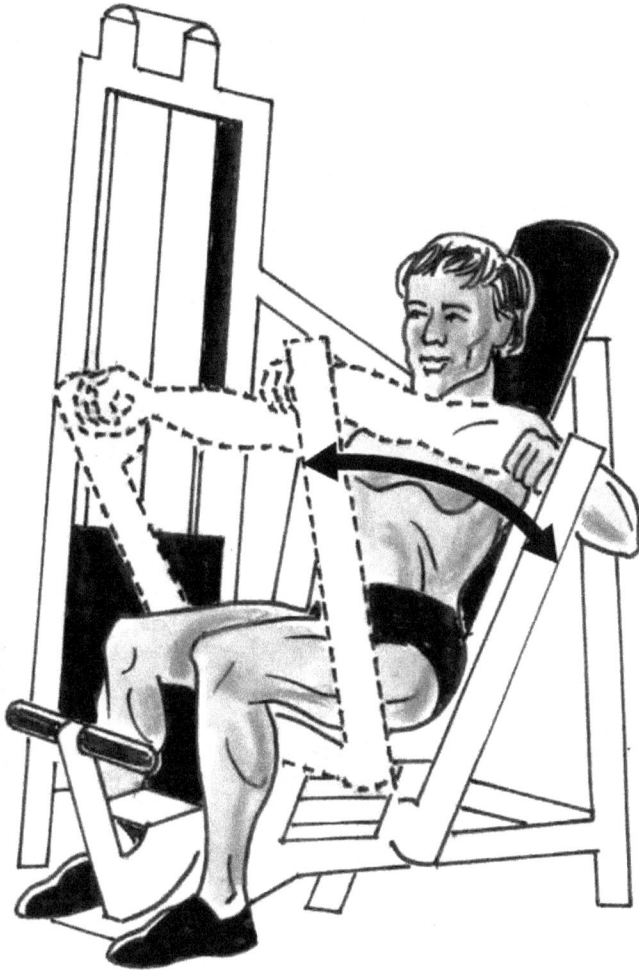

CHEST PRESS – Pectorals

- Sit on seat, feet flat on floor.
- Hold hand grips about 6" wider than shoulder width.
- Fully extend resistance in front of body.
- Return hand grips towards chest.
- Keep elbows out, chest high.
- Move resistance with complete control, making a definite pause at the chest.
- Keep back firm against support; do not arch too sharply.
- Do not raise hips off seat.
- Inhale in, exhale out.

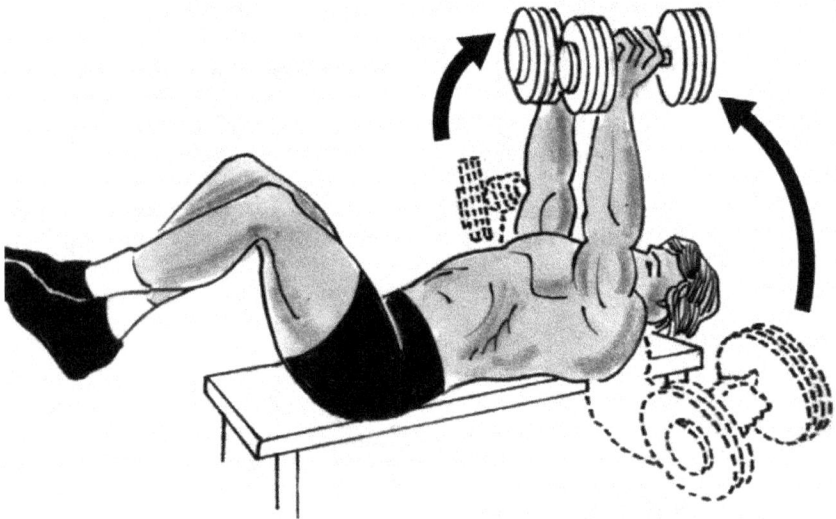

FLAT DUMBBELL FLY – Pectoralis Major

- Lie on bench.
- Hold dumbbells together at arm's length above shoulders, palms facing each other.
- Slowly lower dumbbells so they are even with chest and about 10" from each side.
- Keep elbows bent at bottom position and in line with ears.
- Angle forearms slightly out of vertical position.
- Return dumbbells to arm's length above shoulders using same path.
- Inhale down, exhale up.

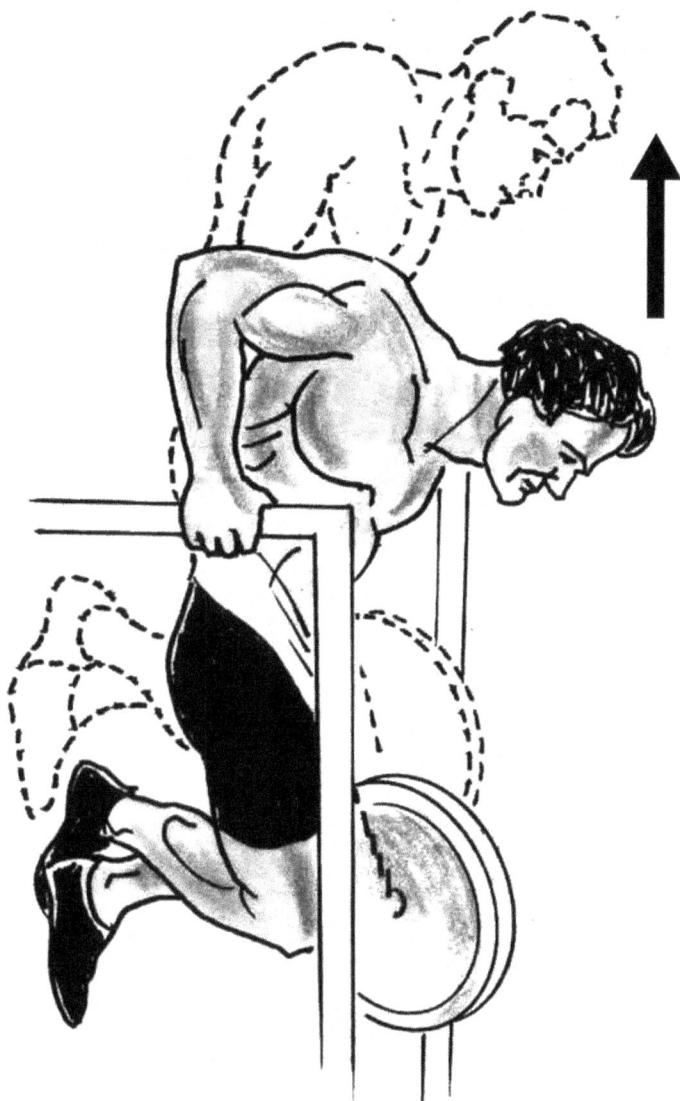

PARALLEL DIPS – Lower Pectorals

- Hold yourself erect on parallel bars.
- Keep elbows into sides, lower body by bending elbows.
- Lower down as far as you can comfortably go.
- Pause, then press back to arms length.
- Do not let body swing back and forth.
- Inhale down, exhale up.

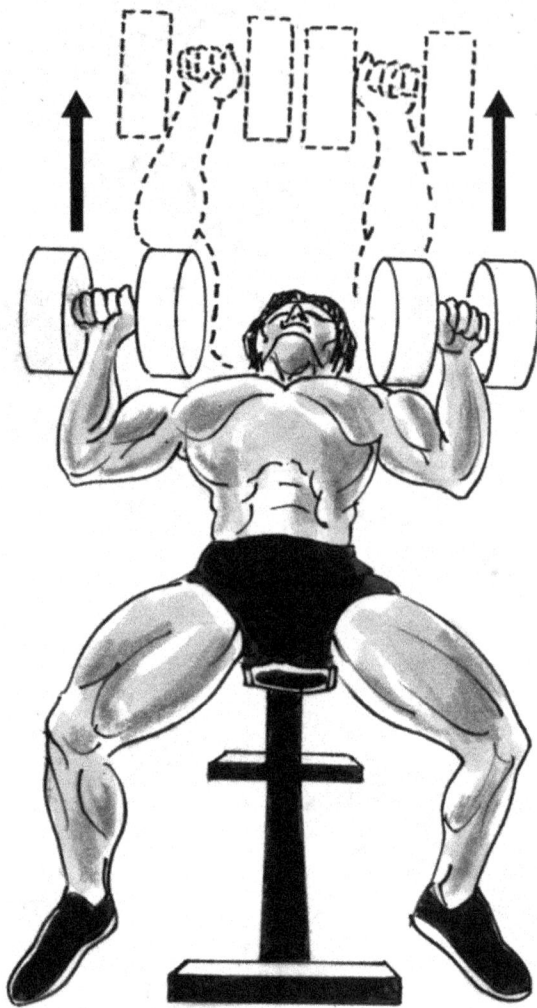

INCLINE DUMBBELL PRESS – Upper Pectorals

- Lie on incline bench.
- Hold dumbbells together at arm's length above shoulders, palms forward.
- Slowly lower dumbbells to sides of chest.
- Keep elbows in line with ears.
- Angle forearms slightly out of vertical position.
- Return to starting position using same path.
- Inhale down, exhale up.

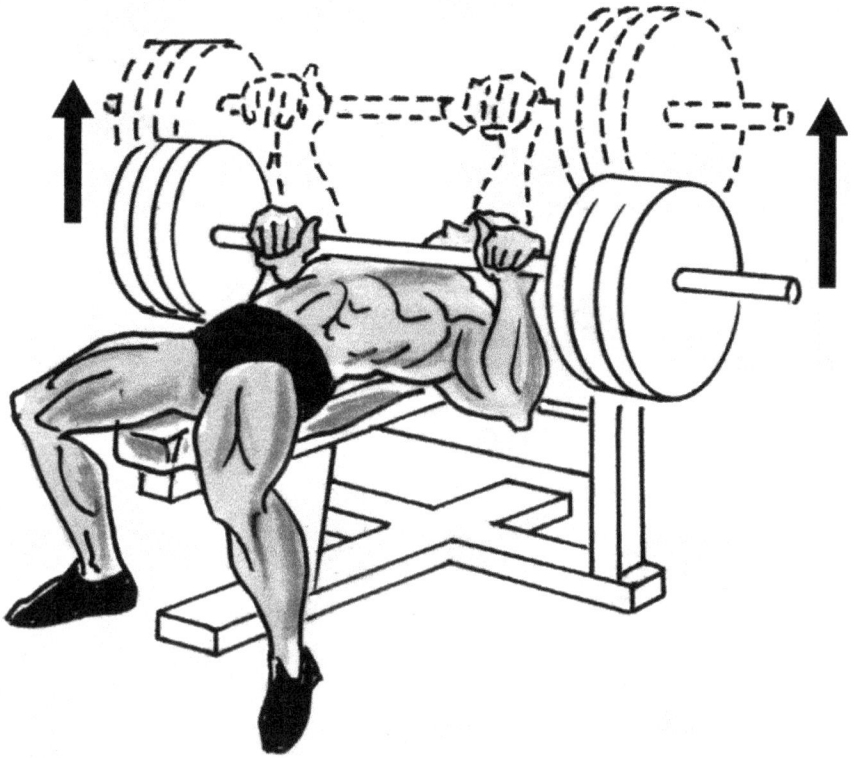

BARBELL BENCH PRESS – Pectorals

- Lie on bench with your feet flat on the floor.
- Raise barbell off weight-rack and hold over your chest with a grip that is about six inches wider than shoulder width.
- Lower barbell to lower portion of chest.
- Push the bar to arm's length.
- Keep your elbows out and your chest high.
- When lowering the weight maintain complete control and pause at your chest.
- Keep your head on the bench, and do not arch your back too sharply.
- Do not raise your hips off the bench.
- Inhale down, exhale up.

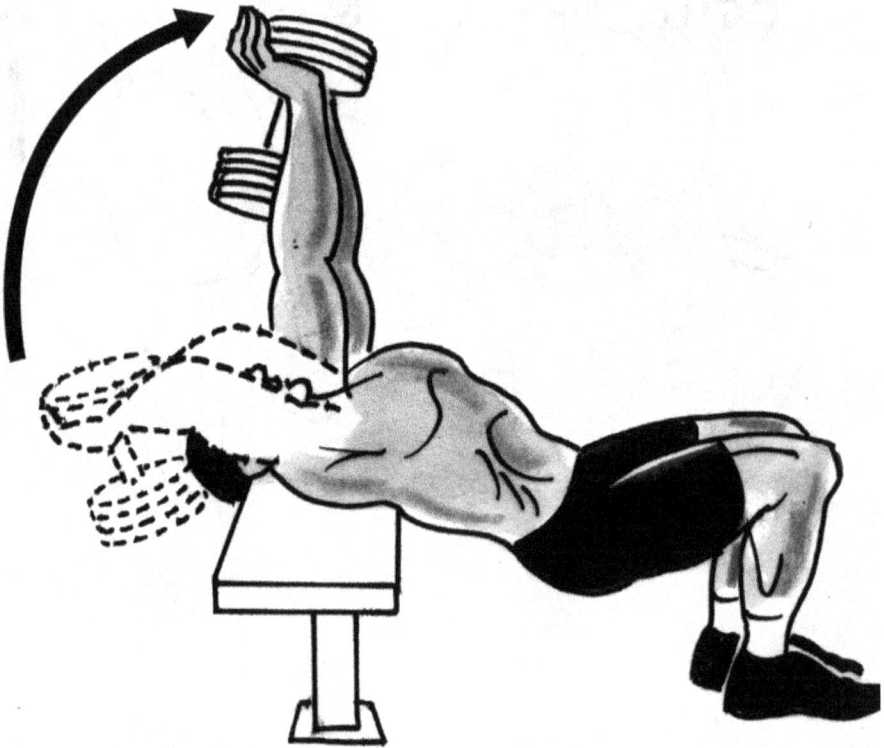

DUMBBELL PULLOVER – Pectorals, Serratus

- Lie across bench, upper back supporting torso.
- Place head off bench, hanging down.
- Keep body and legs nearly straight, drop hips to raise ribcage.
- Hold dumbbell, hands flat against inside weight-plate, at arm's length above chest.
- Keep head down and do not raise hips.
- Breathe deep and lower dumbbell in semicircular motion behind head as far as comfortable.
- Return to starting position, elbows locked.
- Inhale down, exhale up.

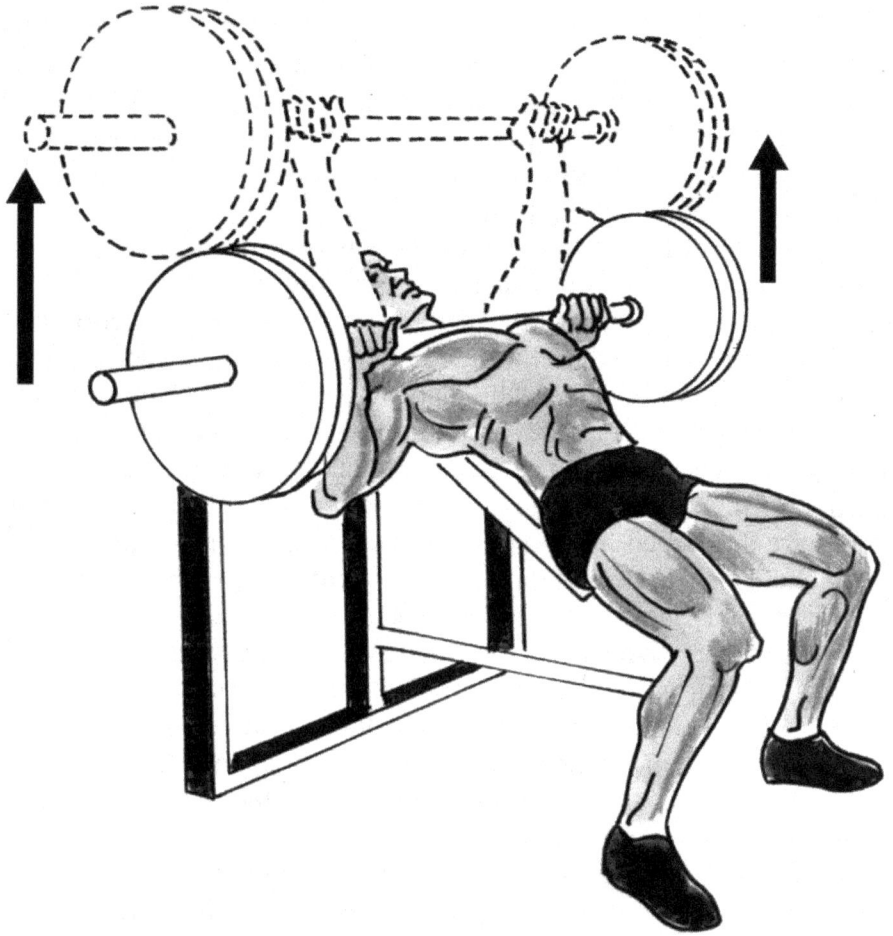

INCLINE BARBELL PRESS – Upper Pectorals

- Lie on incline bench, feet flat on floor.
- Hold barbell about 6" wider than shoulder width.
- Lower bar to upper chest.
- Raise bar to arm's length.
- Keep elbows out, chest high.
- Lower weight with complete control, pause for a moment at chest.
- Keep head on bench; do not arch back too sharply.
- Do not raise hips off bench.
- Inhale down, exhale up.

SHOULDERS

The deltoids are one of three muscle groups, along with the calves and abdominals, which help to create the appearance of a symmetrical physique. They are an important component to developing a winning physique since they are viewed from all angles. When training the deltoids it is important to develop all three heads proportionately. Let us look at the anatomy of this muscle group.

The deltoid region consists of the anterior, lateral, and posterior muscles. All three sections attach to the humerus. The anterior and lateral heads originate on the collarbone, while the posterior head originates on the scapula. The anterior deltoids are the muscles that are visible just to the outside of the upper pectorals. The lateral deltoids are located on the outside portion of the shoulder. The posterior deltoids are located on the back of the shoulder, near the bottom/outer portion of the upper trapezius muscle. When the lateral and posterior heads are developed proportionately, they can give the appearance of wide shoulders. If the anterior head is overdeveloped, it can give the appearance of narrow shoulders. Because the deltoids are exposed more often than most body parts, bodybuilders tend to give this muscle group plenty of work. The one problem that is constantly seen in the gyms is that the anterior deltoid is developed to a greater degree than either the lateral or the posterior portion of the deltoid. This is caused in great part from the direct stimulation the anterior deltoid receives from the chest pressing movements. Therefore, it is imperative that bodybuilders study their deltoids in a mirror and in photos to see how well this muscle group is balanced. If one of the three heads is not proportioned to the others, the overall shoulder group will look lopsided and take away from the physique's symmetrical balance.

The shoulder's deep rotator cuff muscles connect from various parts of the thoracic region to either the front, side, or rear of the humerus. The function of the rotator cuff is to help stabilize the arm during movements and to rotate the arm in or out. The function of the deltoid muscle is to move the arm away from the body. Each section of the shoulder girdle has individual functions. The anterior deltoid brings your arm forward and inwards. The lateral deltoid brings your arm out to the side. The posterior deltoid brings your arm back and helps to rotate it out.

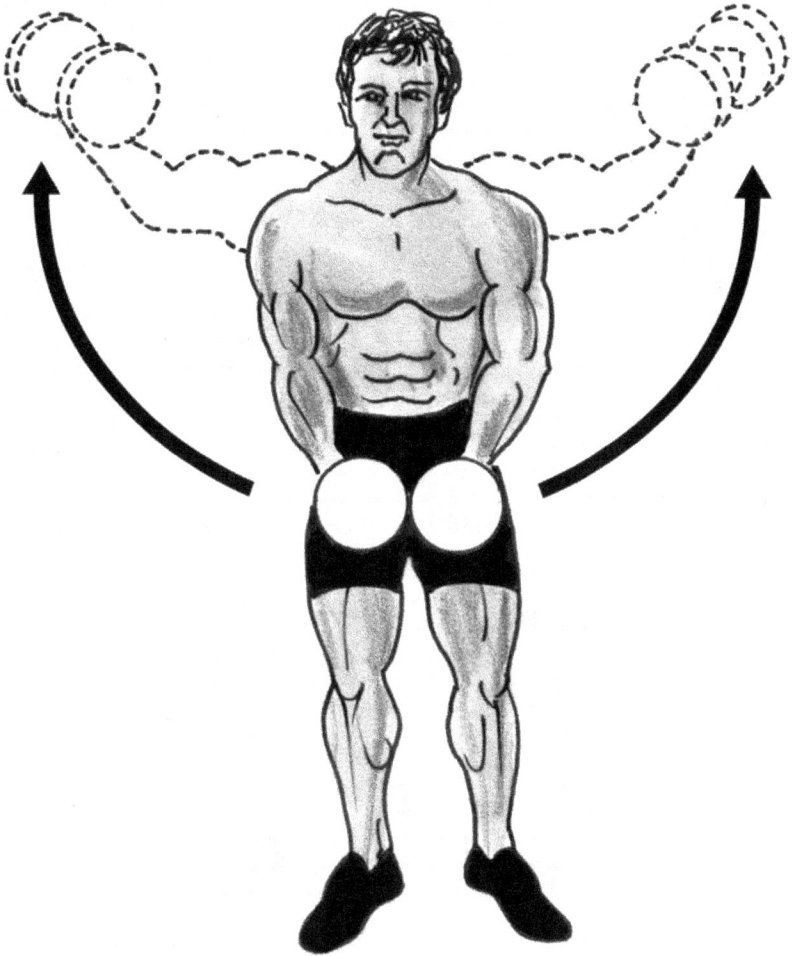

STANDING SIDE LATERAL – Lateral Deltoids

- Stand with your feet firmly on the floor, about 16" apart, and a dumbbell in each hand, with your hands hanging down at your sides and your palms facing your thighs.
- Inhale and maintain a slight bend in your elbows as you exhale and raise the dumbbells outwards in a semicircular motion until they are slightly above shoulder level.
- Pause at top and then inhale as you lower the dumbbells to the starting position.
- Return the dumbbell to the starting position.

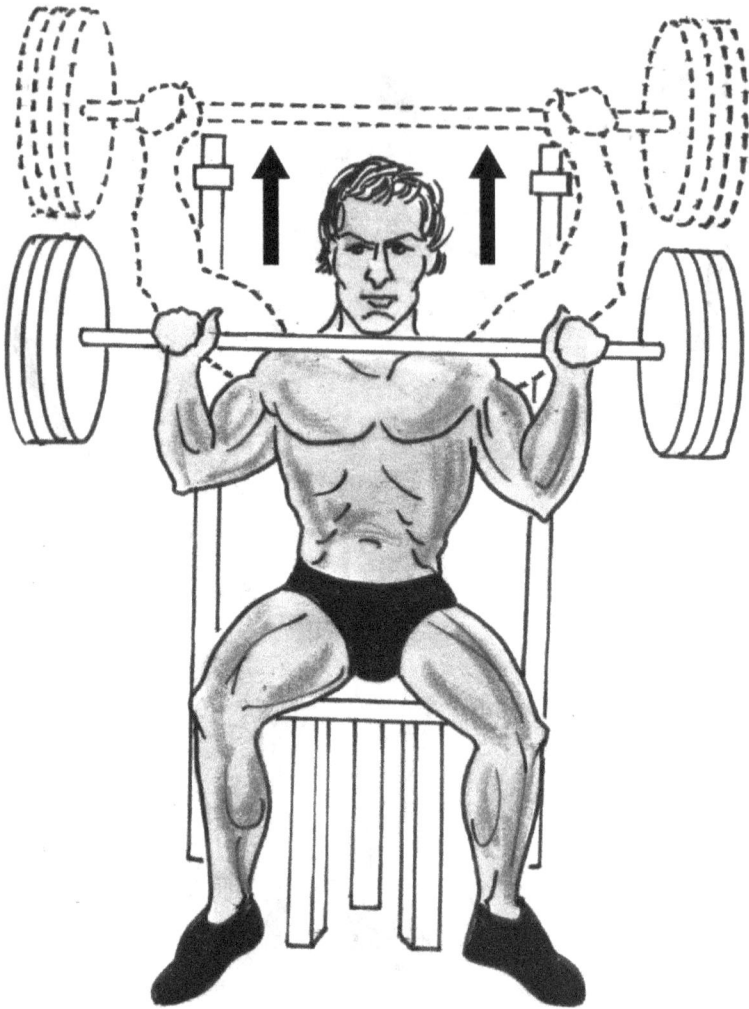

SHOULDER PRESS – Anterior Deltoid

- Hold barbell on upper chest, hands slightly wider than shoulder width.
- Sit on bench with feet firmly on floor and hips solid.
- Keep elbows in, slightly under bar.
- Press bar to arm's length overhead.
- Lower bar to upper chest.
- Be sure bar rests on chest and is not supported by arms between reps.
- Hold chest high.
- Inhale down, exhale up.

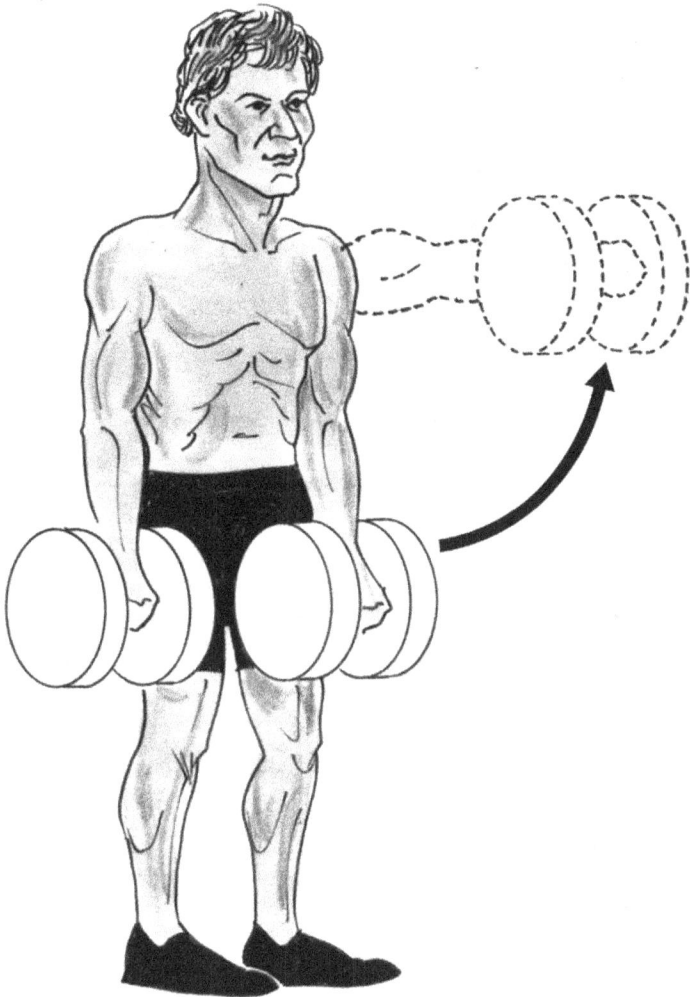

ALTERNATE FRONT DUMBBELL RAISE – Anterior Deltoids

- Hold dumbbells in front of thighs with palms facing body.
- Stand with your feet firmly on floor and have the legs and hips in a flexed position to help keep your back straight.
- With the dumbbells hanging at arm's length, raise right dumbbell forward in a semicircular motion until it is just above parallel with your shoulders.
- Lower to starting position and raise left dumbbell in same manner.
- Inhale while lowering dumbbells to thighs.
- Do not unlock your elbows during movement.

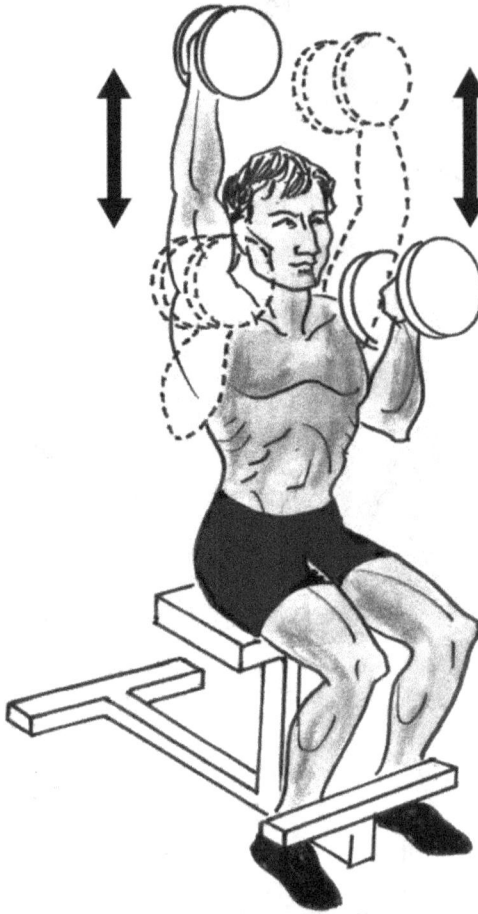

ALTERNATE DUMBBELL PRESS – Anterior, Lateral Deltoids

- Sit at end of bench, feet firmly on floor.
- Raise dumbbells to shoulder height.
- Press one dumbbell straight up to arm's length, palm facing in.
- Lower dumbbell to starting position and press other dumbbell up.
- Keep body rigid.
- Perform all work with shoulders and arms.
- Do not lean from side to side.
- Inhale down, exhale up.
- Can also be done with palms facing out.

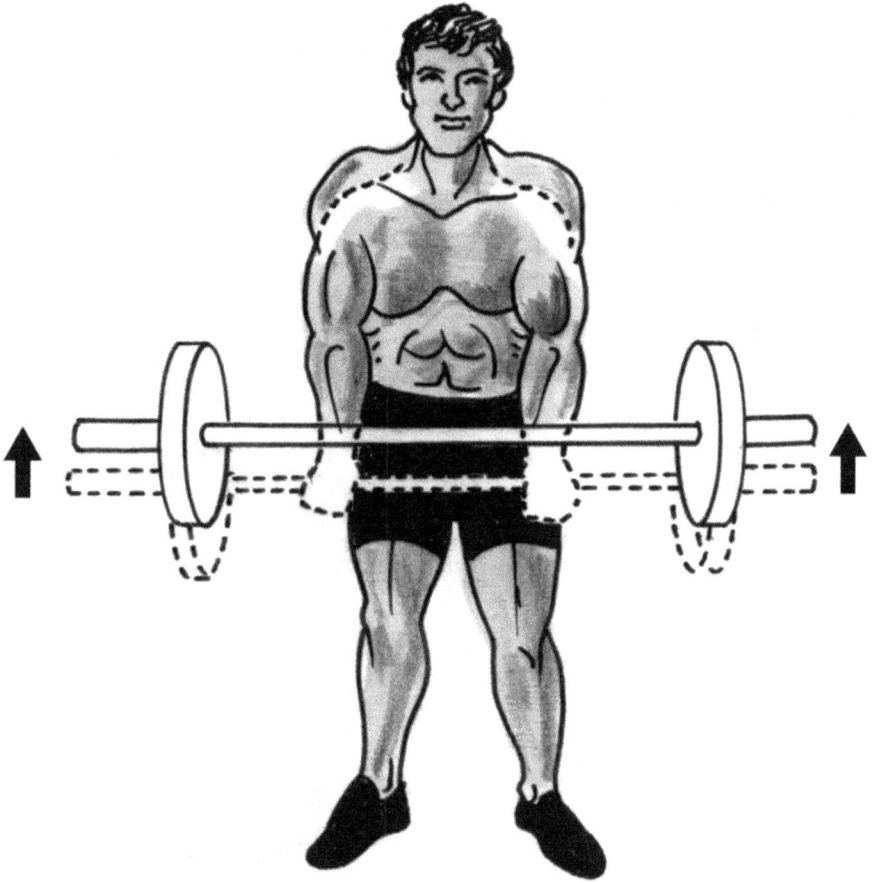

BARBELL SHRUG – Trapezius

- Hold barbell, palms down, hands shoulder width apart.
- Keep feet firmly on floor.
- Stand erect, bar hanging at arm's length.
- Lower shoulders as much as possible.
- Raise shoulders up as high as possible then return to starting position.
- Inhale at beginning, exhale at end of repetition.

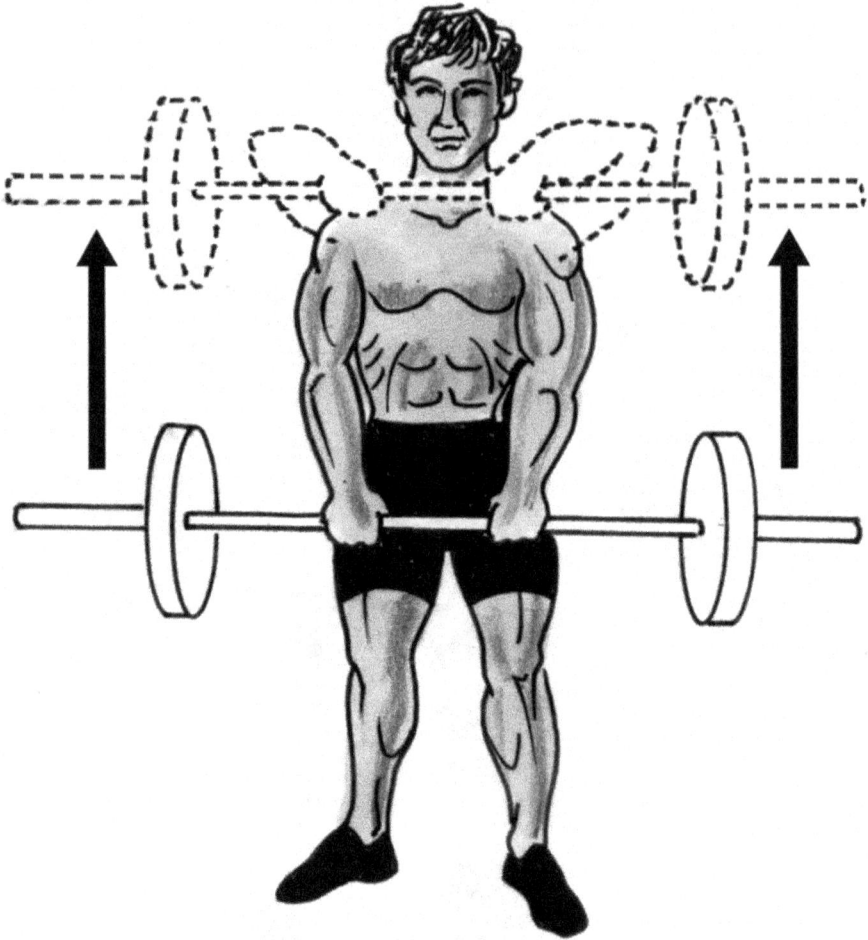

UPRIGHT ROW – Lateral Deltoids, Trapezius

- Grip barbell with your hands 6-8" apart.
- Pull the bar straight up until it nearly touches your chin.
- Allow your elbows to go out to the side and as high as your ears on the upward movement.
- Pause shortly at the top before you lower the bar back to the starting position.
- Concentrate on your deltoids as you raise and lower the weight.
- Inhale up, exhale down.

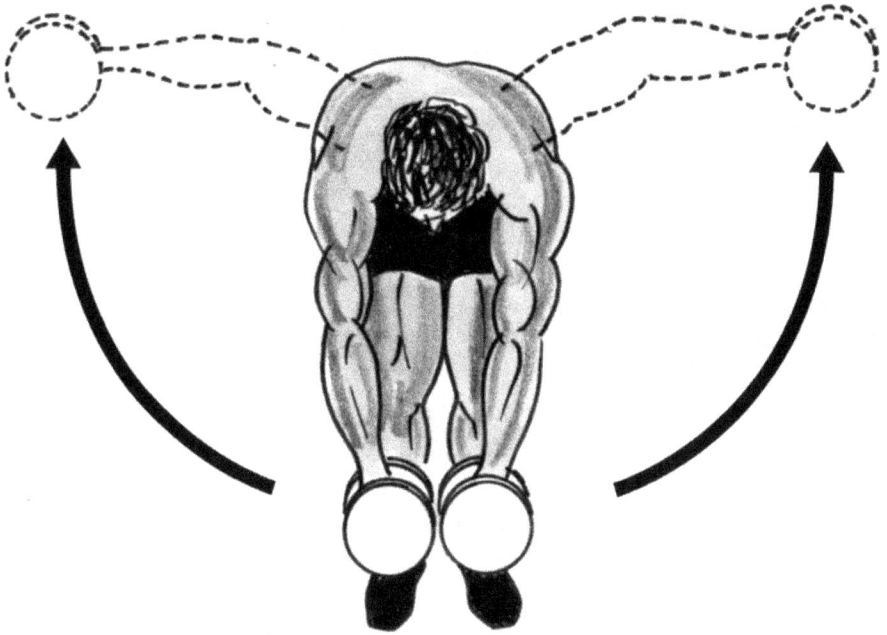

BENT-OVER LATERAL RAISE – Posterior Deltoids

- Hold dumbbells with palms in.
- Feet firmly on floor, back straight.
- Bend forward until chest is nearly parallel to floor.
- Hang dumbbells, elbows slightly unlocked.
- Raise dumbbells outwards in a semicircular motion until parallel to floor, even with ears, and with pinky finger high.
- Lower in same path.
- Inhale up, exhale down.

ARMS

Biceps

When someone asks you to flex your muscles, they are referring to your biceps. The biceps have become universally symbolic for muscles. They are the first body part most bodybuilders ever focus on. The biceps receive a lot of indirect stimulation when we train our backs and only require a limited amount of work to reach their fullest potential. The biceps brachii is a round, two-headed muscle located on the front of the upper arm. It originates at the scapula, attaching itself to the forearm bone called the radius. The primary function of the bicep muscle is to move the forearm towards the shoulder. This is called elbow flexion. A secondary function of the biceps is supination of the forearm. Curling and pulling movements are performed with the help of the bicep muscle.

Triceps

This muscle accounts for most of our upper arm mass. The triceps brachii has three heads, which connect the humerus and scapula to the forearm bone (ulna). These heads are known as the lateral, medial, and long heads. The lateral head has a horseshoe shape and is located on the outward facing side of the humerus. The medial head is located towards the midline of the body. The longhead is the largest head and is located along the bottom side of the humerus. The triceps function is to allow the forearm to extend from a bent position to a straight position. Pressing and pushing movements are performed with the help of the triceps.

Forearms

Given their composition, the muscles of the forearm are very complex and respond best to exercises that allow for a full contraction. The upper part of the muscle consists of the brachioradialis and the extensor carpi radialis. The brachioradialis is the thick cord-like muscle that is best viewed when the forearm is fully extended. These muscles travel the outside length of the forearm and are best developed with reverse curl type movements. The muscles located on the bottom of the forearm are the flexor muscles. The flexors travel the length of the inner forearm and are the most notable forearm muscles in terms of size conveyance. Wrist curling movements (palms up) best develop this body part.

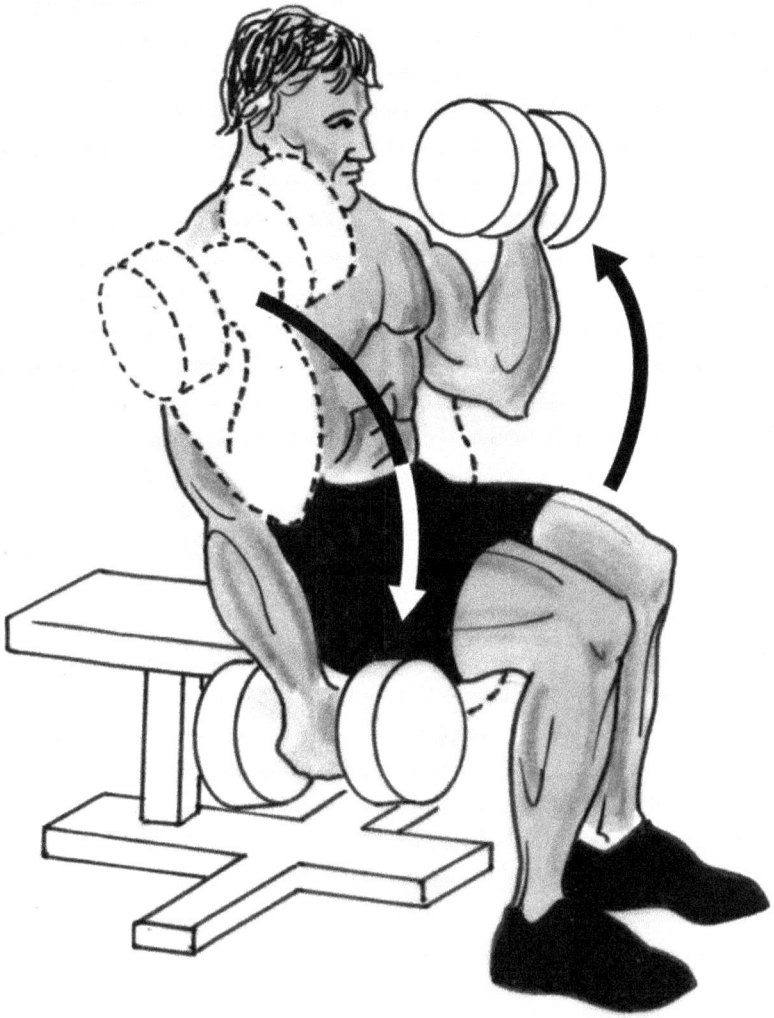

SEATED DUMBBELL CURL – Biceps

- Hold dumbbells.
- Sit on bench, feet firmly on floor, close together.
- Start with dumbbells at arm's length, palms in.
- Begin curl with palms facing in until past upper thighs, then turn palms up for remainder of curl to shoulder height.
- Keep palms up while lowering until past upper thighs, then turn palms in.
- Keep upper arms close to sides.
- Inhale down, exhale up.

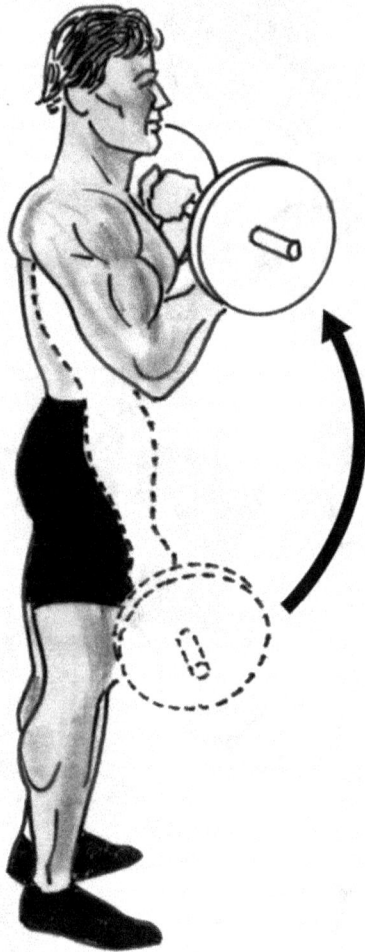

BARBELL CURL – Biceps

- Hold barbell with both hands, palms up, shoulder width apart.
- Stand erect, back straight, head up, feet firmly on floor.
- Start with bar at arm's length against upper thighs.
- Curl bar up in semicircular motion until forearms touch biceps.
- Keep upper arms close to sides.
- Lower to starting position using same path.
- Do not swing back and forth to help lift bar.
- Inhale down, exhale up.

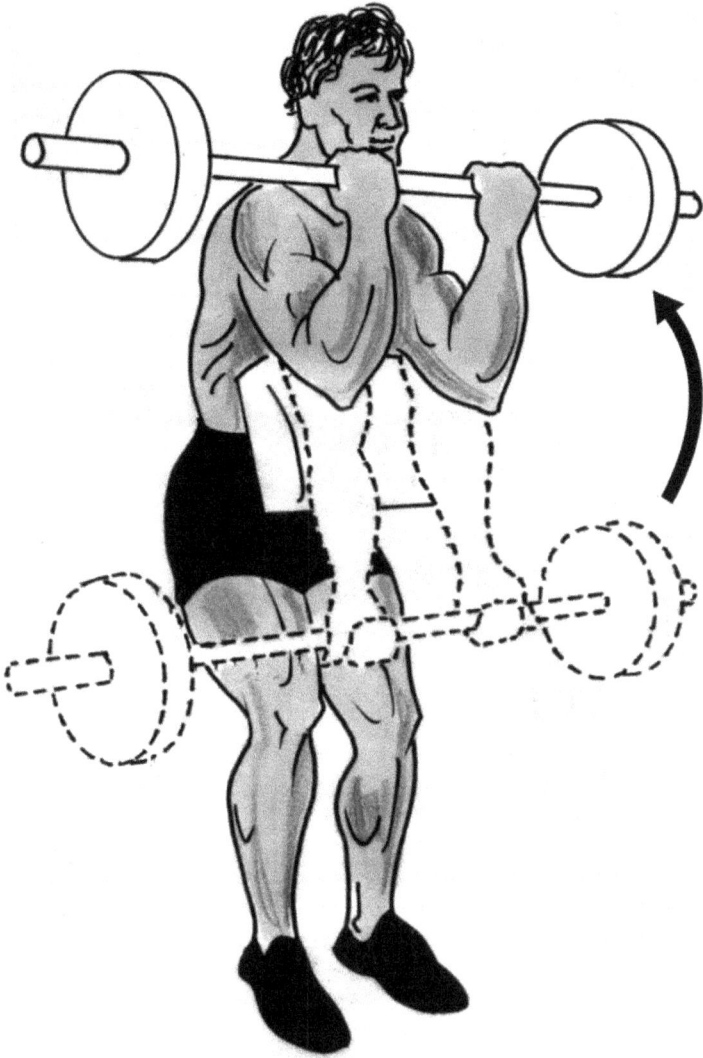

BARBELL SCOTT CURL – Biceps

- Hold barbell with palms up.
- Sit on bench, arms resting on angled support.
- Curl barbell up in semicircular motion until forearms touch biceps.
- Keep elbows inward.
- Return to starting position using same path.
- Inhale down, exhale up.

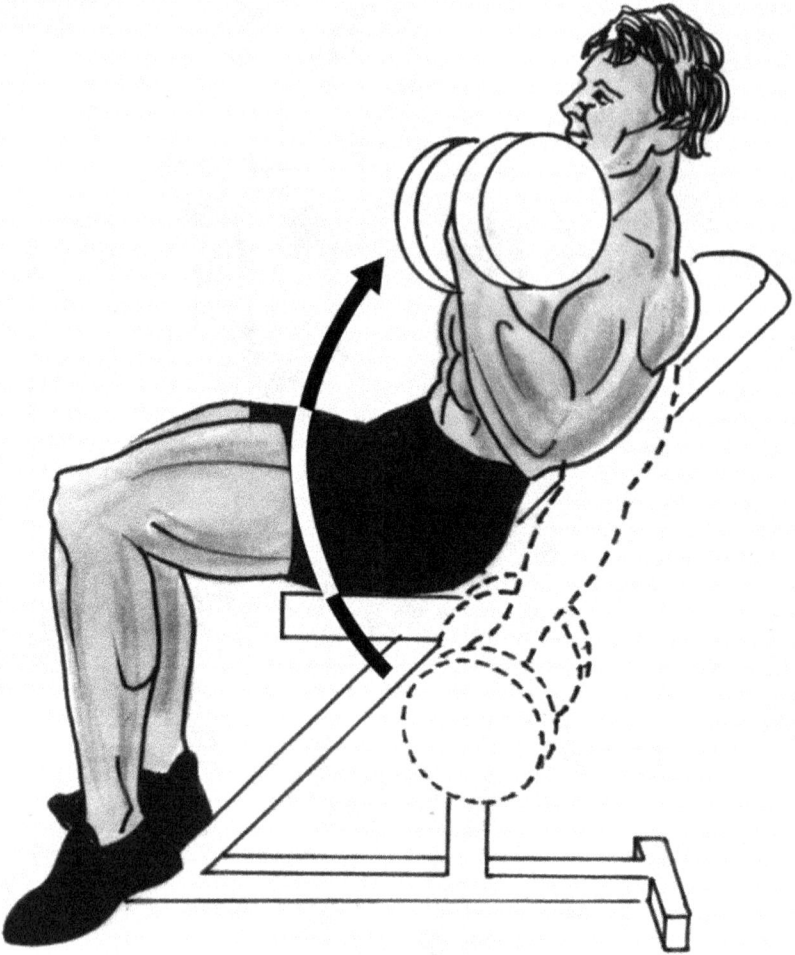

INCLINE DUMBBELL CURL – Biceps

- Hold dumbbells.
- Lie back on incline bench.
- Start with dumbbells at arm's length, palms in.
- Begin curl with palms in until past upper thighs and then turn palms up for remainder of curl to shoulder height.
- Keep palms up while lowering until past upper thighs, then turn palms in.
- Keep upper arms close to sides.
- Inhale down, exhale up.

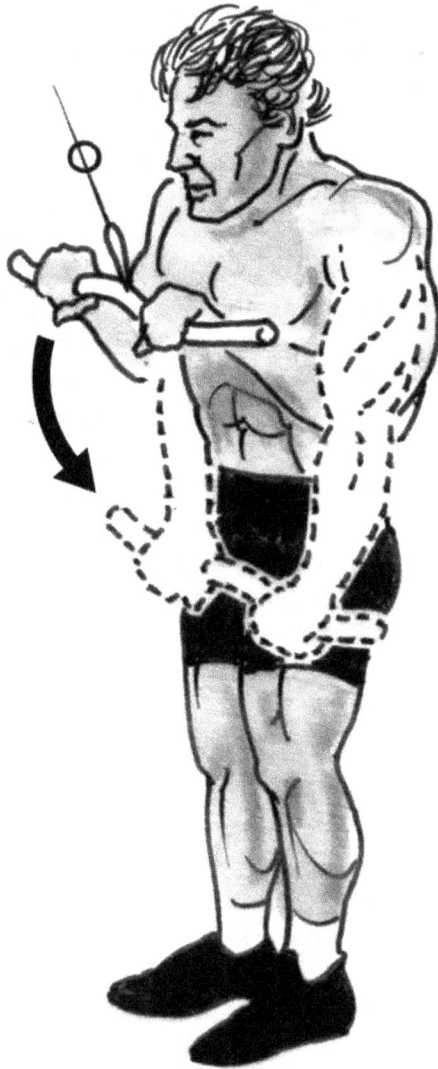

TRICEPS PUSH-DOWN – Triceps

- Stand erect, head up, feet firmly on floor.
- Hold bar with hands 8" apart, palms down.
- Bring upper arms to sides and keep them there.
- Start with forearms and biceps touching.
- Push bar down in semicircular motion to arm's length.
- Return to starting position.
- Inhale up, exhale down.
- Can also be done with reverse grip.

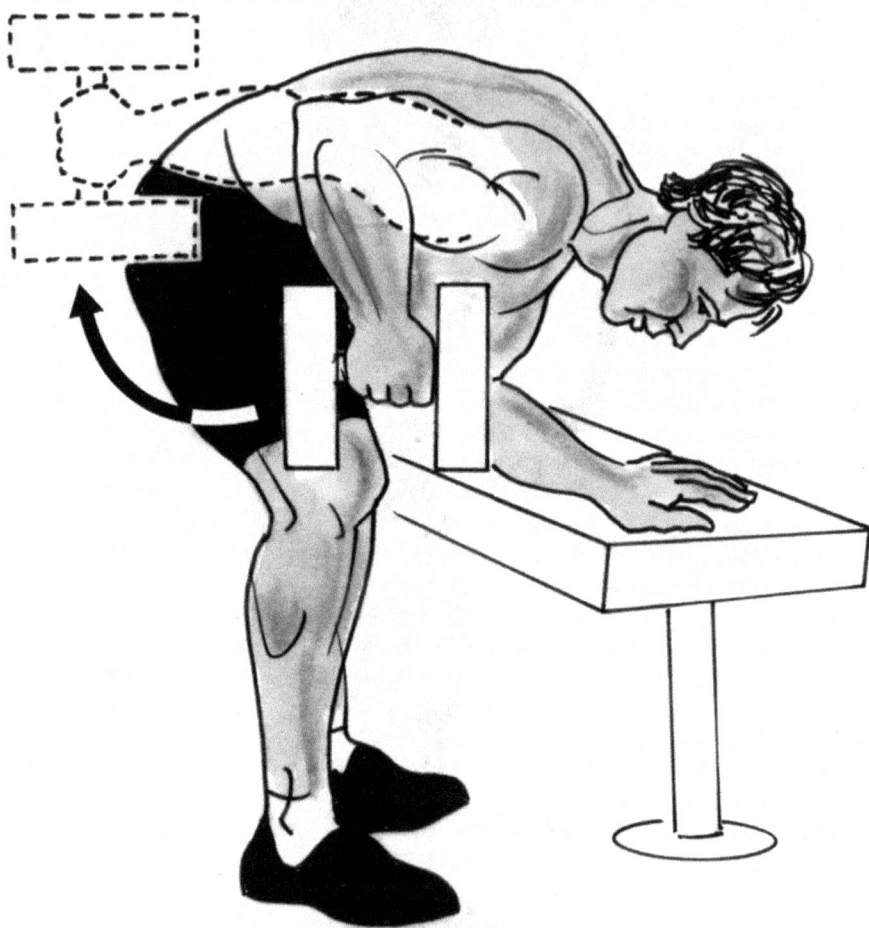

DUMBBELL TRICEPS KICKBACK – Triceps

- Hold a dumbbell in right hand, palm in.
- Bend over until upper body is parallel to floor.
- Place left hand on bench, right leg back.
- Place right upper arm at side while keeping lower arm vertical.
- Extend dumbbell backwards in semicircular motion until entire arm is parallel to floor.
- Briefly hold dumbbell at top of movement.
- Lower slowly to starting position.
- Inhale down, exhale up.
- Repeat with opposite arm.

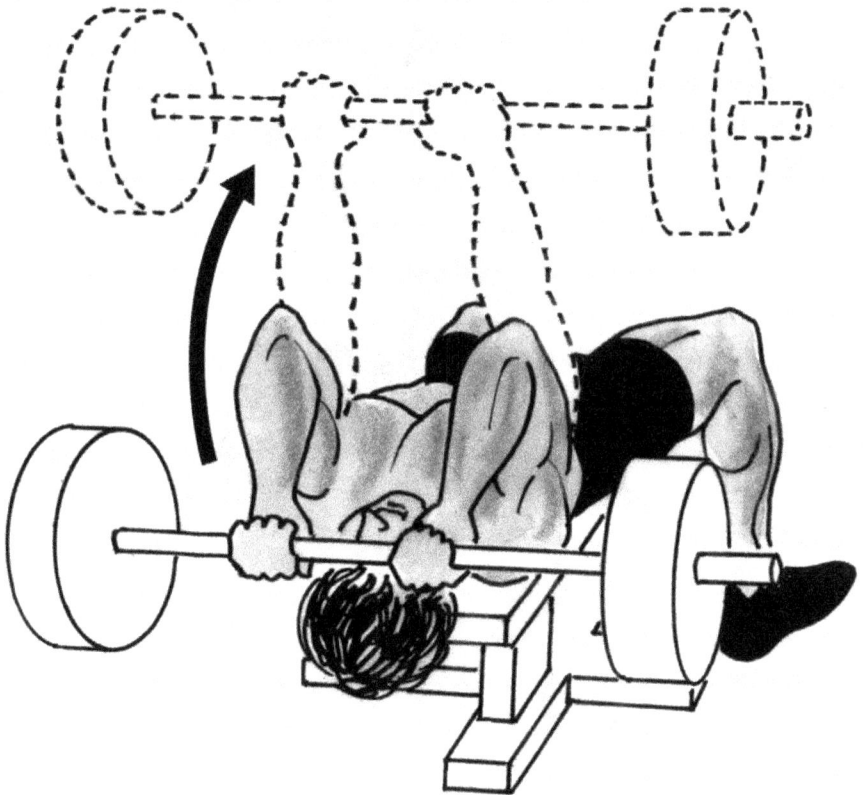

LYING TRICEPS EXTENSION – Medial Head of the Triceps

- Lie on flat bench, barbell over your head, hands about 8" apart.
- Head should be slightly hanging off bench.
- Elbows should be locked and palms facing upward.
- Slowly lower barbell by bending arms at the elbow joint.
- Bar should lower behind head, do not hit skull.
- Extend barbell back up into locked position overhead.
- Inhale down, exhale up.

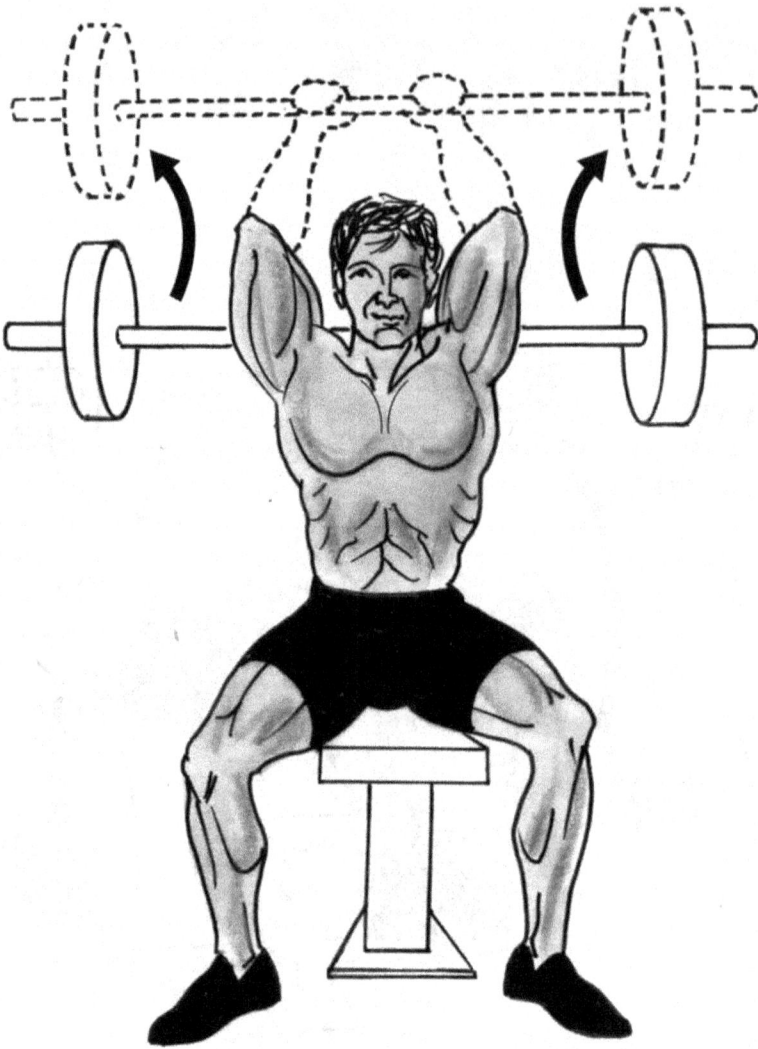

OVERHEAD TRICEPS EXTENSION – Long Head of the Triceps

- Hold barbell with hands about 8" apart.
- Raise overhead to arm's length.
- Sit erect, head up, feet firmly on floor.
- Keep upper arms close to head, elbows facing upward.
- Lower barbell in semicircular motion behind head until forearms touch biceps.
- Return to starting position.
- Inhale down, exhale up.

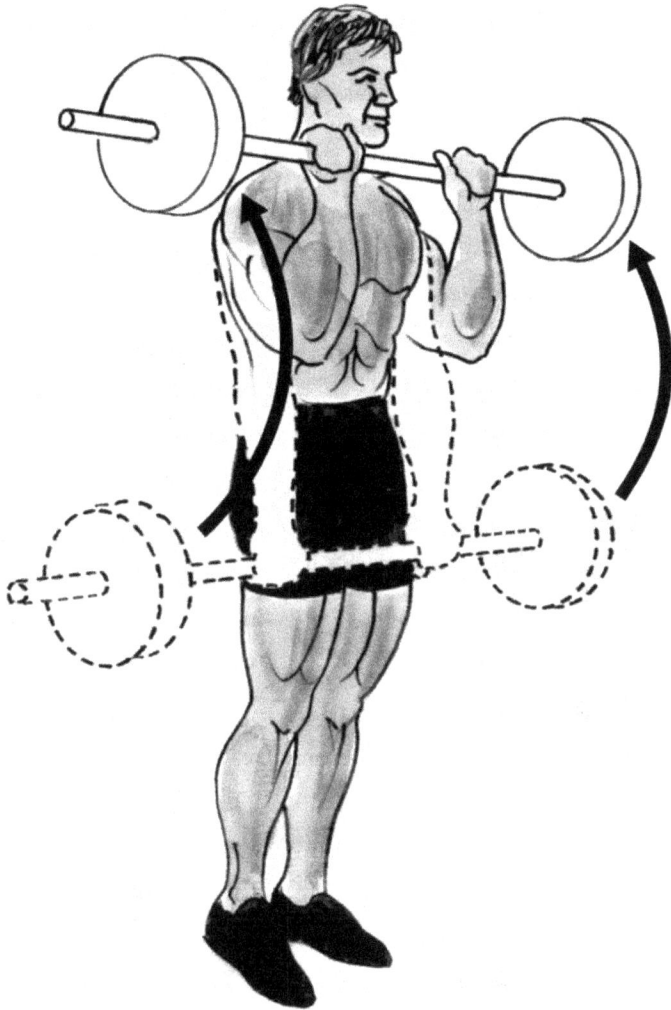

REVERSE BARBELL CURL – Brachialis, Extensor Muscles

- Hold barbell with both hands, palms down, 18" apart.
- Stand erect, back straight, head up, feet firmly on floor.
- Start with bar at arm's length against upper thighs.
- Curl bar up in semicircular motion until upper forearms touch biceps.
- Keep upper arms close to sides.
- Lower to starting position using same path.
- Do not swing body back and forth to help lift bar.
- Inhale down, exhale up.

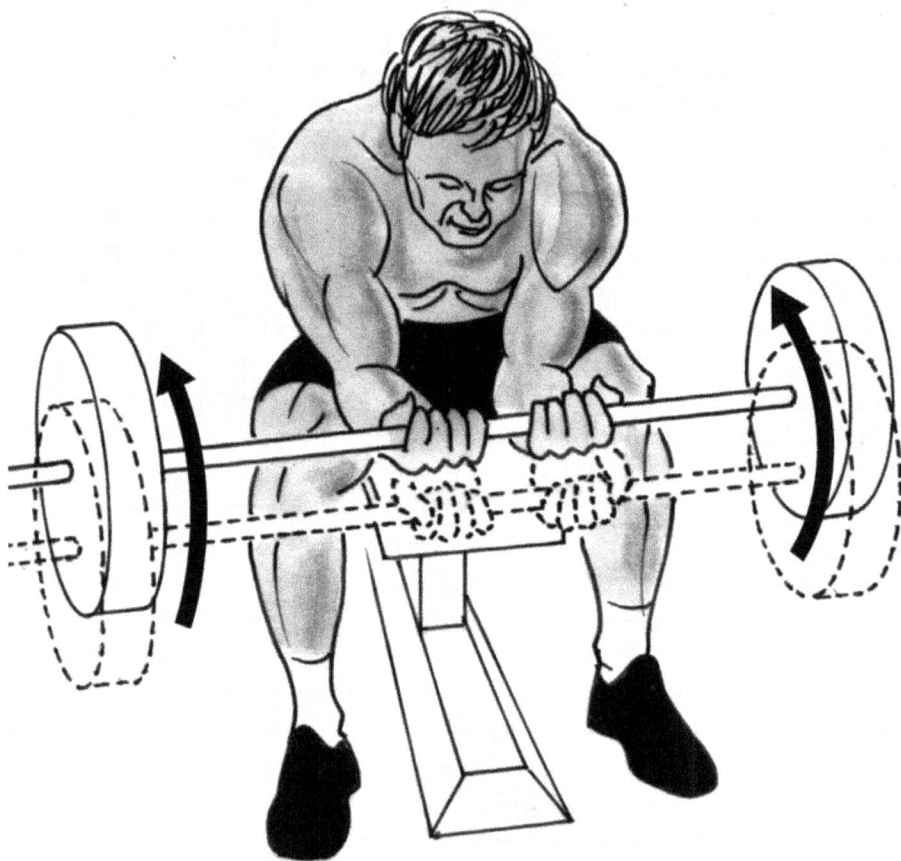

WRIST CURL – Flexor Muscles of Forearms

- Hold barbell with both hands, palms up, hands 16" apart.
- Sit at end of bench, feet firmly on floor.
- Lean forward, place forearms on bench or upper thighs.
- Let wrists hang over bench or knees.
- Lower bar as far as possible, keeping tight grip.
- Curl bar as high as possible.
- Do not let forearms rise up.
- Inhale up, exhale down.

ABDOMINALS

One muscle group that competitive bodybuilders can be seen training hard in the gym is the abdominals. Located in the center of the body, the abdominals are the first area to be noticed on a physique stage or at the beach, and along with calves and deltoids, are vital to creating a symmetrical physique. While attaining prize-winning definition requires dieting, it is first the development of these muscles, through direct exercises, that will create that rugged six-pack look. To better understand this let us look at the anatomy of the abdominals.

The abdominal group consists of several muscles, the rectus abdominus, transverse abdominus, external oblique, and the internal oblique. These muscles are located on the front and sides of the lower half of the torso. They originate along the ribcage and attach along the pelvis. The abdominals help to provide postural support as each muscle has its own specific function. The rectus abdominus flexes the spine as it brings the ribcage closer to the pelvis; an example of this motion is the Abdominal Crunch. When the movement is reversed, the rectus abdominus brings the pelvis closer to the ribcage; an example of this motion is the Vertical Leg Raise. The rectus abdominus is also what gives us that six-pack effect. There are varying degrees of deepness within the abdominal region. The transversus abdominus is the deepest layer, as it wraps laterally around the abdominal area and acts as a support to keep your insides secure by keeping them firm and strong while providing postural stability. Both the internal oblique and external oblique help to stabilize the abdomen area by allowing for angled movement as well as helping with torso rotation and lateral flexion of the spine. To develop the abdominal muscles completely, you must train all areas of its region thoroughly and consistently.

The flexion of the hip is an important factor that relies on two main iliopsoas muscles, which are the iliacus and the psoas major. The iliacus originates on the pelvic crest and attaches to the femur. The psoas major, which is the longer of the two muscles, originates on the lumbar vertebrae and attaches to the femur. The function of the iliopsoas is hip flexion, which means bringing the thigh up towards the abdomen, ex, Knee Pull-In. The hip flexors are also active when the abdomen is being moved towards the thighs, ex; Incline Bent-Knee Sit-Up.

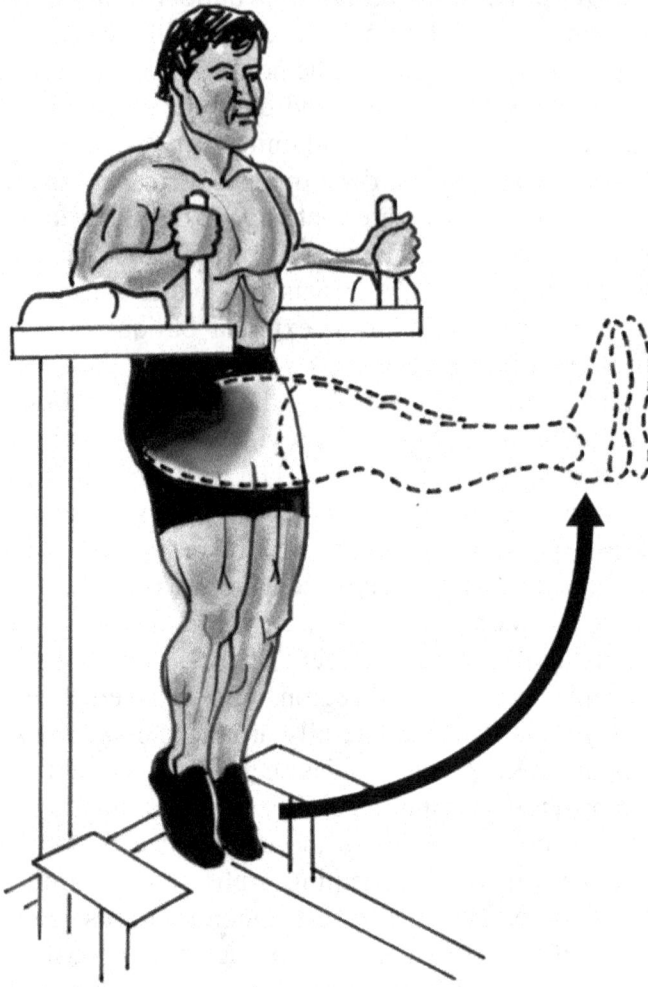

VERTICAL LEG RAISE – Rectus Abdominus

- Grasp the handles of the leg raise apparatus to support your body.
- Elbows resting on pads, legs locked.
- Hang your legs straight down.
- Raise legs until parallel to floor.
- Keep knees locked.
- Return to starting position.
- Inhale down, exhale up.

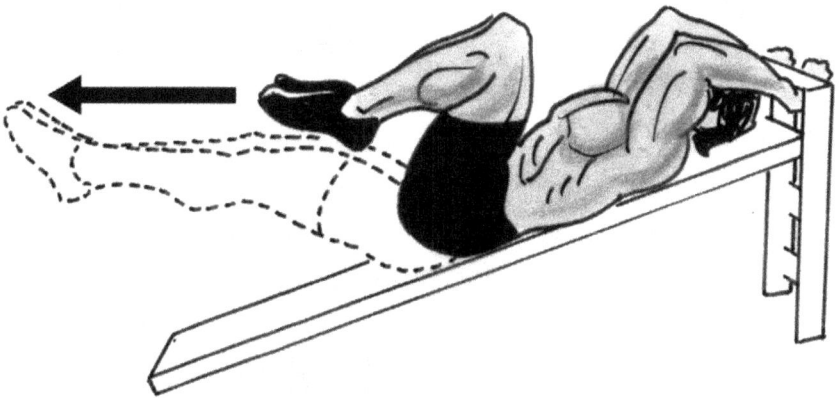

INCLINE KNEE PULL-IN – Rectus Abdominus, Iliopsoas

- Place incline board at desired angle.
- Lie with head at top of board.
- Hold bar behind head.
- Bend knees, pulling upper thighs into midsection.
- Return to starting position.
- Do not let feet touch board once exercise has started.
- Concentrate on lower abdominals.
- Inhale down, exhale up.

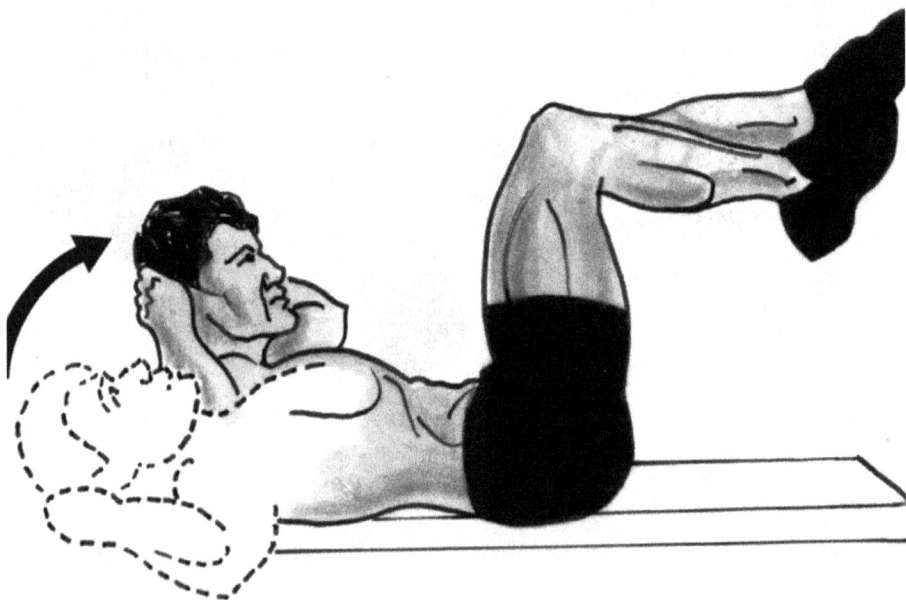

ABDOMINAL CRUNCH – Rectus Abdominus

- Lie on bench on your back.
- Raise feet off bench, knees bent.
- Place hands behind head.
- Pull torso up as far as possible.
- Return to starting position.
- Inhale down, exhale up.

394

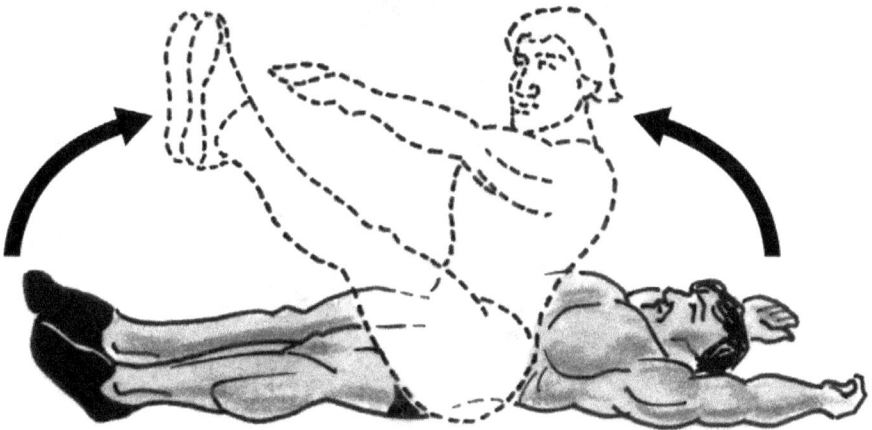

LEG AND BODY RAISE – Rectus Abdominus

- Lie on your back, using a bench or floor for support.
- Place arms straight back behind head.
- Bend at waist while raising legs and arms so both upper and lower limbs meet.
- Lower arms and legs to starting position.
- Inhale down, exhale up.
- Keep elbows and knees locked.

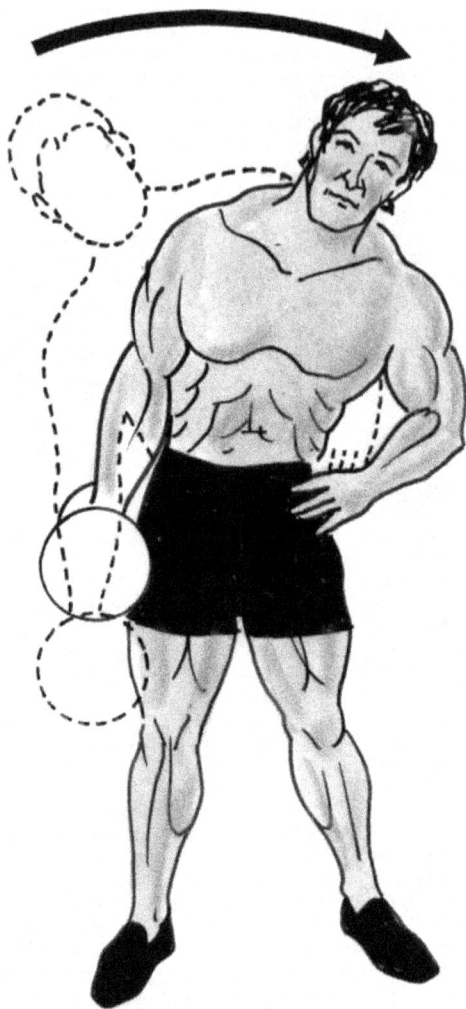

DUMBBELL SIDE BEND – Obliques

- Stand erect, feet 18" apart.
- Hold a dumbbell in your right hand, palm in.
- Place left hand on waist.
- Keep back straight.
- Bend to right as far as comfortable and then bend to left as far as comfortable.
- Place dumbbell in opposite hand and repeat movement.
- Bend at waist only, not at hips or knees.
- Inhale while bending, exhale on return.

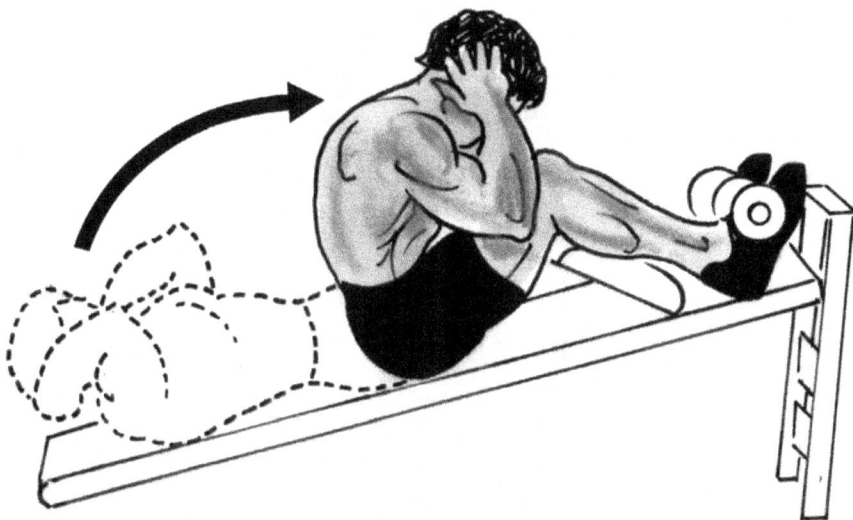

INCLINE BENT-KNEE SIT-UP – Rectus Abdominus

- With the sit-up board set at desired angle, hook your feet under foot support.
- Place hands on sides of head.
- Lower your upper body until your back touches the board then return to the starting position.
- Keep your knees bent throughout the exercise.
- Inhale down, exhale up.

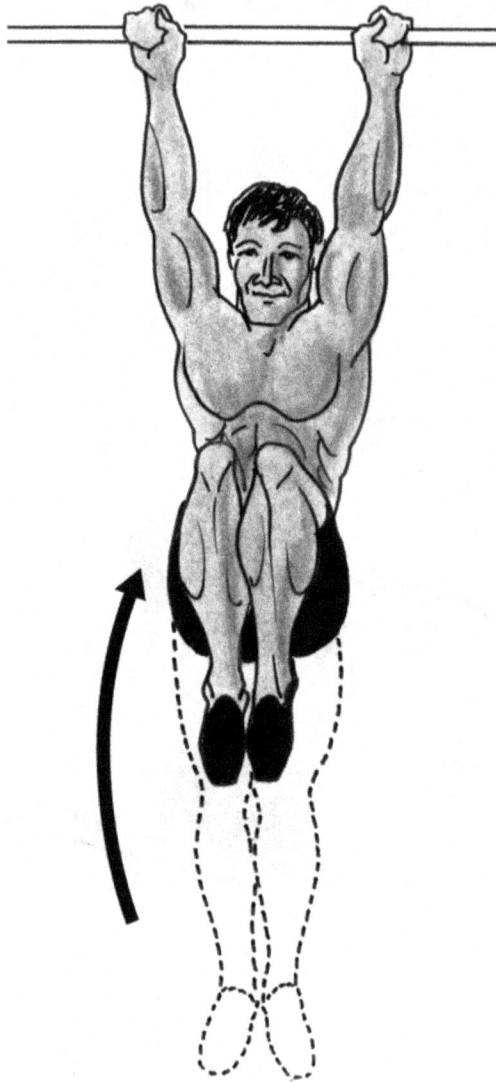

HANGING KNEE PULL-UP – Rectus Abdominus, Iliopsoas

- Grip high bar and hang, legs straight.
- While hanging pull your knees towards your chest.
- Do not sway upper body.
- Slowly lower legs to starting position.
- Inhale down, exhale up.

Please consult with your physician before starting any of the exercise or nutritional programs within this book. Have your physician give you a complete medical checkup and seek his or her advice on following any such prescribed fitness orientated programs, especially if you are overweight, have not exercised for a while, have had any health problems, or if there is any history of health problems. I also recommend that you visit your physician on a regular basis and report any problems that may occur.

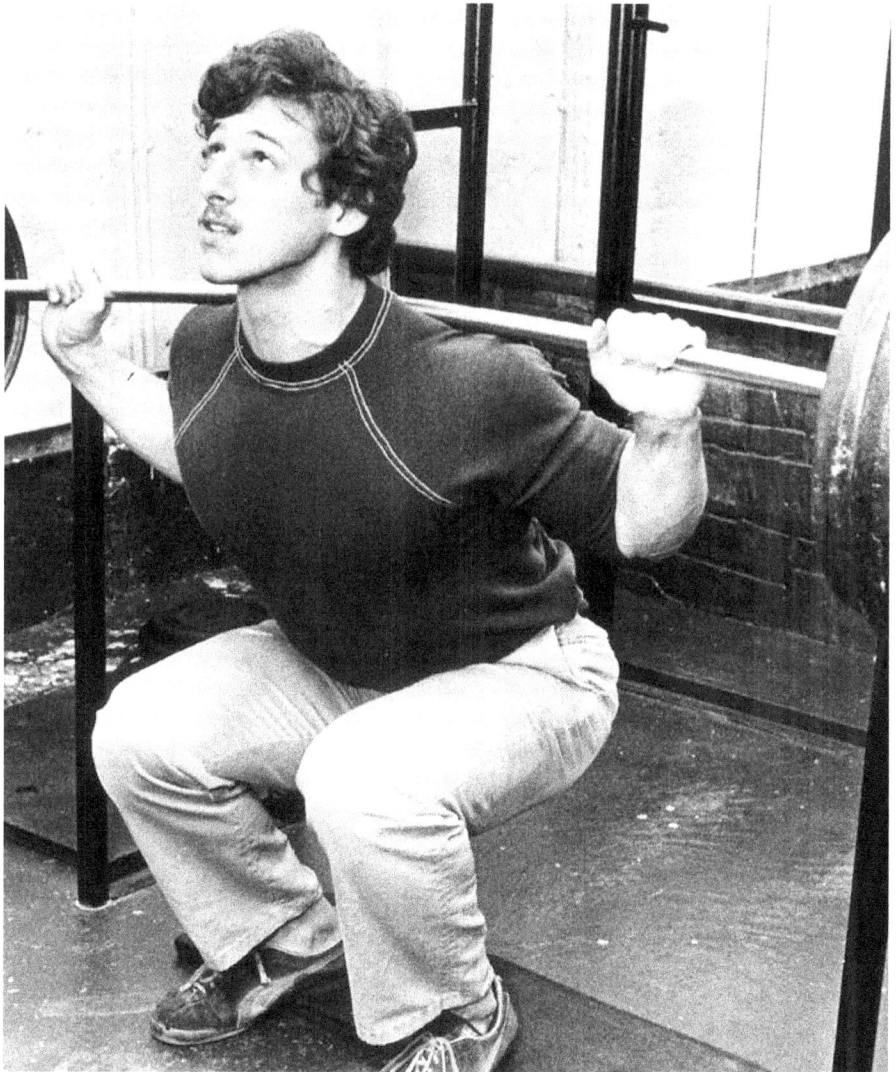

Weight training exercises are the tools we use to increase mass and strength

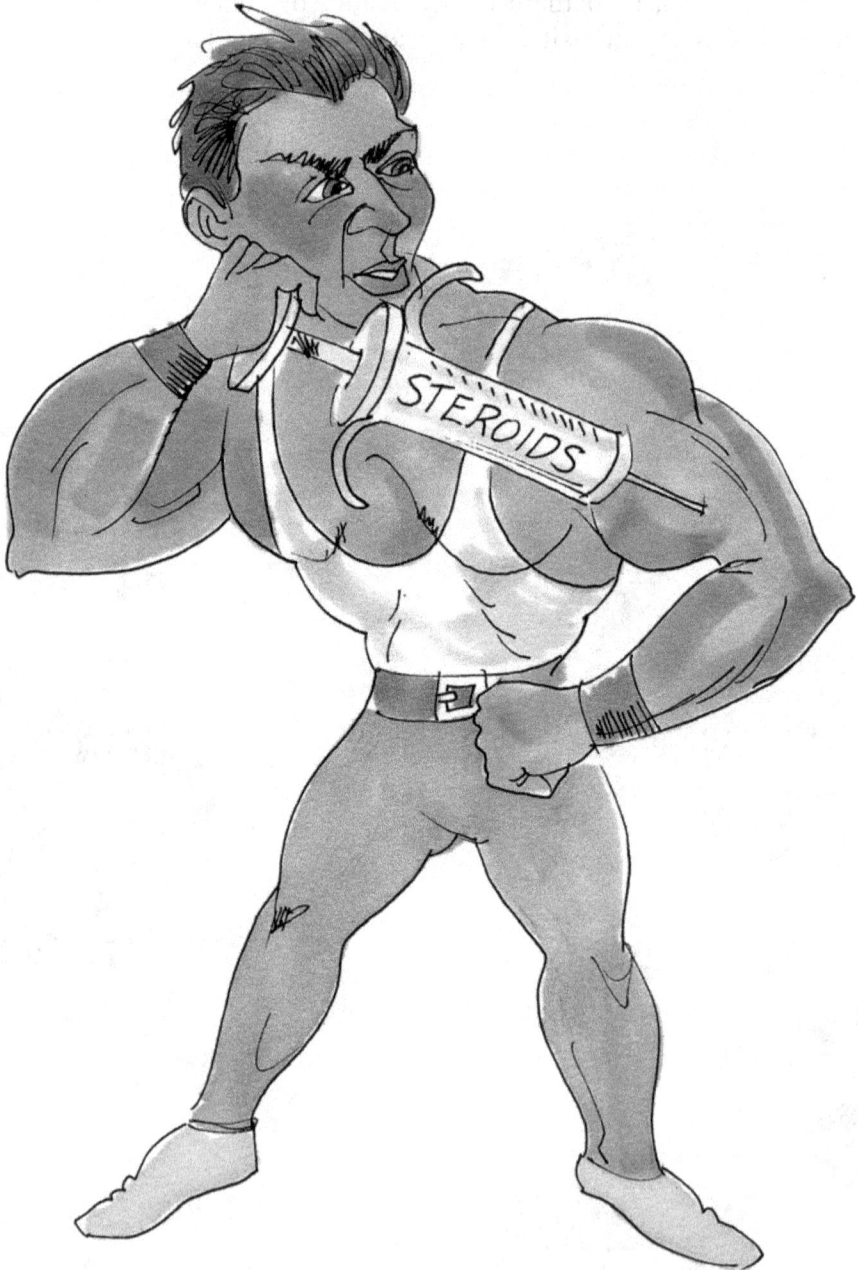

PART 3

INVASION
OF THE NATURAL
BODYBUILDERS

ANABOLIC REVOLUTION

Throughout the centuries, the concepts of physical culture have evolved from the raw Grecian theatres of the 600 B.C. era, where stone trained athletes such as boxers, wrestlers, and strongmen would compete against one another, to the modern day physique man, whom science and technology has provided the latest state-of-the-art fitness centers and nutritional know-how to create huge muscular physiques with power to match. In the 20th century, bodybuilding came of age in America. With its roots as a sideshow attraction, to becoming a billion dollar industry, it has branched out to become a staple of the American culture. Today, bodybuilding can be found not only on the physique stage, but also in many endeavors of society, such as entertainment, sports, politics, and the medical field. What began as a noble effort towards health and fitness by some, slowly evolved into a drug-laden sport filled with lies, deceit, illness, and even death!

In 1977, while participating as a judge in Dan Lurie's WBBG World Bodybuilding Championships at New York City's Madison Square Garden, I had the good fortune to be sitting in front of the honorary guest of the evening, Mr. Steve Reeves. During the intermission, I introduced myself and broke into a conversation with the legendary Hercules. One of the topics I recall Steve Reeves being passionately against was the use of anabolic steroids in the sport of bodybuilding. That evening, Steve Reeves told me that the sport of bodybuilding would split into two different philosophies (this was long before the evolution of natural bodybuilding ever took hold). He also stated that bodybuilders who continued the use of chemical agents to enhance their physiques risked not only impairing their health but death as well. Decades later, the predictions of this Herculean legend came true, as many amateur and pro-bodybuilders alike died long before their time, leaving a trail of dead bodybuilders across the globe.

Today, reports of drugs in some professional sports have become a common occurrence. The hypocrisy of major league baseball and professional wrestling early in the 21st century served as a wakeup call for an American culture that indulged in reckless living by risking its health through fast foods, alcoholic beverages, smoking, recreational drugs, and the like. Even the entertainment industry became shadowed by the dark anabolic cloud, when accusations of prescribed shipments of steroids and injectable human growth hormone were discovered to have made their way to several private residences, hotels, and production studios. Medical experts claimed that the entertainers were being prescribed the drugs under the pretense that the chemicals could enhance their looks, strength, speed, slow aging, and aid healing. One well-known actor actually went on record saying, "Testosterone to me is so important for a sense of well-being when you get older; everyone over 40 years old would be wise to investigate it because it increases the quality of your life. Mark my words. In ten years it will be sold over the counter."

Before we can ever hope to see bodybuilding return to its roots in physical culture, we will first have to witness a 'new way of life' throughout our society. There will have to be a loud cry from the public for an end to the nonsense and an awakening to the fact that drugs are ruining not only the health of many Americans but also destroying our culture as well.

Since the early days of physical culture, modern man has been searching for the elusive Fountain of Youth. The promise of radiant health, enduring strength, and a Herculean physique has drawn millions on this quest for physical perfection. Arguably, the first physical culturist in America was Bernarr MacFadden. MacFadden, who is often referred to as the Father of Physical Culture, was internationally-known during his lifetime. He authored many fine articles and books on the positive effects of weight training as it related to mental health and fitness. A muscle builder from the late 1800s, MacFadden became renowned throughout the world as a pioneer in physical culture and muscle building. His philosophy was among the first to plant the seeds of what would one day become the sport of bodybuilding.

Through the early decades of bodybuilding, the forefathers of physical culture established basic guidelines for the muscle enthusiast to follow. Natural foods, resistance training, plenty of rest, and a positive outlook on life were the primary ingredients for achieving one's goals. Gradually, as the interest in physical culture increased, the demand for knowledge on how to become a he-man would result in millions of booklets being sold by mail order, while magazine stands and bookshelves were continually being restocked with the latest 'muscle building secrets.' With this quest for knowledge, tons of steel and exercise equipment would also find its way into the homes of thousands of Americans all across our nation. Eventually, health clubs and iron gyms would sprout up in local neighborhoods and towns, while physique competitions were held to determine who the best in the land was. The strong roots of physical culture were taking grip in our society, and the mighty oak of bodybuilding would soon branch out through every city in America.

A new way of life became a reality for many as the "body beautiful" movement swung into high gear. For decades, the much-traveled road to Muscledom kept its promise. Then, in the early 1960s, what seemed pure and natural took a wrong turn as the course of modern bodybuilding changed direction and headed towards a dead end. The introduction of anabolic steroids into the sport would usher in a new era of super-sized and equally strong muscular physiques that would attract millions of young men who desired to achieve the same goals, but was unattainable naturally.

Along with the growth of the sport, the physiques continued to become bigger and increasingly vascular as the bodybuilders experimented with "stacking" the latest in designer muscle enhancing pharmaceuticals. Magazine and ticket sales were at a peak and bodybuilding competitions were seen regularly on network TV. The popularity of the sport was soaring high. Then, what could have been mostly prevented by not promoting and rewarding individuals whose physiques were chemically-altered became a reality as the widespread use of drugs in the sport of bodybuilding became relevant.

Words such as steroids, cycling, and growth hormones became commonplace in our gyms and *juicing* no longer meant enjoying your favorite health drink. Reports of bodybuilders on dialysis and with heart ailments became a frequent occurrence, while the eventual death of several competitive pros hit home hard. What had been a dark cloud over a sport with such great potential turned into a storm that spread its vast shadow on a culture that once shined with pride.

During my Staten Island Bodybuilding Club's first few years of existence, I was somewhat naive to the widespread use of steroids in bodybuilding. Although I knew they existed I never gave much thought to the matter. Back in the 1970s, my gym was somewhat isolated from the metropolitan area and the steroid scene. We believed that in order to get huge you had to train big and eat right. You had to get your rest and be consistent at the gym. We never considered the use of drugs for the purpose of building muscle and gaining strength. To us, it was not only unhealthy but also a means of cheating.

Eventually, the steroids did make their way into Staten Island's gyms and my club was no exception. It would not be until early 1980 that some of my members began to experiment with the chemicals. As much as I and other members preached about the dangers of steroids, our good intentions went in one ear and out the other. The steroid scene on Staten Island became so bad that when new members joined my club the first thing they would ask was, "What steroids should we take for maximum results?" It was a new generation of bodybuilders on the Island. They wanted results overnight and did not care about what ill effects stood before them. The battle had begun!

Results that took natural bodybuilders years to accomplish were now being realized in a relatively short period, with less pain and sweat to show for the gains they displayed. I saw gym members become massively huge and extremely powerful practically overnight. I also saw some of the early side effects that such practices brought. It did not matter to the muscle-heads. To them, life was about the moment and they weren't concerned about the future or living a long healthy life. I even had the unfortunate circumstance of learning that a couple of my members were trying to sell drugs right out of my gym. To say I became a little violent with them would be an understatement, but such action was needed to serve as a warning to those who would dare push that crap in my establishment.

Since the early 1990s, the sport of bodybuilding has been plagued with a succession of tragedies and near calamities that cannot be excused as mere statistical coincidences. Our once great and noble sport has reached a time in its history that must not be ignored. Because of the use of chemical agents in the sport of bodybuilding, many muscle builders, both pro and amateur alike, have become walking time bombs with the sad prospect of a future lived in ill health and possibly an untimely death. When you consider the use of enormous amounts of anabolic steroids, growth hormones, and insulin;

combined with an exotic array of "get high" substances and narcotic pain killers; along with consuming huge quantities of food every couple of hours to add mass; followed by a competitive lifestyle that requires losing up to fifty pounds of bodyweight and then peaking on the day of a physique competition by means of diuretics, so as to be bone dry and severely dehydrated on the competitive stage; you don't have to be a rocket scientist to realize that such a regimen is a formula for disaster.

At the beginning of the 21st century, muscles that were once a sketched representation of an artist's wild imagination finally became a reality, as the proportions of the pro-bodybuilders grew into freakish, cartoonish dimensions that were seen in lineups throughout the competitive bodybuilding world. By 2008, the use of performance enhancing drugs in America became so prevalent that our win-at-all-cost culture became the subject of the limited theater-released documentary *Bigger Stronger Faster*. The film, which gives an objective view of the steroid argument, takes an in-depth look at our society that rewards speed, size, and above all else winning: winning in sport, in business, and at war. It examines the reasoning why so many of America's *heroes* are on performance-enhancing substances and how their practice has influenced new generations to follow in the same manner. The very existence of such a film says volumes about how deep the roots of steroids are within the core of our society. I am afraid it will be many decades before the anabolic tree rots and the sun once again shines on the sport of bodybuilding.

To save certain athletes from themselves, and to save the sport of bodybuilding, an overhaul of how physiques are judged must take place at many bodybuilding competitions held in America and throughout the world. The powers that be must make a commitment to return competitive bodybuilding to a celebration of life, not a shortening of it.

In 1979, while once again participating as a judge for Dan Lurie's WBBG World Bodybuilding Championships, I had the pleasure to meet the ambassador of natural bodybuilding, Mr. Chet Yorton. Chet was a renowned physique champion who, in 1975, created the Natural Bodybuilder's Association (NBA), the first federation to test for drug use at all of its competitions. Earlier in his competitive career, Yorton was introduced to steroids by a top bodybuilder who advised him to take the muscle building pharmaceuticals. Hesitantly, Chet first spoke to a doctor who warned him about the possible side effects of these dangerous drugs. Chet took the doctor's words to heart and immediately began a lifelong crusade against the use of drugs in bodybuilding. By 1981, the former Mr. America and Mr. Universe legend became deeply entrenched in his cause when he published the magazine *Natural Bodybuilding*. The magazine educated the public on the dangers of steroids while also providing media exposure for bodybuilders who chose not to use the physique enhancing substances. Chet Yorton (see photo) was a visionary who pioneered the sport of natural bodybuilding. Decades ago, he saw that bodybuilding was headed in the wrong direction and chose to create a new path for modern day physique artists to follow, as they too, would eventually inspire others to embrace this new way of life. Early in the 21st century, this senior pioneer of the natural bodybuilding movement not only continues to promote the sport that he loves, but also continues to shine as an example of the benefits of healthy living.

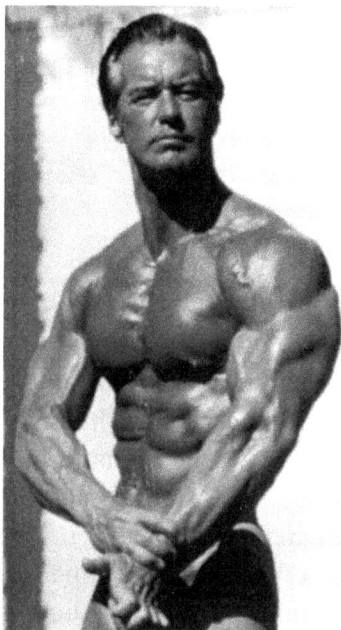

Today, the battle against drugs in the sport rages on as many organizations dedicated to natural bodybuilding and healthy living have responded with an Anabolic Revolution, by calling for a return to the ideals set forth by the forefathers of physical culture. On the physique stage, promoters throughout the U.S. and across the globe have created natural bodybuilding competitions so athletes can compete on a level playing field without running the risk of ruining their health. Publications featuring natural bodybuilders are now widely read as the gospel of healthy living (through proper nutrition and exercise) is communicated to the masses. The televised media has joined in the fight by broadcasting natural bodybuilding and fitness programs to inspire future generations of muscle builders. Today, with the age of cyber space upon us, the Internet has become a learning resource for concepts and advice, and a place for bodybuilders to express their views. The new millennium is here, and those dedicated to physical culture have begun to prevail, as the radiant beacon of light from the torch of natural living begins to shine through the storm.

THE STEROID GURU

Probably the most popular steroid proponent in the history of bodybuilding was the self-proclaimed Steroid Guru of Venice. While his name and widely-publicized book are not worth mentioning, he nevertheless had a dramatic influence on the sport of bodybuilding. In the early 1980s, this proponent of drugs in bodybuilding published a how-to-take steroids book that led untold numbers of bodybuilders and athletes down the wrong path. His book also opened up the floodgates for other self-proclaimed geniuses to jump in and promote their own special formulas on how to take and cycle these dangerous sports enhancing pharmaceuticals. The Steroid Guru of Venice believed in what he preached. So much in fact, that he conducted experiments on himself by taking large doses of steroids to test his twisted theories. Since he was not happy with his limited genetic structure, the drugs in his view represented a way for him to gain acceptance into the Venice Muscle Beach scene.

When he first published his steroid book, it sold for just a few dollars. It was half a how-to-manual and half a drug catalog. The heart of the book detailed nearly thirty drugs in all. Each drug listing had a review and often a suggested price while describing the effect each chemical agent delivered. At first, a small ad marketing the book ran in a single physique publication and was successful enough to receive several hundred orders. As future ads ran, thousands of additional requests began to flood the mailbox of this anabolic guru. His book was so successful that in its first year of publication it sold tens of thousands of copies, which netted him and his cohorts nearly half a million dollars.

I remember one day early in 1983, when a member of my gym brought this how-to-take steroids book to my club. I first heard about the book through the physique publications and was disgusted with the openness of how it was being marketed. When my member handed the book to me, initially it did not seem like much. However, as I thumbed through its pages I realized that this journal was poison in the hands of the young egomaniacs who wanted to be big and strong instantly. From what I remember, it was a thin paperback book and amateurishly written, but what it represented was a new era in the evolution of bodybuilding. What had been a misunderstood science of physique enhancement by the bodybuilding community became common knowledge thanks to this self-proclaimed steroid guru. After skimming through the book's pages, I tore it into several pieces and told its owner to stay away from drugs, while at the same time warning him never to bring that kind of material to my club again. As I threw the shredded papers into the trash, I thought to myself that this was the end of physical culture, as I knew it.

In 1980, when the Steroid Guru of Venice first entered the California bodybuilding scene, he was a wannabe actor looking for a stage. By January of 2000, he was someone who had served time in federal prison for selling steroids, had aged badly, and was now suffering from a serious kidney disease. He became a shadow of his former fit self and stopped caring about his life and health. When I heard of his passing that same winter, I felt no sorrow for the 48-year-old drug promoter. This was the person responsible in large part for the popularity of anabolic steroids in America. The Steroid Guru of Venice had planted a seed in the bodybuilding culture that mushroomed into a giant monster. Today, his legacy continues to grow as modern day bodybuilding gurus follow in his path, pushing their steroids, growth hormones, insulin, and diuretics in much the same manner as the once-famed Steroid Guru of Venice.

OF ALL THE SENSES COMMON THE LEAST COMMON IS COMMON

THE BATTLE RAGES ON

In early 2008, I received a disturbing e-mail from a visitor of my Web site saying how disgusted he was with the availability of anabolic steroids on the Internet and how the misinformation being posted on the various pro-steroid Web sites was negatively influencing youths and young adults. The e-mail also went into detail about a major Internet search engine that was planning to align itself with a person in the bodybuilding community that was very pro-steroids and who went by various aliases. After reading the e-mail, I searched online and became very alarmed at what I found. Although I knew these pro-steroid Web sites existed I had never really given them much thought. I had better things to do than to look at pictures of anabolic androids and read about how they built their bodies through cycling and stacking. Without giving any pro-steroid Web sites some undeserved publicity, there was one in particular that rattled my bones. This site boasted 100,000 plus members and seemed oblivious to the immoral and illegal practices it was preaching. It also made available a wide spectrum of anabolic steroids to accommodate the specific needs of those who wanted to take such dangerous drugs. There were pages on the history of steroids, black market prices, anabolic effectiveness charts, steroid laws, steroid abuse, side effects of steroids, steroid profiles, steroid cycling, steroid detection time, steroid forums, etc. While reading some of the rants of the Web site's editor, it was obvious that his thinking was slanted in the wrong direction. It was remarkable how blatant he was about the promotion of steroids and the position his Web site took in acting as a resource for the sale of these very dangerous and illegal drugs. I thought for a while about what I should do about this Web site as well as the others that were helping to destroy bodybuilding. I came up with the conclusion that it would be a waste of my time to go after each one directly. There were just too many of them! Besides, it would have been foolish to get into a shouting match across cyber space with those who were ignorant in their misguided views. Only a fool argues with another fool!

My Web site and its related blog were already promoting the truth about the dangers of muscle-enhancing drugs, and the last thing I needed was to give those jerks added publicity. Thanks to *MarioStrong.com* and the other Web sites that promote natural bodybuilding in America, the fight has been blazing in this venue called the Internet for some time now and thankfully, those in the trenches for truth are realizing positive gains. The best example I have to show that natural bodybuilding is the only course to take is my own flesh and blood. Not only am I a natural for life bodybuilder, but also something of a physical culturist with a heavy slant towards longevity. If I can build quality muscle and power to last a lifetime, then so can others who choose to make natural bodybuilding their way of life. For me, this is a much better way to win over some young minds than to throw explicative comments across the Internet with those who believe in the very poisons they spew. The Internet has become a wonderful tool in providing endless amounts of information to viewers throughout the world. It has also opened the floodgates for those who take advantage of its format for their own personal greed and gain. Sadly, the anabolic battle will rage on throughout the 21st century. I will continue the fight alongside those on the side of health and longevity, as this battle of chemical warfare in the sport of bodybuilding marches on.
5

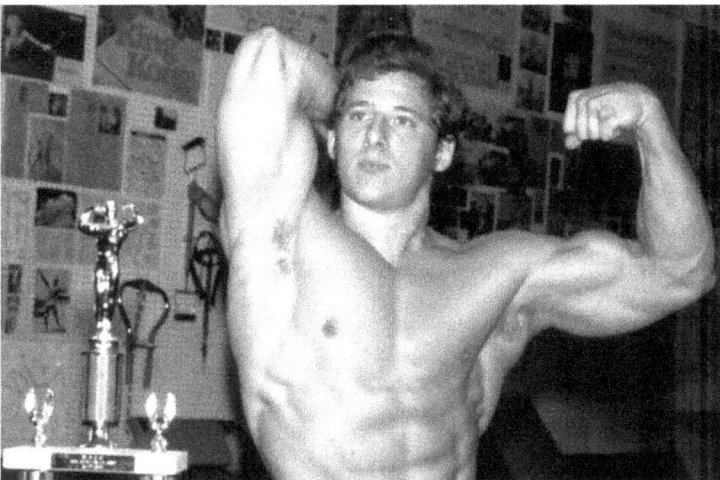

BANNED SUBSTANCES

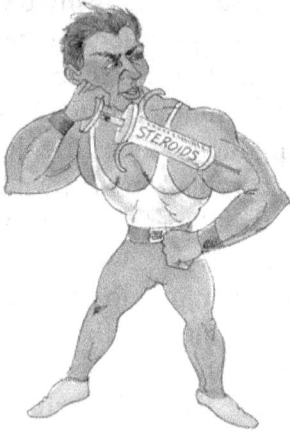

There are several types of approaches to the sport of bodybuilding. One approach is called *natural bodybuilding*, which is building muscle without the use of performance enhancing substances such as anabolic steroids and growth hormones. These dangerous pharmaceuticals, along with many others, are banned from natural bodybuilding organizations in the United States. In natural physique contests, bodybuilders are routinely tested for these illicit substances and are banned from competition if the test proves that any forbidden sports enhancing pharmaceuticals were used. Although testing can be done on urine samples, the less expensive polygraph test is the choice of most show promoters. What qualifies as an illegal substance varies between some natural federations and does not necessarily include only substances that are illegal under the laws of the relevant jurisdiction.

The eligibility requirements to compete in a natural bodybuilding competition vary from one year drug-free to natural for life. Even more important than the time element is what is actually banned by some natural federations. Quasi-supplements such as pro-steroids, anti-estrogenics, thermogenic aids, prohormones, and hormonal products border the line of what is allowed in natural bodybuilding competitions. When trying to decide on a natural bodybuilding organization to join, choose one that bans such *supplements* and all illicit sports-enhancing drugs as well as recreational substances.

The following is a brief introduction on drugs and substances that have found their way into some sports arenas, and are banned by most natural bodybuilding organizations, whether through means of blood doping, pharmacological, chemical, or physical manipulation.

ANABOLIC AGENTS

Testosterone and substances that are related in structure and activity are found in the anabolic androgenic class. Anabolic steroids are synthetic derivatives or chemically altered versions of the hormone testosterone. They were developed in an effort to minimize the androgenic effects while retaining the anabolic properties of testosterone. In males, testosterone is the main androgenic hormone. The hormone plays a major role in the development and maintenance of masculine secondary sexual characters. Anabolic steroids also influence certain other secondary sexual characters, such as hair growth pattern and voice quality. Chemically-enhanced bodybuilders primarily use testosterone to increase both muscle mass and strength. Because anabolic steroids increase a person's masculine properties they tend to magnify the biological factors associated with these male hormonal qualities. Although the use of these drugs has been shown to increase both muscle mass and strength, the more dramatic results are witnessed when they are used in conjunction with resistance training. Because of this, steroids have become the drug of choice. However, no amount of exercise or drug use, no matter how long a period they are used for, will ever enable anyone to throw 1,000-pound boulders. There is a limit to what training and steroids can and cannot do.

Throughout the decades, many different synthetic derivatives of the testosterone molecule have made their way into the sport of bodybuilding. All of these versions have had varying degrees of androgenic and anabolic potencies. The stronger androgenic versions have been demonstrated to have more anabolic characteristics and thus more effectiveness for the purposes of increasing muscle mass and strength. Anabolic steroids can be taken orally, sublingually, or by injection. Oral steroids usually act faster than their oil-based injectable counterparts do. Injectable steroids such as Deca-Durabolin have been designed to reduce the androgenic characteristics and can stay in the body much longer than oral steroids such as Dianabol. Dianabol travels quickly to the liver where it is broken down to a large degree. This type of steroid stresses the liver and can lead to some very serious illnesses.

The side effects of anabolic steroids vary depending on individual physiological characteristics and gender. The degree of negative reactions depends on age, dosage, and duration of time these powerful drugs are taken. Anabolic steroids promote aggressiveness and an inner confidence to succeed. In the brain, steroids can affect other chemicals, such as serotonin and dopamine, leading to depression or impulsive behavior. They also might send the user into a hormone fueled violent outburst known as *roid rage*. Many bodybuilders, who take large doses of steroids to build strength and muscle mass, are not able to control the violent outburst they display because of these dangerous drugs. The use of steroids may also lead to psychosis and other anti-social behaviors. As stated previously, a psychological dependency can occur because many steroid-laden bodybuilders fear the loss of the strength and physique attained by using these illicitly-abused drugs. Some other possible side effects of anabolic steroids include: torn muscle tissue and tendons, acne, liver damage, testicle shrinkage, erectile dysfunction, decreased sperm count, an increase in men's breast size (gynecomastia), high blood pressure, abnormal cholesterol levels, jaundice, male-pattern baldness in both men and women, and the growth of facial hair in women. Some examples of anabolic agents are Anadrol, Winstrol, and Dianabol.

HUMAN GROWTH HORMONES
Human Growth Hormones (HGH) are very powerful substances used by bodybuilders, athletes, and high profile individuals. HGH has a synergistic effect with testosterone and has its own intrinsic muscle building and fat loss properties. This may be why many pro-bodybuilders and athletes use it in combination with their steroid cycle regimen. One of the more notable side effects of too much HGH in the body is acromegaly, which is an overgrowth of the bones and connective tissue, causing a protruding jaw and eyebrows. Bodybuilders who take HGH sometimes have facial features similar to that of the prehistoric Cro-Magnon man. They may also display an abdominal region that is distended, along with hands and feet that are abnormally large. Changes to the internal organs, including the heart, are irreversible. Liver, thyroid, insulin levels, and life expectancy may also be affected by the use of this powerful drug. Some examples of human growth hormones are Chorionic Gonadotrophin (HCG - Human Chorionic Gonadotrophin), Corticotropin (ACTH), and Growth Hormone (HGH, Somatropin).

DIURETICS

Diuretics are among the most dangerous drugs a physique competitor can use. This has been witnessed on several occasions, when severe dehydration and electrolyte imbalance has caused serious medical issues and even death among those who abuse these powerful pharmaceuticals. Sadly, since diuretics lower subcutaneous water concentrations to produce that super-ripped look, many of today's muscle artist rely heavily on them. It is extremely difficult for a natural bodybuilder to compete against the androids that use diuretics to polish their physiques. That alone is reason enough to compete only in drug-free competitions. Some serious side effects of diuretics include dizziness, cramping, vomiting, diarrhea, fainting, and circulatory disturbances. Furosemide, Acetazolamide, and Spironolactone are types of diuretics.

STIMULANTS

Stimulants are drugs that temporarily increase alertness and awareness. When this activity increases, it sends signals throughout the body that may raise blood pressure, heart rate, and breathing. Stimulants usually have increased side effects with increased effectiveness. The abuse or misuse of these dangerous drugs can cause serious medical issues including irregular heartbeat, heart failure, seizures, or even death. The most common side effects from stimulants are insomnia, anorexia, irritability, weight loss, abdominal pain, and headaches. Some stimulants may also lead to serious behaviors, such as hostility, distortion, and paranoia. Some examples of stimulants are Amphetamines, Cocaine, and Ephedrine.

NARCOTICS

Narcotic agents are potent analgesics that alleviate physical pain, suppress coughing, alleviate diarrhea, and induce anesthesia. Analgesics are selective central nervous system depressants used for such reason. Even in therapeutic doses, narcotic analgesics can cause respiratory depression, nausea, and drowsiness. Long-term administration produces tolerance, psychic, and physical dependence called addiction. Natural narcotics are derived from the Opium poppy, and synthetic narcotics are made to act like the major constituents of Opium. Some examples of narcotics are Methadone, Morphine, and Hydrocodone.

OTHER MEANS OF ENHANCEMENT

When it comes to the alteration of the physique, bodybuilders are quite resourceful in accomplishing their goals. Aside from using drugs for gains in size and strength, bodybuilders also rely on others means to enhance their appearance. Let us look at a couple.

SYNTHOL

A substance that has become commonplace on today's physique stage is Synthol. This substance is now as much a part of the hardcore bodybuilding scene as steroids, growth hormones, and diuretics. In the 1990s, Synthol became a jackpot for thousands of anabolic bodybuilders who were dissatisfied with the size of their arms, delts, and calves. Today, it's commonplace to see the results of Synthol in bodybuilders that have injected the substance directly into any of these small muscle groups. Bodybuilders use Synthol because it gives some additional size and fullness in whichever body part the bodybuilder desires to enhance. Synthol is composed of 85% medium-chain triglyceride oils (fatty acid), 7.5% lidocaine (painkiller), and 7.5% benzyl alcohol. The preparation is injected deep into the muscle where it is encapsulated between the fascicles. The more injections a bodybuilder takes the more oil builds up inside his muscles, forcing them to expand in much the same way as a balloon filling up with air. The body metabolizes about a third of what is injected. The rest remains lodged in the muscle where it breaks down very slowly over several years. While steroids do help anabolic bodybuilders increase both size and strength, the muscle builders still need to perform resistance training in order to build maximum muscle mass. Not so, because Synthol acts primarily as a muscle inflammatory agent, and therefore anyone who injects the chemical directly into a small body part will show large increases in muscle fullness with little effort. Makes the term bodybuilding take on a new meaning, doesn't it?

CALF IMPLANTS

A practice that seems to be widely accepted in the sport of bodybuilding is calf implants. Since many bodybuilders find it very difficult to develop their calf muscles because of inferior genetics, they opt towards the quick and easy way to increase the mass of this stubborn muscle group. By no means is the implantation of a foreign object into the calf muscle a new procedure. Like breast implants, this relatively simple operation has been around for decades. Getting a calf implant does not necessarily guarantee a perfectly-balanced diamond shaped calf either. Sometimes they can seem too large and round when compared to the thigh, and can protrude outwards too much, making them look constantly flexed, even when the bodybuilder is sitting or standing. The implants themselves come in varying sizes and are made of a solid, but pliable, inert material. The primary goal is for the implants to look as if they actually belong on that body. The standard procedure consists of two average-sized implants placed in each leg over the heads of the gastrocnemius. In my book, calf implants should be classified as cheating in any physique competition, since judges are supposed to be comparing physiques composed of muscle, not implanted hunks of silicone that required no effort to attain. Unfortunately, in physique competitions they are often overlooked, as are breast implants.

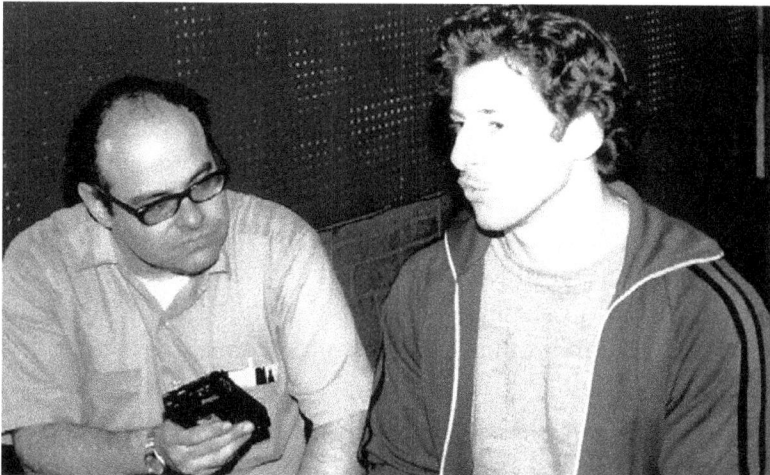

Mario discusses steroid abuse with bodybuilding author Bob Gruskin - 1980

STRONG REMARKS

Maybe it's just me, but after reflecting on the previous two chapters, I wonder how any rational being could ever put any of the mentioned chemical enhancers into his or her body for the purpose of bodybuilding. Drugs take the body further than nature ever intended it to go. When bodybuilders take drugs for the purposes of building muscle, gaining strength, losing fat, dropping water, getting high, blocking pain, or whatever, without the sound medical supervision of a qualified MD, they are participating in a reckless behavior that could have some serious consequences. Life is short enough and risking it to such senseless practices says a lot about those who partake in such self-destructive behavior. Over the decades, I have seen thousands of pill poppers come and go in our sport and I am sure I will continue to see many more in the future. To endure in bodybuilding and enjoy a full, radiant life, you have to make health your number one priority and not destroy it with irrational acts.

Unfortunately, many newcomers to the sport of bodybuilding look at some of these "champions" in awe and disbelief. They read the muscle magazines and go to the muscle shows, and soon learn that they want to emulate their newfound heroes. They become motivated and inspired by these superhuman men and women and want the same naturally unattainable goals. So what do they do? They hook up with the local gym pusher. Just about every muscle gym has one. These drug merchants who seem to be able to come up with every form of anabolic steroid and other performance enhancing substance ever created. These rodents of the iron game spend most of their time in the club locker room, making a living selling these dangerous drugs right out of their gym bags. I have personally have encountered such individuals through the decades and when necessary have had to use physical force to rid their sorry asses away from the young bodybuilders.

When a bodybuilder starts using steroids, he or she experiences relatively quick gains in both muscle mass and strength. As the gains are realized, some bodybuilders experience painful muscle tears, pulls, strains, and debilitating injuries; partly because the steroids they took did little in the way of strengthening their tendons and ligaments. Another problem for anabolic bodybuilders is that they develop a tolerance for the muscle building chemicals and soon find themselves requiring larger doses of the drugs to maintain their already ill-gotten gains. Soon, they become dependent on the sport's enhancing substances, not only physically, but also psychologically. They watched their bodies become muscular and powerful with the aid of the drugs and the last thing they are going to do is stop taking them and chance losing some of their artificial gains. Instead, they begin swallowing and injecting even larger doses in hopes of adding greater muscle mass and strength, and soon learn how to stack and cycle the various pharmaceuticals at their disposal. They become hooked on the deadly chemicals and head straight down a dead end. Eventually, they crash and crumble from the poisons poured into their formerly healthy bodies.

On a local level, in the 1980s there was a popular Staten Island bodybuilder who went by the nickname of Dr. Big (he wasn't a real doctor, but acted as such). Dr. Big trained at another gym on the Island and whenever we met, we would both get into a heated debate on the use of anabolic steroids for the purposes of building muscle and gaining strength. Dr. Big actually believed that drugs were the way to go and that the possible side effects were minimal. Although he trained hard and was consistent at the gym, he relied greatly on chemicals for his enormous size and power. During this time, Dr. Big was injecting various substances into his body, while also preaching to others how pharmaceuticals were needed to make gains. Unfortunately, Dr. Big did influence some naïve bodybuilders who followed his example and risked destroying their health by taking the sports enhancing substances he prescribed. Again, it came as no surprise to me when one day I received a phone call from a friend stating that Dr. Big had died of a massive heart attack. He was only in his early forties and had a whole life in front of him. Sadly, he became just another statistic on an endless list of preventable tragedies.

Throughout the decades, I have witnessed many bodybuilders I knew personally, take ill, or even die, because of anabolic steroids and I find it sickening. Not too long ago, a member of a gym I train at informed me that he was suffering from liver disease. This fellow holds some national powerlifting records and is pleasant to talk to. He was also very muscular and had enormous strength because of the drugs. Several times over the years, he stated to me that he was going to get off the chemicals. Nevertheless, every time he tried, he lost his gains and returned for his fix. Unfortunately, he returned to the syringe one too many times and now has not only lost everything he has trained so hard for, but may lose his life as well. Another local Island muscle builder who fell under the spell of the dark cloud years ago is now paying the price for his ill-gotten gains. Now in the prime of his life, when he should be enjoying the benefits of all the hard work he put in the gym, he is instead suffering with degenerative bone disease and rotted tendons throughout his entire body. His future looks very bleak, as he may one day need to permanently trade in his crutches for a wheelchair. Certainly, their temporary gains weren't worth all the pain and disease. When you take illicit drugs for the purposes of building muscle and gaining strength, you take your body further than nature ever intended it to go and you put your life at risk.

THE BOTTOM LINE

America awards those that are bigger, stronger, and faster. This is a fact that cannot be denied. We have professional athletes who have made fortunes because of their enhanced athletic abilities, and many who have even gained fame on an unimaginable scale. As well publicized as the abuse of drugs in sports is, we as a nation continue to applaud the chemically-driven accomplishments of the artificial champs by filling stadiums with fans and purchasing products they endorse. Our homes, workplaces, and schools are filled with those wanting the same glory as the athletes whose images constantly appear in the media outlets. These wannabes train hard for their teams and for themselves. Some even have aspirations of grandeur when it comes to emulating the champions they believe in. Unfortunately, there comes a time when the trainees are pressured by their teammates, goals, and desires. Many take the high road and stay away from sports-enhancing substances, but sadly, many more do not. Because of these pressures to succeed, is it any wonder why the use of these substances has become so abused and prevalent among our population, especially the young?

However, as prevalent as these drugs are in the sports arenas, they pale in comparison to the multi-billion dollar tobacco and alcohol conglomerates. These mainstream corporations spew out their well documented, health destroying products by the ton on an American public that has witnessed the horrors of what these legal items can bring. Nevertheless, as much pain and suffering as these products have brought, they are still used in great deal by those that know better.

We are a nation on drugs! I'm not only referring to the feel good or sports enhancing substances. We rely on all sorts of goodies to get us through our day. Go to any local pharmacy and you will find many varieties of tranquilizers, pain relievers, beta-blockers, anti-inflammatory agents, allergy relievers, decongestants, and even some drugs for improved sexual performance. They're all there, some by prescription, some over-the-counter. The point is that our society has become chemically-dependent and it should come as no shock that many muscle builders find it easy to include sports-enhancing substances into their regimens.

Living in the free society we do enables us to make choices to fulfill our wants and needs. Those lucky enough to be born with a sound mind and healthy body have the opportunity to live a long, radiant, and full life. Unfortunately, some of the choices we make can come back to haunt us. The use of alcohol, cigarettes, exotic drugs, and performance-enhancing substances, among other things, has been well-documented in leading many promising lives down a dead end road. The drive to satisfy some egotistical warped visions of grandeur within our sports-minded-culture is just mindboggling. I will never understand why anyone would risk destroying their most important possession, their health. The purpose of this chapter is not to judge those who use enhancers, but rather, to give warning to the possible side effects that these dangerously powerful drugs can bring. Many decades ago, I made my choice towards health and longevity, and never looked back. Each one of us gets just one shot at life. Once our story is written and played out, our script is placed on a shelf, forever. Some of us have many chapters in our lives. Some unfortunately, just a few pages. I am going to do my best to make my story a lengthy and honorable bestseller. How about you?

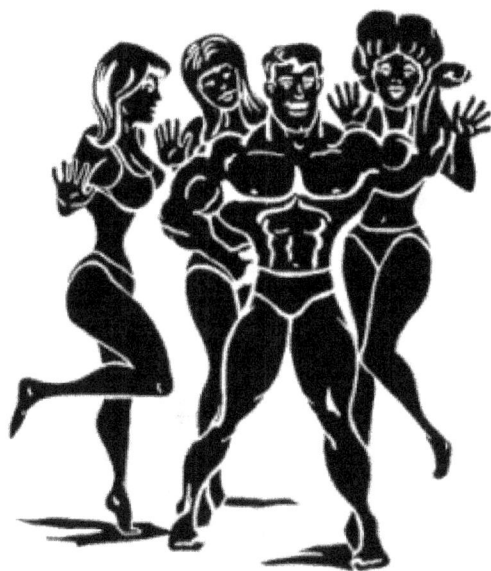

MARIO STRONG.COM

For those who
dare to be...NATURAL!

NO PAIN NO GAIN

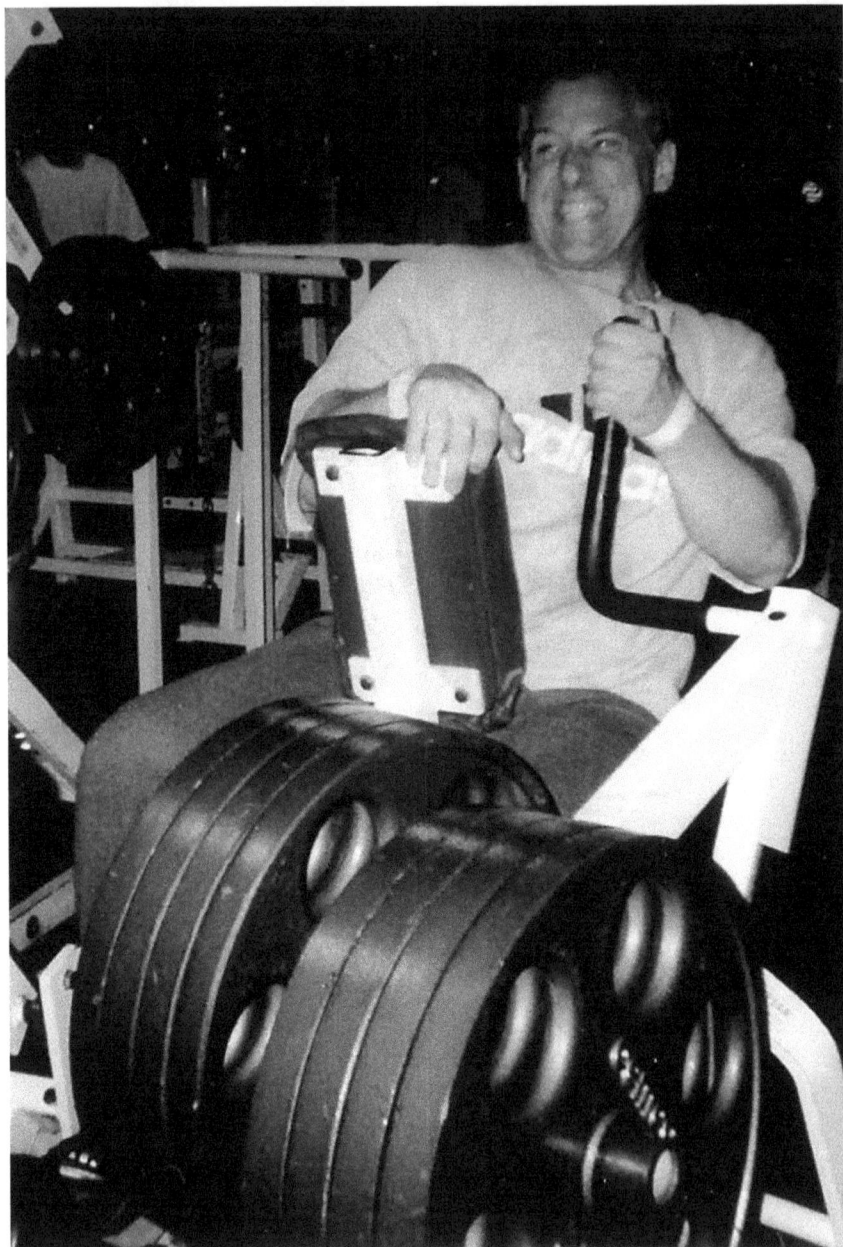

Mario Strong training like there is no tomorrow - 2006

AFTERWORD

I have set down in this book some of my reflections from the world of bodybuilding over the past four decades. The information, programs, and advice that are provided within these pages come from my many years of experience, both through my own personal life and that of the thousands of students I have trained. Natural bodybuilding is a process that brings out the best in us. Not only in physique, but in mind and spirit as well. The athlete that realizes harmony along his journey in our sport has found the balance that comes from hard work, perseverance, and fortitude. It is my hope that in some small way this book will not only enhance your time in the gym but your lifestyle as well.

Mario Strong

INDEX

A

Anabolic 413-14
Anabolic Revolution 402, 407
Anabolic Steroids 44, 102, 132, 141, 149-51, 161, 402, 404-5, 409-10, 412-
    14, 418-20
Anadrol 414
Analgesics 415
Andersen, Neil 139
Anello, Vince 136
Animal Room 74, 84-6, 111
Ann, Sally 69
Annual AAU Eastern Classic 89
Arnold 14, 20, 32, 45-6, 82-4, 86, 112, 114, 137, 173, 228-9, 288
Arnold Schwarzenegger Classic Expo Weekend 136
Art of Muscle Building 113, 168
Arteries 192, 204
Athletic Abilities 250
Atlanta 113-14
Atri 128-9
Attitude, Positive 34, 83, 140, 185, 226, 233-4, 266, 338-9
Auld Lang Syne 88
Austrian Oak 83, 229
Aversa's 80

B
B-Vitamins 197
Badel, Tony 22
Baglio, Joseph 137-8, 152
Balboa 57, 146
  Rocky 143, 145-6, 148
Balboa's 147
Baltimore Orioles 327
Barbarian 228
Barbell Bench Press 281, 288, 369
Barbell Curl 10, 225, 259, 261, 278, 282, 312, 336, 382
Barbell Front Lunge 259
Barbell Reverse Curl 10
Barbell Row 263, 283, 311, 362
Barbell Scott Curl 284, 310, 383
Barbell Shrug 281, 309, 377
Barbell Squat 263, 293
Barbell Squats
  Completing 263
  Regular 259

D

Dais, Posing 33, 35, 74-5, 89, 244
Dan 22-4, 38, 44
Dan Lurie Barbell Company 22
Dan Lurie Moon Bench 81
Dan Lurie's Crash Weight Gain Formula 14
Dan Lurie's Muscle Training Illustrated 2, 22, 61
Dangerfield, Rodney 85-6
Dan's World Body Building Guild 154
Dawn 101
Deadlift 286, 295, 313
Deaths 55, 87, 99, 128, 151, 175, 182, 217-18, 323, 334, 402, 404-5, 415
DeBella, Lou 59
Deca-Durabolin 413
Decembre's 80
Declaration of Independence 146
Decreased risk of Osteoporosis 245
Deep Vein Thrombosis 220
Dehydroepiandrosterone 240
Delayed Onset Muscle Soreness 291
DeLuca, Patrick 2, 99
Denie 42, 141
Denise 27, 69, 117
Denise's 117
Dennis 50-1, 54, 76, 78
DHEA 240-1
Diabetes 192-4, 216, 218-20
Diamond Head Crater 177
Dianabol 12-13, 413-14
Dickerson, Chris 23, 114
Diet
  Perfect 26-7
  Restricted 308
  Sample 268, 270, 272
Dietary fiber 193
Digest 187, 193, 195, 200, 212-13, 269, 301
Digestion 196, 210, 212-13
District Attorney 152
DNA 205-6
Dolphin Fitness Center 100-1
Dolphin Fitness Center on Staten Island 105, 125
Domenic 1, 11, 15, 65, 80, 88, 106, 113, 121, 124, 159
Donna 53

K

L

N

P

Pacino's 152
Palms Fitness Center on Staten Island 108
Pain 8, 10, 27, 31, 33, 38, 40, 84-6, 101-3, 119, 137, 170, 259-60, 262, 290-1, 420-1
  real 86-7
Pancreatitis 220
Pantothenic Acid 206
Parallel Dip 281, 286, 292, 311, 313, 364
Paralysis 232
Patricia 69
Patrick 99
Peanuts 205, 207-8
Pearl 64, 94, 158, 160, 293
  Bill 55, 64-5
Pectoral Avulsion 291
pectorals 28, 31, 113, 162, 291, 316, 359, 364-5, 369-70
  Upper 368, 371-2
Pentagon 127
Performing Hyperextensions 262
Perine, Shawn 136
Phil 131, 153
Philadelphia Museum of Art 145-6
Philip 88, 91-3, 106-7, 131
Physical Culture 2, 94, 132, 140-1, 222-3, 335, 402-4, 407, 409
Physique Publications 1, 19, 30, 32, 35, 42, 68, 82, 158, 409
Physique Stage 16, 20, 32, 34, 43, 46, 52, 61, 79, 89, 91, 122, 127, 138, 148, 163
Pink Grapefruit 204
Planet Earth 182
Planet Hollywood in Waikiki 326
Platz 83
Plaza Theater 31
Plaza Theater in Manhattan 31
Popcorn 207
Posture 250
Power Clean 313
Power of Positive Thinking 234
Powers, Larry 30
Power, Recuperative 237, 240, 242, 275, 284, 289, 308, 326
Preston, Jeff 137
Procrastination 222

Protein   14, 26, 161, 183, 185-7, 192-3, 199-200, 205, 209, 211-13, 249-51,
        269-72, 300-1, 303-4, 306, 338-9
  High Amounts of   199, 250
  Large Amounts of   200
Protein Breakdown   240-1
Protein Foods   212-13
Protein Requirements   200-1
Protein Sources   187, 201, 213
Protein Supplements   201, 203
Pumpkin   204
Pumping Iron, Bodybuilding Documentary   55, 67

Q

Quadriceps   323, 336, 344-8, 350-1
Quads   83, 113, 344-5

R

Raisins   207
Rapacciulo, Frank   2, 57
Rate, Metabolic   252, 302, 312-13
Raw Almonds   271, 304
Rectus Abdominus   391-5, 397-8
Rectus Femoris   344
Red Berries   205
Red Meat   205
Reeves, Steve   22, 24, 44, 402
REM   237
Renal Cell Cancer   220
Reps   25, 28, 47, 103, 108-9, 161-2, 176, 227, 231-2, 253-4, 261-3, 274,
        286, 288, 336, 364
  Forced   285-6
Resistance Training   29, 243, 253, 341, 404, 413, 416
Rest & Recuperation   236
Reverend Norman Vincent Peale   234
Reverse Barbell Curl   282, 312, 389
Reverse Curl   259, 265, 278
Rheumatoid Arthritis   220
Richmond County   122
Rick   92, 148-50
Rivera, Joe   2
R&J   81
R&J's Bodybuilding Gym   32
Robby   63

U

Uncle Sal   13
Unger, Kathy   123
Unsaturated fats   186
Upright Row   281, 311, 313, 378
Uric   201
Urinary Stress Incontinence   220

V

Vada Kempo   80
Valente, Jerry   2, 30, 81
Venice   82, 408-9
Verrazano Bridge   53, 100
Vertical Leg Raise   391
Vinny Venditti   98
Vitamins   14, 71, 183, 186, 199-200, 203-6, 208-9, 216, 218, 241, 268-70, 302, 338
Vitamin B-1   205
Vitamin B-2   205
Vitamin B-3   205
Vitamin B-6   205
Vitamin B-12   205
Volleyball   315
Votinelli, Rocco   51

W

Wagner College Seahawks on Staten Island   13
Waikiki   125, 182, 298
Waikiki Beach   177
Warren   162
Warren Lincoln Travis   136
Washington Irving High School in Manhattan   33
Washington Monument   146
WBBG (World Body Building Guild)   23, 33, 35, 37, 42, 50, 56, 58, 73, 82
WBBG Eastern American Bodybuilding Championships   55
WBBG Hall of Fame   67
WBBG World Bodybuilding Championships   24
Web Site MarioStrong.com   164
Weider   19, 29
  Joe   19, 113-14
Weider Headquarters   19
Weight Loss   222, 299-300, 306, 318, 415
Weight-Plates   8, 22, 47, 75, 94, 105, 107, 110, 176, 370

Weight Room 14, 153
Weight Train 10, 70, 233, 258, 308, 312, 321
Weight Training 3, 14, 17, 27, 30, 44, 63, 100, 103, 105, 108-9, 119, 153,
    256, 261-2, 293-4
Weight Reduction 314
Weightlifting Hall of Fame Museum 135-6
Wheat Germ 204, 208
White, Jimmy 129
Wide World of Sports 19
Williams, Charlie 116
Winstrol 414
Winter Squashes 204
WNBF 123
WNBF Fitness Team 123
Woodland Hills 19
World Body Building Guild *see* WBBG
World Body Building Guild Championships 44
World Bodybuilding Championships 402, 406
World Gym 82-3, 100
World Gym in Venice 82
World Gyms in Venice 228
World Health Organization 218
World Series 11, 215, 327
World Trade Center 121, 127
World Trade Center in Manhattan 128
World War 22, 175
World Weightlifting 135
Wrist Curl 310, 390

Y

Yankees 152
Yates, Dorian 114
Yeast 206
YMCA 30
York Barbell 29, 135-6
York Barbell Company 103, 135
Yorton 406
  Chet 2, 406-7

Z

Zane 158
  Frank 1, 23, 67, 81-2, 114
Zinc 207

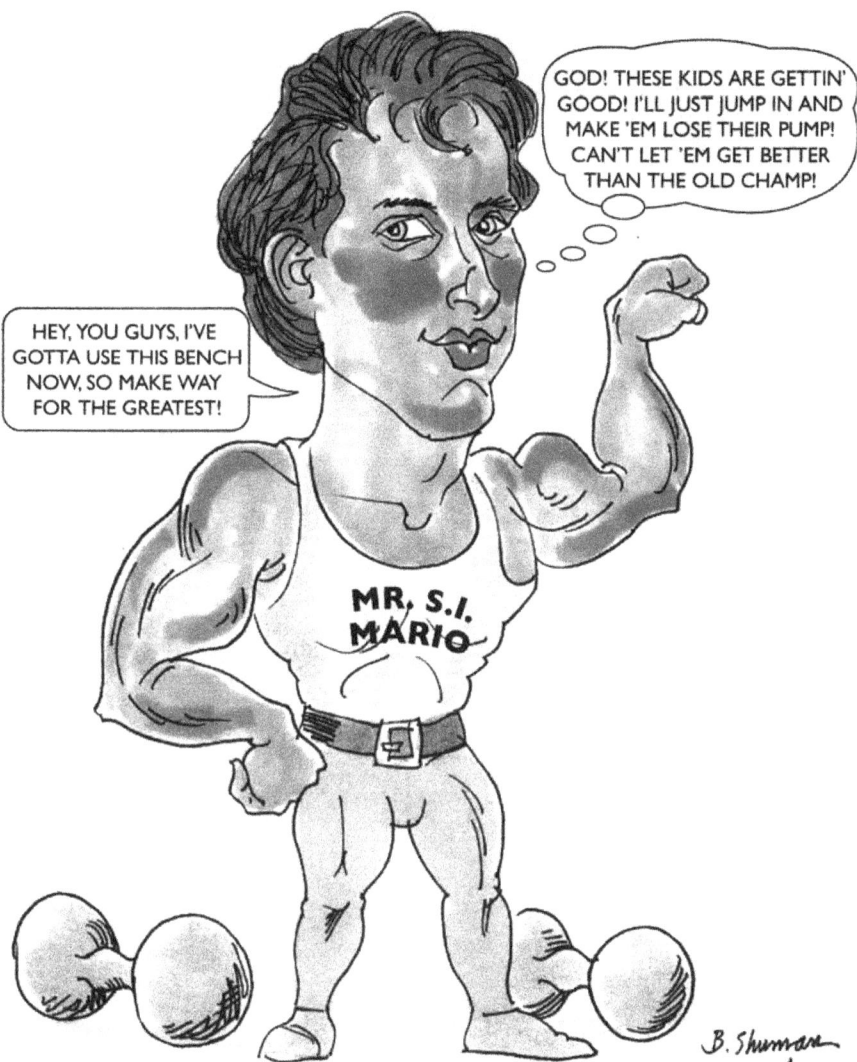

ABOUT THE AUTHOR

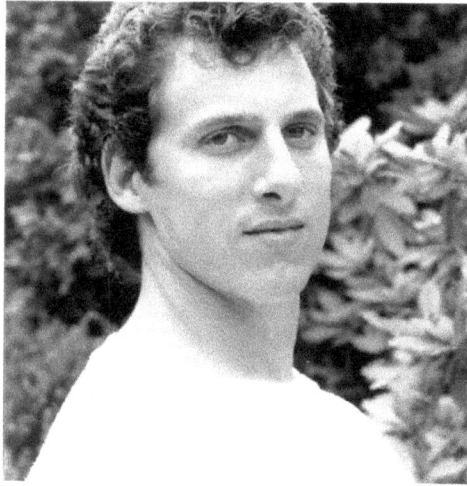

Mario Strong is one of the most respected and knowledgeable natural for life bodybuilders on the scene today. For decades, his passion for excellence has inspired thousands of bodybuilders to reach their muscle building goals quickly and safely without the use of illicit or unhealthy drugs. Mario Strong is a bodybuilder that practices what he preaches!

Since 1976, Mario Strong has been a dedicated proponent of natural muscle building in America. He is a nationally recognized author who has promoted numerous bodybuilding competitions, trained countless natural champions, and has served as judge to World class athletes. Mario Strong has also championed the physique stage and is the founder of the once famed Staten Island Bodybuilding Club.

Today, Mario continues to strive for excellence while focusing much of his time and energy on helping future generations of natural bodybuilders.

Mario lives in Staten Island, New York.

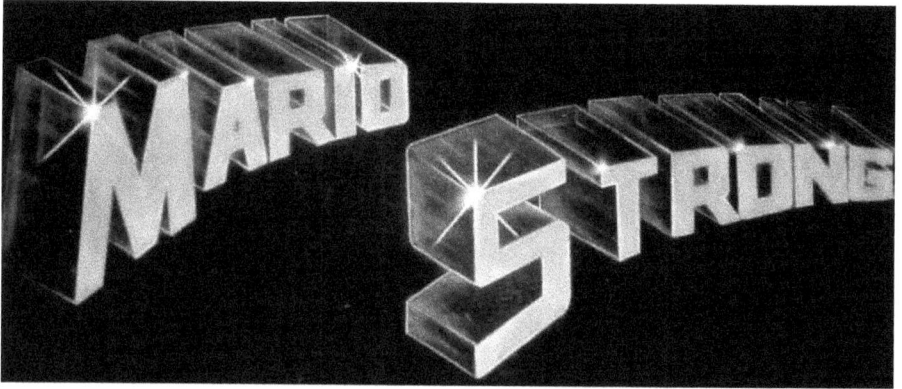

LIVE LONG AND BE STRONG…NATURALLY!

www.ingramcontent.com/pod-product-compliance
Lightning Source LLC
Chambersburg PA
CBHW071219290326
41931CB00037B/1452